Your Career as a
Physical Therapy Aide

Your Career as a Physical Therapy Aide

Roberta C. Weiss, LVN, Ed.D.

Allied Healthcare Curriculum Specialist
Vocational Education Teacher
Trainer UCLA Education Extension Division

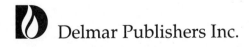 Delmar Publishers Inc.

NOTICE TO THE READER

Cover design by: Pompeo Designs

Delmar Staff

Executive Editor: David Gordon
Associate Editor: Adrianne C. Williams
Project Editor: Carol Micheli
Production Supervisor: Teresa Luterbach
Art Supervisor: Judi Orozco
Design Coordinator: Karen Kemp
Electronic Publishing Supervisor: Lisa Santy

Copyright © 1993
by Delmar Publishers Inc.

printed in the United States of America
published simultaneously in Canada
by Nelson Canada, a division of The Thomson Corporation

1 2 3 4 5 6 7 8 9 10 XXX 99 98 97 96 95 94 93
Library of Congress Cataloging-in-Publication Data

Weiss, Roberta C.
    Your career as a physical therapy aide / Roberta C. Weiss
        p. cm.
    Includes index.
    ISBN 0-8273-5110-0
    1. Physical therapy – Vocational guidance.   I. Title.
    [DNLM: 1. Allied Health Personnel. 2. Career Choice. 3. Physical
Therapy. WB 460 W432y]
RM701.W45 1993
615.8 ' 2 ' 023 – dc20
DNLM/DLC   92-23403
    for Library of Congress   CIP

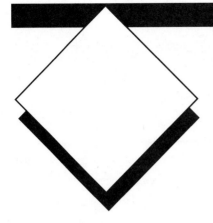

Contents

Preface

This text is written in simple, yet comprehensive, language, and is accompanied by photographs and basic illustrations in order to provide the reader with a well-rounded introduction to the principles and techniques involved with working as a Physical Therapy Aide.

While the author firmly believes that there are many adequate textbooks currently in use that provide information for the advanced learner studying physical therapy, it is the goal of this text to present a manual that meets the very distinct and unique needs of the Physical Therapy Aide or Assistant.

The text is made up of 25 chapters and covers such information as anatomy and physiology of the musculoskeletal, nervous, cardiovascular, and nervous systems, physical therapy modalities, therapeutic and range of motion exercises, and turning, positioning, transferring, and ambulating patients.

To assist readers in their understanding of the subject matter, each chapter is accompanied by behavioral objectives and key words at the beginning and a summary outline and review questions at the end. The four appendixes are included to provide the learner with additional information, such as musculoskeletal terminology, a practice evaluation test, and anatomy and physiology plates of the musculoskeletal system, body directions, and correct postures for standing, sitting, and lifting objects.

Roberta C. Weiss, LVN, Ed.D.
North Hollywood, California

Acknowledgments

I would like to extend my deepest gratitude and appreciation to all those who have assisted me in the preparation and development of this text book, including:

Ms. Sandy Watson, LPT, Director of the Physical Therapy and Rehabilitation Department at Huntington Memorial Hospital, Pasadena, California, and all the members of her wonderful and caring staff, for the time, energy, and expertise they provided in the preparation of this text.

The individual patients receiving physical therapy treatments at Huntington Memorial Hosptial's Physical Therapy and Rehabilitation Department, for all their help and time in providing assistance and a "personal touch," allowing their photographs to be used in this text.

Ms. Marla Keeth, LVN, Coordinator of the Health Careers Academy at Blair High School, Pasadena Unified School District/Los Angeles County Regional Occupational Programs, for her assistance and continued support, in providing time for her health career students to be photographed and work with actual patients, for the preparation of this text.

The many individual Blair High School Health Careers Academy students, for their time, expertise and participation in being photographed and kept available for the many hours needed for the photography session involved in the preparation of this text.

Boyd Flinders, II, M.D., orthopedic surgeon and concerned medical practitioner, for his input and knowledge, in the preparation of this text.

Robyn Gilmore, a talented artist, and friend of many years, who worked many hours helping to formulate sketches for future illustrations and photographs for this text.

Bill Ahern, Sales Representative for Delmar Publishers Inc., for all his help and fortitude in finally bring my work to the "right" people at Delmar Publishers.

Finally, I would like to thank Ms. Adrianne C. Williams, Associate Editor for Delmar Publishers Inc., for all of her help, understanding, cooperation, and particularly, the willingness and time she spent with me in preparing a high quality textbook.

♦ ♦ ♦

Dedication

This book is lovingly and respectfully dedicated to my friend and teacher, Phyllis V. Stilson, RN, whose enduring support and friendship continue to provide me with the vision and skill necessary to develop quality materials for prospective allied health care professionals.

SECTION I

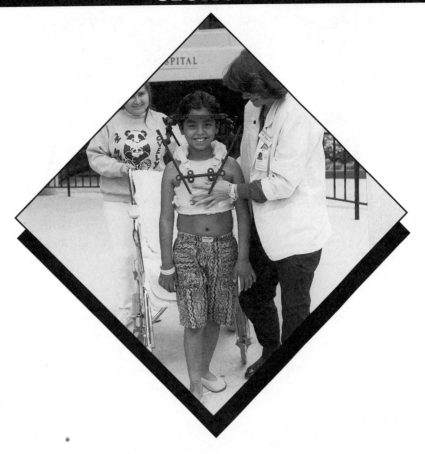

INTRODUCTION TO PHYSICAL THERAPY

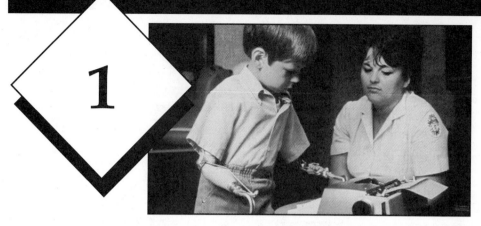

The Profession of Physical Therapy

Objectives

After studying this chapter, you will be able to:

1. Describe the evolution of physical therapy in the United States from the early 1900s to present day.

2. Discuss how physical therapy became a new occupation.

3. Briefly describe the role Mary McMillan played in the evolution and history of physical therapy.

4. Explain the impact of World War I and World War II on the field of physical therapy.

5. Define the major focus of the rehabilitation team.

6. List the different members of the rehabilitation team and describe the function of each.

7. Discuss the role of the physical therapy aide as it relates to working with patients with physical disabilities.

VOCABULARY

Learn the meaning and the correct spelling of the following words and abbreviations:

Physical therapy
Physical therapist
Physical therapy aide
Physical therapy assistant
Occupation
Occupational therapist
Practitioner
Vocational
Rehabilitation
Physical medicine
Disability
Athletic director
Recreation therapist
Recreation aide
Exercise physiologist

♦ HISTORY AND EVOLUTIUON OF PHYSICAL THERAPY

The evolution of physical therapy during the twentieth century can best be grasped by comparing its earliest definition from the 1920s, when the field was first introduced to those definitions and concepts widely used and accepted by modern day practitioners.

During the 1920s, the physical therapist was referred to as a trained assistant to the established medical profession. They were only allowed to work in agencies that catered to muscle training, therapeutic massage, hydrotherapy, and mechanical, electro, and, light therapies, and they could only practice under the prescription of a licensed physician. In comparison to the early

role of the physical therapist, today's therapist is described as a practitioner who, where permitted by law, is responsible for the evaluation, treatment, preventive care, and consultation of patients requiring his experience or expertise in the field of physical therapy (see Figure 1-1).

Physical Therapy: A New Occupation

In the United States, the use of physical therapy as a specialty area of therapeutic intervention, dates as far back as the late ninteenth century, with a sudden increase in its application occurring in the early 1900s. At that time, the use of physical modalities and procedures applied for therapeutic purposes were first used systematically in the United States during the 1890s, in the early treatment programs for infantile paralysis. By 1914, numbers of persons stricken with the disease rose so high, that in an attempt to provide treatment and follow-up care to patients, teams of non-

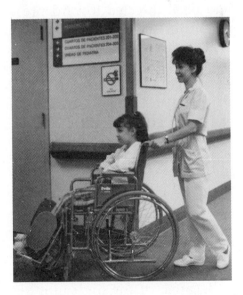

Figure 1-1 Physical therapy aide transporting a patient in a wheelchair. (From Hegner and Caldwell, *Nursing Assistant: A Nursing Process Approach*, 6th edition, copyright 1992 by Delmar Publishers Inc.)

physician workers were organized under medical direction to provide care to those stricken with the disease. Among the non-physician personnel on these teams were those who came to be known as physical therapists.

Even though the occupation of physical therapy was not, at that time, a distinct entity, the foundations were being laid for its acceptance as such. By World War I, which forced attention on the use of restoring physical function in injured members of both the military forces and the civilian work force, the specialty of physical therapy was becoming more widely accepted. Through recognition of the application of physical therapeutics to the needs of military personnel, the specialty branch of medicine known today as physical therapy received a major impetus for becoming a clearly identifiable occupation.

During the earliest years in the evolution of physical therapy, the preservation of human resources was of great importance. During World War I, attention had been directed toward preserving, restoring, and maintaining a fighting force. By the end of the war, however, physical therapy was directed back to preserving and maintaining the work force, in the industrial society from where it emerged.

Formalized Training for Early Practitioners

Mary McMillan, recognized as the first physical therapist in the United States, received her training in England, before returning to the United States in 1915. Because of the high number of personnel needed to provide care to members of the military forces during World War I, other early practitioners in the United States provided the needed services without formal training specific to physical therapy. Preparation for the expanded use of physical therapy fell under the guidance of people whose backgrounds were similar to those practitioners who played a significant role in the early treatment efforts for patients with infantile paralysis. Marguerite Sanderson, a graduate of Wellesley College and the Boston Normal School of Gymnastics, was one of those practitioners who assisted in the planning and organization of activities that would eventually make physical therapeutics a part of the care provided for military personnel. By 1918, because of Sanderson's work, outlines for a course of study had been developed, and cooperative efforts between the military and personnel in civilian institutions were underway to prepare practitioners who would serve, in a civilian capacity, as Reconstruction Aides in special Reconstruction Hospitals.

A New Title for the Practitioner

As a result of these newly-developed training programs, individuals who completed the courses of study were given the title of Reconstruction Aide. In addition, individuals who had prior experience in using physical therapeutics in civilian life were recruited for service with the military as Reconstruction Aides. Practitioners rendering similar service in civilian facilities were referred to as Physiotherapy Aides, Physiotherapy Technicians, Physiotherapy Technicians and, in some cases, Physician's Assistants. Those individuals who were called "Assistant" were personally trained by a physician to work in his or her private office.

Physical Therapy: 1920 to Present

Therefore, a national crisis and the usual pressures of an industrial society spawned and supported the development of the occupation of physical therapy during the early twentieth century.

As a result of the great efforts made toward the training of personnel during World War I, greater numbers of physicians and non-physicians became knowledgeable about the benefits of physical therapeutics. The use of physical modalities as a means to alleviate dysfunction and promote movement, spread through the country. By the 1940s, the value of physical therapy would once more be tested through circumstances reminiscent of those that had led to its initial recognition: the polio epidemic and World War II. The challenges were met by once again combining the forces of the military and civilian sectors, and the practice of physical therapy was propelled through a major period of growth.

As a result of treating survivors of World War II, major new concepts in physical therapy, began to emerge. Two of these were rehabilitation services, both vocational and emotional, and the investigation by neuroscientists of the application of neurophysiologic principles in body movement.

During the years immediately following World War II, a new medical specialty, focusing on the use of physical therapeutics, emerged. This new specialization, called "physical medicine", concentrated on caring for the patient through the use of physical properties such as light, heat, cold, water, electricity, massage, manipulation, exercise, and mechanical devices for physical therapy in the diagnosis and treatment of disease.

The rehabilitation concepts that emerged during World War II fostered the growth of the new specialty of physical medicine. The title would eventually become interchangeable with rehabilitation and rehabilitative medicine.

Emergence of the Occupation

Physical therapy as an occupation in the United States, is clearly an occupation of the twentieth century. It emerged from a need for a specific kind of health service related to the restoration of locomotor function of the human body. Today, physical therapy is listed routinely among the occupations related to health care and is often referred to as an "emerging" profession. The evolution of physical therapy reflects the society in which the occupation has evolved and includes the establishment of standards for education and practice, efforts toward clarifying the scope of practice, and finally, endeavors toward professionalization of the occupation.

At times, progress in the growth of physical therapy has been slow, but it has never halted. At times, its focus may have been diminished, but it has never once been obscured. With each and every renewal of focus on understanding human movements as a basis for alleviating and correcting movement dysfunction, the services of the physical therapy team have been enhanced and the contributions of the individual physical therapy worker has been magnified.

◆ THE REHABILITATION TEAM

How does physical therapy fit into today's health care environment, that is,

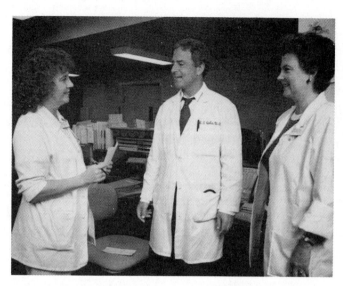

Figure 1-2 Members of the health care delivery team include the physical therapy aide. (From Hegner and Caldwell, *Nursing Assistant: A Nursing Process Approach,* 6th edition, copyright 1992 by Delmar Publishers Inc.)

how it is used in the rehabilitative process? To explain how physical therapy has become the valued profession it is today, we must first begin with the people who work within this rehabilitative process. These individuals are part of what is referred to as the rehabilitation team (see Figure 1-2).

The major focus of the rehabilitation team is rendering care to patients after they have begun recovery from an acute or debilitating illness. However, some rehabilitation services, such as special breathing exercises or exercises that help to maintain the patient's range of motion to a specific joint, may be rendered during the acute phase of the illness. After the acute phase of the disease has subsided and the risk to life has passed, many patients face partial or complete loss of function to an extremity or damage to a part of the nervous system which may affect normal body movement and the ability to function in the daily environment. It is important to remember that it is mainly damage to a part of the nervous, vascular, or skele-

tal system, that is most frequently responsible for causing physical disabilities (see Figure 1-3).

Oftentimes, patients are not able to return to their homes or places of employment unless they are able to regain some of the functions they have lost. Simple tasks that most of us take for granted, such as being able to walk up and down stairs or dress and undress ourselves, may become monumental stumbling blocks to the patient who has sustained a physical disability. Every day we perform innumerable functions with our arms and legs without necessarily concentrating on them. After one loses some function in part or all of an extremity or joint, one becomes acutely aware of how important each part of the body really is. The loss of motion to an ankle or the loss of function in a hand brings about the patient's need for treatment. Such treatment, extensibly, is done by members of the rehabilitation team; the same team that was made up of "reconstruction aides" who only worked as trained assistants

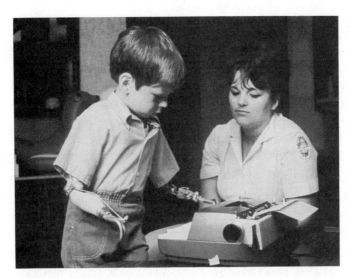

Figure 1-3 The rehabilitation department helps patients return to maximum levels of self care. (From Hegner and Caldwell, *Nursing Assistant: A Nursing Process Approach,* 6th edition, copyright 1988 by Delmar Publishers Inc.)

to physicians. And not only is the team responsible for caring for the patient's physical needs, but, just as important, it is responsible for helping the patient deal with his or her emotions.

The loss of bodily function sometimes brings with it feelings of inadequacy or despair, and oftentimes, an unwelcome dependence on others. Therefore, a major goal of the rehabilitation team is to assist the patient in minimizing the disability and to help in planning a way of daily living that is optimal for the individual.

Members of the Rehabilitation Team

In addition to the physician-in-charge, there are generally seven key individuals in the rehabilitation team. These include a physical therapist, physical therapy assistant, physical therapy aide, athletic trainer, recreation therapist, recreation therapy aide, and an exercise physiologist. Some teams also include a psychologist or social worker and an occupational therapist.

Physician. The physician in charge is responsible for outlining the rehabilitation program for the patient and for ordering any special physical therapy treatments. This individual has attended medical school and has generally secured a specialty in physical or rehabilitative medicine, often with a secondary specialization in psychiatry.

Physical Therapist. The physical therapist has graduated from a four-year-college program with a bachelor's degree, and, in addition to studying physical therapy, has received a postgraduate master's degree in the health sciences. In order to practice, the physical therapist must also be licensed or registered by a state.

The role of the physical therapist is quite extensive and comprehensive. In addition to performing treatments which require special training in therapeutic exercises, hydrotherapy, and electrotherapy, this practitioner is also required to perform procedures dealing with individual muscles and muscular movement.

The physical therapist is also responsible for evaluating the patient and designing an individual therapeutic program. Physical therapists are generally employed in home health agencies, hospitals, nursing homes, fitness centers, and orthopedic offices.

Physical Therapy Assistant. The physical therapy assistant is a graduate of a two-year associate of arts or applied sciences community college program. This individual works under the direction of the physical therapist and is responsible for assisting with patient care and performing selected treatments such as ultrasound. The physical therapy assistant, who is usually employed by home health agencies, nursing homes, hospitals, fitness centers, and orthopedic offices, may also be called upon to assist the physical therapist in evaluating the patient's progress during the treatment.

Physical Therapy Aide. The physical therapy aide is generally responsible for carrying out the non technical duties of physical therapy, such as preparing treatment areas, ordering devices and supplies, and transporting patients. Working under the direction of the physical therapist, the physical therapy aide may be employed in home health agencies, nursing homes, hospitals, fitness centers, and orthopedic offices. Usually the physical therapy aide receives his or her training in a health occupational education (HOE) program, vocational school, or on-the-job training program (see Figure 1-4).

Athletic Trainer. The athletic trainer has graduated from a four-year college program with a bachelor's degree and may or may not be state licensed or nationally certified, depending upon the individual state in which he or she is employed. Most athletic trainers are employed by athletic teams in high schools and colleges, sport teams, and fitness centers and are primarily concerned with preventing and treating athletic injuries and providing rehabilitative services to athletes. The athletic trainer may also be responsible for teaching proper nutrition, assessing an athlete's physical condition, giving advice on exercises, and taping or padding players in order to protect body parts from injury.

Recreational Therapist. The recreation therapist uses recreation and leisure activities as a means of treating patients' symptoms and thereby improving their physical and mental well-being. This is generally accomplished by the recreational therapist's planning of activities for the patient and then evaluating the patient's progress. Most recreational therapists graduate from either a two-year associate of arts program or a four-year bachelor of science program, and state licensure varies according to type of employment. Recreational therapists may be employed by amusement parks, cruise ships, hospitals, mental health facilities, nursing homes, and rehabilitation centers.

Recreational Therapy Aide. The recreational therapy aide is generally trained on the job, and works under the direct supervision of the recreational therapist; they are responsible for carrying out activities the recreational therapist has assigned. This individual, who is most often employed by amusement parks, cruise ships, hospitals, nursing homes, and rehabilitation centers, is most often responsible for noting and reporting patients' responses and progress to the

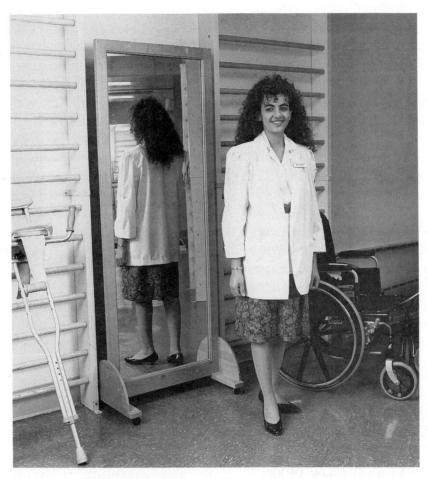

Figure 1-4 The physical therapy aide.

recreational therapist. Recreational therapy aides also maintain supplies and equipment, in good working order and schedule activities for recreation.

Exercise Physiologist. The exercise physiologist designs a physical activity program that is tailored to the specific needs of the individual participant. Educational requirements for the exercise physiologist vary with the position, and employment for this member of the rehabilitation team is usually in hospitals, fitness centers, industry, hotels, research, resorts, and free-lance consultations.

Occupational Therapist. An occupational therapist is a graduate of a school for occupational therapy and

has acquired expertise in making special equipment in order to facilitate the performance of a patient's daily activities. This person is responsible for analyzing bodily maneuvers, step-by-step, and for training the patient in such a manner that she is able to compensate for weakness or paralysis of a limb. It is the occupational therapist who is responsible for teaching the patient how to get in and out of a bathtub, or how to set the table for dinner if one arm is damaged, or how to use a weakened arm in order to support the good arm for bimanual activities. The occupational therapist may also design special equipment in order to compensate for the patient's loss of range of motion to a joint.

Social Worker or Psychologist. The social worker or psychologist is also essential for the effective functioning of the rehabilitation team. This person, who has completed either a postgraduate program in medical social work or a doctorate in clinical psychology, has been trained in analyzing patients' emotional needs and reconciling these with the means that their community, or society as a whole, can offer. This individual is also responsible for assisting both patients and the family members of patients in obtaining rehabilitation services or financial support from state or federal agencies, as well as assisting in making arrangements or appropriate referrals for visits by visiting nurses or help from other home-bound services.

♦ THE ROLE OF THE PHYSICAL THERAPY AIDE AS A MEMBER OF THE REHABILITATION TEAM

As a physical therapy aide, you are considered an essential member of the health care delivery system. A great part of that responsibility is your actual involvement with the rehabilitation team. Medical rehabilitation is a specialty that concerns itself with the overall improvement of the functional capacity of patients who, for one reason or another, have been left with impaired motion of an arm or leg, or with impaired balance or coordination.

As we have already discussed, the physical therapy aide works under the direction of the physical therapist and may be assigned any number of nontechnical tasks. These may include both clinical and administrative functions, and they are always assigned by the supervising physical therapist. The aide may be asked to teach the patient how to walk with crutches or, after having received proper training, may be directed to apply a heating modality to the patient. The physical therapy aide may also be asked to make appointments, complete insurance billing, or clean the physical therapy equipment.

In order to teach a disabled person how to perform a physical task, the aide must realize that such a task is very challenging for the person. Teaching requires much compassion and patience. Patients may be elderly and the physical impairment may seem unsurmountable to them. They may need much encouragement, and they may have to return to their home and friends in order to be successful. As a physical therapy aide, you must never allow yourself to become disappointed when patients do not show any gratitude for all the efforts you have extended to improving their condition. Physical disabilities may arouse bitterness in patients toward their environment. Patients may feel that not enough has been done for them. You may often hear patients say, "I worked all my life and now this happens to me. Why do I have to be a cripple?"

Some of the patients you may encounter may also have some impairment of speech. The decrease in their ability to express themselves may cause patients to feel great frustration and to exhibit feelings of inadequacy. Such a patient may have to write down on paper or use some form of sign language in order to communicate. As a healthcare professional, your patience and understanding may be challenged. It is in this critical situation that you have to call on your human qualities. Show patients that you are concerned and compassionate, but do not become so personally involved that you lose your objectivity and professionalism.

Because patients will look to you for guidance, you must be very careful of what you say in their presence. You should always make sure you are clean and neat, with your uniform or lab coat well kept. You should always be well groomed and appear dignified. It is not only your technical skill but also your personality and appearance that have a beneficial and positive effect on a patient's course of treatment. You should also remember that you may not achieve any improvement in your patient right away, and he or she may become easily discouraged. It will be during this time that the patient will look to you as a professional.

Some patients may ask you questions for which you do not have the answer. In the event that this happens, you should feel free to say so and explain to the patient that you have to confer first with the physical therapist. Never feel compelled to render a therapeutic regimen that you are not familiar with or not accustomed to, or that you are not certain you should do at this particular time. Speak first with your supervisor. If you are asked by a patient to do something that is contrary to the rules of the institution by which you are employed or are in direct conflict with his or her treatment regimen, do not involve yourself. Inform the patient that you are not permitted to do what has been asked. It would not increase the patient's estimation of you if you acted contrary to the rules. If you feel an exception has to be made, you are much better off to first discuss the matter with your immediate supervisor.

As previously stated, a physical disability may change a patient's attitude toward surroundings or toward friends or family members. In some instances, such as patients suffering from Parkinson's Disease, the patient may become very timid. Such a person may need a little extra encouragement. Each activity this patient engages in may take a little longer time and more effort than does the same activity in a patient free of disease, therefore, never try to hurry a patient along. You will find greater rewards for your patience and effort as you see the Parkinsonian patient, or any patient for that matter, liven up under your care and their course of treatment.

Always remember that the aim of assisting patients with physical disabilities is bringing them back to the greatest state of health they can achieve. Such involvement on your part includes aiding the patient to achieve ambulation or completely restore normal strength. Remember, the most important part of your job is to make the patient able to function in his or her home environment without assistance or with minimal assistance from other persons. Your goal, then, is to accomplish the most optimal improvement possible for the specific disability.

Finally, it is important to remember that one of the single most important responsibilities you have is to make patients feel secure and good about themselves. Above all, always try to preserve the patients' dignity and self-esteem. Show patients the same courtesy and dignity you would expect shown to yourself if the roles were reversed.

It is a difficult, yet very rewarding, task to improve the physical disability of another person. One would have to search high and low in order to find a nobler job than that of helping another and easing the burdens of the disabled and physically challenged.

◆ ◆ ◆
SUMMARY OUTLINE

History and Evolution of Physical Therapy
- Introduction of the field of physical therapy
- Physical therapy as a new occupation
- Physical therapy in the early 1900s
- Formalized training for early physical therapy practitioners

- Physical therapy: 1920 to present
- Emergence of the occupation

The Rehabilitation Team
- Major focus of the rehabilitation team
- Members of the rehabilitation team

The Role of the Physical Therapy Aide as a Member of the Rehabilitation Team
- Clinical and administrative functions

CHAPTER REVIEW QUESTIONS

A. Short Answer

1. Who is considered the founder of physical therapy?
2. The use of physical modalities and procedures applied for therapeutic purposes was introduced during 1914 to combat what crippling disease?
3. Who was most responsible for assisting in the planning and organizational activities that eventually made physical therapeutics a part of the care provided for Army personnel?
4. What was the first title given to an individual who completed the newly developed physical therapeutics training classes?
5. What is the specialty of medical rehabilitation concerned with?
6. What is the major focus of the rehabilitation team?

B. Matching

Match the correct answers in Column A with its appropriate response in Column B:

Column A		Column B
physician-in-charge	___	teaches patient to work equipment and assist ADL
physical therapist	___	responsible for outlining patient's care and treatment
occupational therapist	___	acquired advanced training in kinesiology
social worker and psychologist	___	analyzes and deals with patient's emotional needs
physical therapy aide	___	assists physical therapist in carring out physical therapy tasks

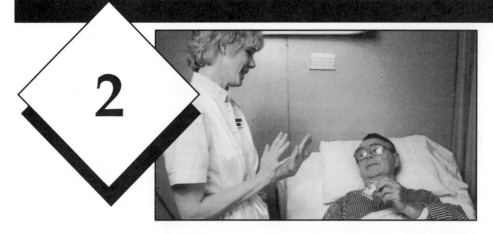

Ethical and Legal Issues Affecting the Physical Therapy Aide

Objectives
After studying this chapter, you will be able to:

1. Describe what the focus was of the American Physio-therapy Association when it was originally founded.

2. Identify the main premise of the American Physical Therapy Association's Code of Ethics.

3. Define morals and moral norms.

4. List the five categories morals are generally grouped into.

5. Define ethics and briefly discuss its relationship to morals.

6. Define what is meant by an ethical dilemma.

7. Briefly explain the concepts of confidentiality, informed consent, interprofessionalism, and justice as each relates to health care.

8. Describe the physical therapy aide's role in relationship to medical ethics.

9. Briefly explain the concepts of negligence and malpractice.

10. Discuss the physical therapy aide's role in the following situations: reporting illegal and dishonest acts, writing or witnessing a patient's will, and applying restraints.

VOCABULARY

Learn the meaning and the correct spelling of the following words and abbreviations:

Code of ethics
Morals
Moral norms
Attitudes
Behaviors
Ethics
Ethical dilemma
Confidentiality
Informed consent
Interprofessionalism
Justice
Negligence
Malpractice

◆ ETHICAL AND LEGAL ISSUES IN PHYSICAL THERAPY

Practitioners involved in the field of physical therapy have always been concerned about the ethics of their profession. The first code of ethics, which was adopted in 1935 by the American Physiotherapy Association, initially focused almost solely on the duties of the physical therapist, while the sophistication and timeliness of the current American Physical Therapy Association code of ethics stands in stark contrast to earlier guidelines set by its predecessors.

The code of ethics originally adopted by the American Physical Therapy Association in May, 1948, and all its subsequent amendments and principles stand firmly on the premise that such a code is important as a set of broad moral guidelines and as a public document professing the group's moral and ethical commitments to the profession and to the patient. The individual practitioner's commitment to upholding high standards are the best indicators of how the profession as a whole will be judged.

Morals and Ethics

Morals, or "moral norms," are the attitudes and behaviors that a society agrees upon as both desirable and necessary in order to maximize the realization of things cherished most in that society. At one end of the moral spectrum are minimum rules designed to keep the society from destroying itself. At the other end, are the ideals toward which members can strive in trying to create a perfect society. By adhering to these rules and ideals, we are helped in preserving and fostering the conditions necessary for living together in peace and harmony. While some rules and ideals have changed, others have stood the test of time and have had exceptional staying power.

Morals are generally grouped into several categories, including duties, rights, responsibilities, character traits, and conditions of justice.

Within the framework of health care, some of the basic moral norms are especially important. This is due primarily to the nature of the health care professional and patient relationship. Among them are duties to do no harm, to keep one's promise to patients, and to tell the truth. Rights include the right of patients to their life and the right of health care professionals to be free to make the best possible judgements. Additionally, there are responsibilities of health professionals, patients, and society as a whole, that ought to be taken

American Hospital Association

AHA Policy — A Patient's Bill of Rights

This policy document presents the official position of the American Hospital Association as approved by the Board of Trustees and House of Delegates.

The American Hospital Association presents a Patient's Bill of Rights with the expectation that observance of these rights will contribute to more effective patient care and greater satisfaction for the patient, his physician, and the hospital organization. Further, the Association presents these rights in the expectation that they will be supported by the hospital on behalf of its patients, as an integral part of the healing process. It is recognized that a personal relationship between the physician and the patient is essential for the provision of proper medical care. The traditional physician-patient relationship takes on a new dimension when care is rendered within an organizational structure. Legal precedent has established that the institution itself also has a responsibility to the patient. It is in recognition of these factors that these rights are affirmed.

1. The patient has the right to considerate and respectful care.

2. The patient has the right to obtain from his physician complete current information concerning his diagnosis, treatment, and prognosis in terms the patient can be reasonably expected to understand. When it is not medically advisable to give such information to the patient, the information should be made available to an appropriate person in his behalf. He has the right to know, by name, the physician responsible for coordinating his care.

3. The patient has the right to receive from his physician information necessary to give informed consent prior to the start of any procedure and/or treatment. Except in emergencies, such information for informed consent should include but not necessarily be limited to the specific procedure and/or treatment, the medically significant risks involved, and the probable duration of incapacitation. Where medically significant alternatives for care or treatment exist, or when the patient requests information concerning medical alternatives, the patient has the right to such information. The patient also has the right to know the name of the person responsible for the procedures and/or treatment.

4. The patient has the right to refuse treatment to the extent permitted by law and to be informed of the medical consequences of his action.

5. The patient has the right to every consideration of his privacy concerning his own medical care program. Case discussion, consultation, examination, and treatment are confidential and should be conducted discreetly. Those not directly involved in his care must have the permission of the patient to be present.

6. The patient has the right to expect that all communications and records pertaining to his care should be treated as confidential.

7. The patient has the right to expect that within its capacity a hospital must make reasonable response to the request of a patient for services. The hosptial must provide evaluation, service, and/or referral as indicated by the urgency of the case. When medically permissible, a patient may be transferred to another facility only after he has received complete information and explanation concerning the needs for and alternatives to such a transfer. The institution to which the patient is to be transferred must first have accepted the patient for transfer.

8. The patient has the right to obtain information as to any relationship of his hospital to other health care and educational institutions insofar as his care is concerned. The patient has the right to obtain information as to the existence of any professional relationships among individuals, by name, who are treating him.

9. The patient has the right to be advised if the hospital proposes to engage in or perform human experimentation affecting his care or treatment. The patient has the right to refuse to participate in such research projects.

10. The patient has the right to expect reasonable continuity of care. He has the right to know in advance what appointment times and physicians are available and where. The patient has the right to expect that the hospital will provide a mechanism whereby he is informed by his physician or a delegate of the physician of the patient's continuing health care requirements following discharge.

11. The patient has the right to examine and receive an explanation of his bill regardless of source of payment.

12. The patient has the right to know what hospital rules and regulations apply to his conduct as a patient.

No catalog of rights can guarantee for the patient the kind of treatment he has a right to expect. A hospital has many functions to perform, including the prevention and treatment of disease, the education of both health professionals and patients, and the conduct of clinical research. All these activities must be conducted with an overriding concern for the patient, and, above all, the recognition of his dignity as a human being. Success in achieving this recognition assures success in the defense of the rights of the patient.

Figure 2-1 A patient's bill of rights. (From Hegner and Caldwell, *Nursing Assistant: A Nursing Process Approach*, 6th edition, copyright 1992 by Delmar Publishers Inc.)

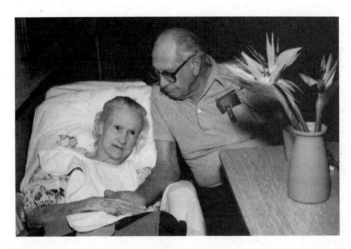

Figure 2-2 The preservation of life is fundamental to the ethical code. (From Hegner and Caldwell, *Nursing Assistant: A Nursing Process Approach* , 6th edition, copyright 1992 by Delmar Publishers Inc.)

into account, and character traits, such as compassion, honesty, and conscientiousness, that are valued.

Ethics is related to morals since it is the study of morals and moral judgments. Ethical theories enable a person to reflect on and find resolution to conflicts of duties, rights, or responsibilities.

In health care, we are continuously bombarded with ethical dilemmas, that question or compromise our own ethical belief system or values. As a physical therapy aide, you can expect, at some point in your career, to encounter one of these "no win" situations. One such example may be the decision to honor a patient's wishes to have information about his condition, knowing full well that to provide it would be in direct conflict with the physician's expressed wish that the patient not be told. Another example maybe a decision to spend an extra fifteen minutes with a patient who really needs attention, even though it will mean cutting corners with the next patient (see Figure 2-1).

Health care practitioners employed in the field of physical therapy face the wide range of moral problems confronting today's health professions. In their professional role, physical therapy aides may not be directly involved in some morally complex situations such as abortion or discontinuing life-support systems; however, they are by no means exempt from many ethical issues affecting the health care industry in general. Most of these issues fall under one of four different areas of concentration: confidentiality, informed consent, interprofessional issues, and issues dealing with justice (see Figure 2-2).

Confidentiality

In the health care setting, one's commitment to honoring confidences should be considered a momentous challenge, especially when a patient is being seen over a long period of time and by a multitude of professionals, which is usually the case for a patient receiving physical therapy treatments. It is important to keep in mind that most patients expect all health professionals to keep secret the harmful, shameful, or embarrassing information the patient reveals to them. While most health facilities continuously process data and information regarding the

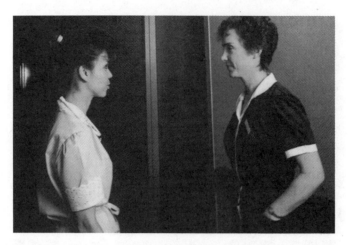

Figure 2-3 Information about patients is confidential and must not be discussed casually with others. (From Hegner and Caldwell, *Nursing Assistant: A Nursing Process Approach* , 6th edition, copyright 1992 by Delmar Publishers Inc.)

patient's state of health from one department to the next, it is always the responsibility of the individual health care worker to be as descrete and protective as possible in order to not defame the patient in any way (see Figure 2-3).

Informed Consent

Mechanisms for securing informed consent, or obtaining the patient's permission for care and treatment are many, but they, like the concepts surrounding confidentiality, are challenged by long-term treatment and the often complex nature of some health care programs. Seldom does the patient consent initially to becoming a part of a particular program. For example, seldom does the patient consent to the many different kinds of intravenous injections that are tried in the over-all goal of rehabilitating him. Today, more than ever, we are seeing physical therapy treatments and evaluation procedures guided more by moral principles and legal con-

straints, thereby leading to the implementation of the mechanism known as informed consent.

♦ **INTERPROFESSIONAL ISSUES**

Issues which fall into this category tend to give rise to other types of moral dilemmas befalling the physical therapy worker. For example, many physical therapists and physical therapy aides are justifiably worried that the practice of working in a physician-managed or other privately owned physical therapy clinic may entail built-in conflicts of interest. Other areas, such as the move by many physical therapists toward practice independent of physician referral, have raised consciousness and concern regarding the effect such an arrangement may have on the physician-therapist relationship. At the same time, all members of the physical therapy and rehabilitation team continue to examine ways in which physician-therapist arrangements can be designed to best preserve intraprofessional integrity while better meeting the needs of the patients.

♦ JUSTICE ISSUES

The physical therapy department and the professionals working within its dimensions are not exempt from being involved in agonizing decisions about how to distribute scarce resources according to an acceptable standard of fairness and equity. More and more, the physical therapy worker is being forced to become involved in policy and government in order to help assure that just policies and practices for the field continue to gain support.

♦ MEDICAL ETHICS AND THE PHYSICAL THERAPY AIDE

As a member of the health care delivery team, one of the areas the physical therapy aide is concerned with deals with the subject of medical ethics and how it relates to his or her job as a physical therapy aide. Ethics, as it relates to medicine, is a set of rules that guides or governs the conduct of all individuals who come into contact with patients. These rules, which are moral rather than legal, have been established for the protection of the patient. When you, as a physical therapy aide, assume the responsibility for caring for a patient, you are also agreeing to live up to the ethical code that protects the patient.

Generally speaking, one of the most basic rules of ethics is that life is precious. Therefore, everyone who is involved in the care of patients must put the saving of human life and the promotion of health above all else. For most health care providers, it is not always easy to keep this rule in mind when you are caring for a patient who may be suffering or dying, especially if you know the patient is in pain or has a limited potential for a productive life.

Living in the 1990s, one might say that, probably at no other time in history have the questions of medical ethics been under such watchful eyes. Frequently questions arise that trigger deep-seeded emotional responses—responses that tend to remove the clinician's objective point of view and replace it with a more , subjective, emotional reaction. When is life gone from a person on a life support system? How much heroic effort should be given in situations where the patient is dying of a terminal illness? How valid and legally acceptable are "living wills" which have been written by a terminally ill patient? These and many other medical-legal questions continuously surround us today and will eventually be decided in a court of law.

Still one fact remains very clear, those of us involved in the delivery of health care share a major responsibility, and that responsibility is to preserve life whenever possible, and make comfortable those whose lives may not last much longer.

Now, you may be asking yourself, as a physical therapy aide, what role or responsibility do I play in fulfilling medical ethics? How do the rules or guidelines which govern the medical–legal ramifications of caring for patients affect me on a day-to-day basis? You must always remember that one of the most

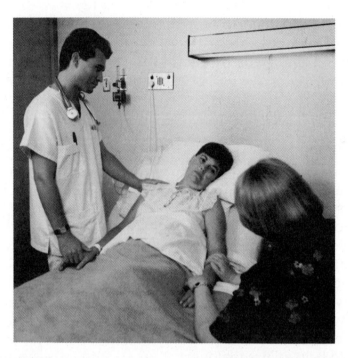

Figure 2-4 A visit from clergy or other members of the religious community can be very reassuring and helpful to the patient. (From Hegner and Caldwell, *Nursing Assistant: A Nursing Process Approach* , 6th edition, copyright 1992 by Delmar Publishers Inc.)

basic rules that you will be expected to follow will deal with confidentiality; that is, whatever you hear or say within the medical environment must always remain within that environment. While individual circumstances will always arise that will tempt you to "talk shop," you must never break the confidence the health care environment has bestowed upon you. Discussing patients with others not involved with their care is considered gossiping and always is considered ethically wrong.

Talking with Others

Patients, and sometimes others, such as visitors and family members, may question you about the patient's condition, treatment, or prognosis. You must learn to evade such questions and inquiries in a tactful and professional manner. Whenever your are asked such questions, you response should always

be the same. You must redirect the inquiry to your supervisor, the nurse, or the physician responsible for the patient's care. Since it is the privilege of each physician to decide how much information should be given to an individual patient, you must never take it upon yourself to answer questions that are not within your realm or scope of responsibility.

Since you may frequently be entering the patient's room, another rule that you are expected to follow is to never discuss a patient's condition while in her hospital room. Even if a patient appears to be unresponsive, she may still be able to hear everything being said (see Figure 2-4).

Tipping

Patients are charged for services they receive while in the hospital; the salary you are paid is included in that charge.

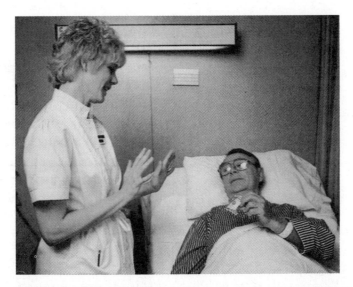

Figure 2-5 Tips must be courteously refused. (From Hegner and Caldwell, *Nursing Assistant: A Nursing Process Approach* , 6th edition, copyright 1992 by Delmar Publishers Inc.)

Therefore, under no circumstances are you to accept monies or gifts for the services you are expected to perform during your daily work. Tipping within the health care environment is never acceptable. If offered, a firm yet courteous refusal of the money or gift is usually all that is necessary in order to convince the patient of your meaning (see Figure 2-5).

♦ MEDICAL ETHICS AND LEGAL ISSUES

While working within the health care environment, there are certain legal issues that you should be familiar with because they will influence your role as a physical therapy aide. These issues

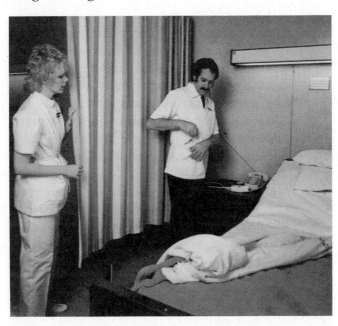

Figure 2-6 Failing to report a dishonest act that you observe makes you guilty of aiding and abetting. (From Hegner and Caldwell, *Nursing Assistant: A Nursing Process Approach* , 6th edition, copyright 1992 by Delmar Publishers Inc.)

deal with negligence, malpractice, reporting illegal and dishonest acts, writing or witnessing a patient's will, and restraining patients— both for their own safety and against their will.

Negligence

When a health care provider fails to give care that is required by the job he has been hired and trained to perform, that provider is guilty of negligence. For example, if the hospital in which you are employed has a policy that states the physical therapy aide cannot ambulate the patient without a waist belt, and you do so, anyway, you would in fact be guilty of negligence, since you did not follow proper hospital policy in carrying out your task. Remember, whether you perform a procedure in the wrong manner or for the wrong reason, you are always accountable for your own actions (see Figure 2-6).

Malpractice

Malpractice occurs when a health care provider improperly delivers care or provides the care without having had proper training or formal instruction. Applying hot packs to a patient without a doctor's order or applying them without proper instruction on how they are to be applied, would be considered malpractice (see Figure 2-7).

Writing or Witnessing a Patient's Will

Sometimes patients ask members of the health care team to write or witness a will. You should note that all matters of this nature should be promptly reported to your supervisor since writing or signing a patient's will is a legal matter for which you are not trained. As a physical therapy aide, you will not have problems if you simply follow the hospital's or medical facility's policies regarding these procedures. Remember, perform only

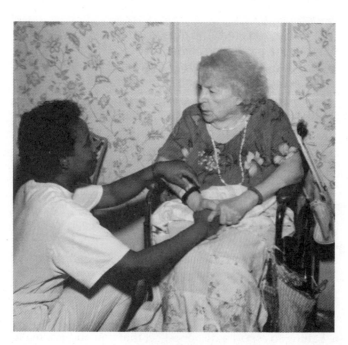

Figure 2-7 Patients have the right to refuse treatment (From Hegner and Caldwell, *Nursing Assistant: A Nursing Process Approach* , 6th edition, copyright 1992 by Delmar Publishers Inc.)

those services that you have been taught and know the proper lines of authority whenever a case arises in which you are asked to do something which is not within your scope of practice.

Restraints

In some instances it may be necessary to restrain the movements of patients. Whenever restraints are employed, always remember that they must be applied in accordance with a specific doctor's order. Such an order indicates the extent of the restraint and the rationale for its application.

As a physical therapy aide, you should not be called upon to apply restraints since they are generally applied by nursing personnel for the sole purpose of protecting the patient or to protect others from the patient. Application of these restraints without the proper authorization or justification can constitute false imprisonment. Whenever you are required to work with a patient who does have restraints applied, always remember to follow good common sense and safety when moving the patient about. If the restraints must be untied or removed during a procedure, always remember to make sure they have been properly reapplied when you have completed your task.

All persons providing care to the patient must voluntarily agree to live up to the medical ethical code. This code protects the patient by prohibiting the discussion of personal matters and by assuring the preservation of life and the promotion of health. Patients receive care based on their need, not their ability to pay: therefore, the acceptance of tips or gifts is never permitted. Remember, as a member of the health care team, you have legal responsibilities— responsibilities that include no toleration of negligence, malpractice, or dishonest acts. There will never be concern about legal complications as long as prudent judgment is exercised and policies are followed.

♦ ♦ ♦
SUMMARY OUTLINE

Ethical and Legal Issues
- American Physiotherapy Association Code of Ethics — 1935
- American Physiotherapy Association Code of Ethics — 1948
- American Physiotherapy Association Code of Ethics — Present Day

Morals and Ethics
- Morals and moral norms
- Ethics

Ethical Issues in Physical Therapy
- Confidentiality
- Informed consent
- Intraprofessional issues
- Justice issues

Medical Ethics and the Physical Therapy Aide
- Role of the physical therapy aide
- Talking with others
- Legal issues

CHAPTER REVIEW QUESTIONS

1. In what year was the first code of ethics adopted by the American Physiotherapy Association?
2. Briefly define what a moral is.
3. List the five categories morals are grouped into.
4. What is the difference between a moral and a moral norm?
5. Briefly define ethics.
6. What are the four main areas of concentration ethics are concerned with in health care?
7. Medical ethics involves rules that are _____, rather than _____.
8. _____ deals with a health care provider failing to give the care expected or required.
9. _____ occurs when a health care provider improperly delivers care or provides care without having had proper training.
10. Not reporting illegal or dishonest acts may be considered _____ _____ _____ the crime.
11. What is always required when restraints are applied to a patient for his or her safety?
12. A medical code of ethics _____ the patient by prohibiting discussion of personal matters related to him or her.

SECTION II

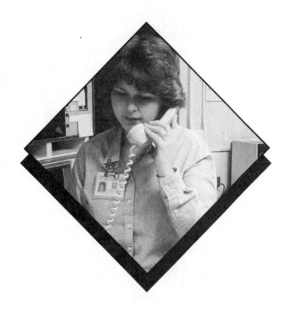

ADMINISTRATIVE SKILLS

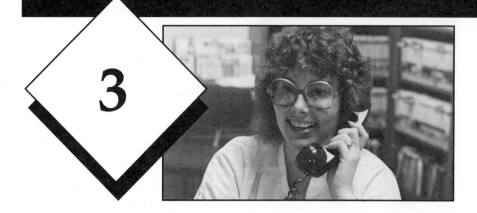

Communicating Effectively

VOCABULARY

Learn the meaning and the correct spelling of the following words and abbreviations:

Atmosphere
Environment
Communication
Empathy
Tact
Patience
Understanding
Verbal communication
Nonverbal communication
Oral communication
Diplomacy
Screening
Etiquette
Appointment book
Appointment log

Depending upon the facility in which you work, occasionally you may be called upon to complete tasks involving the administrative or clerical duties necessary in caring for patients receiving physical therapy treatments. While the majority of skills you undertake generally take place in the clinical setting, you may also be asked to perform basic administrative tasks such as greeting patients, screening and answering the telephone, and appointment scheduling. Whether you are asked to perform a clinical task or one that requires an administrative skill, you must always remember that at the base of all patient or office-oriented duties is the most basic skill of all— effective communication.

Before we discuss the actual mechan-

ics of effective communication, however, we must first take a look at how communication occurs.

Do you remember the very first time you walked into a room of strangers, yet, for some reason, you felt as though the people gathered there seemed to care about you? Did the warmth and feelings of friendliness from the others radiate to you? As a member of the health care team, the atmosphere just described is as much a responsibility of the physical therapy aide as it is all the other members of the team. In order to create an environment in which the patient feels at ease and comfortable, in which she feels a genuine sense of interest and understanding, the key ingredient, effective communication, must be achieved.

In health care, communication is based upon interpersonal skills, or interaction among people. It is a way in which we relate to one another, in which we are able to empathize, reassure, and offer comfort in stressful situations. It is also a way in which we are better able to help one another feel good about themselves.

Communication in the health care environment usually takes many forms and it generally involves projecting concern for others through one's tone of voice, words, and actions. Because patients sometimes experience a high degree of stress when they see a doctor or therapist for treatment, words of friendliness, encouragement, and courtesy help put them at ease. Because emotional sensitivity is often higher when a person is sick or incapacitated, it is important that you project a positive attitude, using good manners and respect for others whenever you are called upon to communicate. Always remember to choose your words carefully, use a soothing tone of voice, and above all, display a professional manner. In the following case scenarios, consider how the words and actions demonstrate that the physical therapy aide cares for the patient.

Case Scenario #1:

"Good morning, Ms. Smith. May I take your coat? I'll put it in this corner so you won't forget it when you leave."

Important Points:
a) The physical therapy aide makes Ms. Smith feel that her coat is important.
b) The physical therapy aide assumes partial responsibility for remembering the coat, which establishes a "we are in this together" attitude that will carry over to other aspects of the patient's care.

Case Scenario #2:

"Good afternoon Mr. Greene. How are you feeling today? I hope the pain in your knee has disappeared. Oh, it's worse today, swollen and inflamed? I'm sorry to hear that, but the physical therapist will check it carefully."

Important Points:
a) The physical therapy aide through words and tone of voice, tells the patient, "I care about you."
b) The physical therapy aide remembers the patient's problem, which makes the person feel important.

c) The physical therapy aide reassures the patient about the care he will receive.

♦ PARTS OF EFFECTIVE COMMUNICATION

For effective communication to occur, the communicator must consider three important concepts. These include the use of empathy, tact, and patience.

Empathy involves the ability to understand another's feelings and the sensitivity to be able to respond to those feelings. Put more simply, it means being able to put yourself in another's place. An empathetic physical therapy aide is able to understand and offer comfort when dealing with relatives or friends of patients because they are worried. Consider the physical therapy aide's behavior in the following case scenarios. Then ask yourself if you believe the physical therapy aide communicates empathy?

Case Scenario #3:

"Mrs. Gomez, I understand how concerned you are because you think Linda has not responded to the treatment. Sometimes it takes several days for improvement to show."

Important Points:
a) The physical therapy aide tries to reassure the parent.
b) The physical therapy aide does not make any promises about the condition improving quickly.

Case Scenario #4:
"Don't worry, Joanne. If you can't do the exercises today, we'll try again tomorrow."

Important Points:
a) The physical therapy aide sets the patient at ease and does not embarrass her because she can not do the the exercises today.
b) The physical therapy aide gives the patient an alternative by indicating that she may do the exercises the next day.

Tact refers to saying or doing the proper thing at the proper time. When a person is tactless, we say that the individual has "put his foot in his mouth." A tactful person is always diplomatic and uses good judgment when working with other people. Most of us would never think of saying to a friend, "your hair does not look good today," or "that outfit makes you look fat." In a physical therapy office, the situations requiring tact may be less personal but are no less important. The patient who owes money must be tactfully reminded to pay; the patient who disturbs the reception area by talking loudly needs to be asked to speak more quietly.

Most people know the difference between tact and tactlessness and therefore strive to be tactful. Unfortunately, however, physical therapy aides who do not understand the effect of tactless comments and actions may jeopardize their jobs. Consider the following case scenarios. Then ask yourself if you thought the physical therapy aide handled the situation tactfully.

Case Scenario #5:
"Mrs. White, could you ask your son, Ben, to play a little more quietly? I'm concerned that his noise may be bothering some of our other patients. If you like, I will get him some books to read.
The parent makes a defensive comment:
"Yes, I know the adults are talking, too, but their conversations aren't very loud. If necessary, I'll ask them to speak more quietly."

Important Points:
a) The physical therapy aide tactfully explains why the child's noise is a problem.
b) The physical therapy aide remains in control while tactfully explaining that other patients will be asked to lower their conversations if necessary.

Case Scenario #6:
"I'll leave the room while you undress, Mr. James. Please remove your slacks and cover yourself from the waist down with this sheet. The physical therapist will be in to check your knee. You may wear your shirt."

Important Points:
a) The physical therapy aide, who is aware of the patient's modesty, leaves the room while he undresses.
b) The physical therapy aide provides the patient with explicit instructions about which clothes should be removed.
c) The physical therapy aide tells the patient the type of examination to expect.

Perhaps no other human relations skill is as important to a physical therapy aide as the third component of effective communication, known as **patience.** Being patient means that you do not become angry or visibly annoyed when a patient blames you for a long wait before an appointment. It also means not being curt when a person asks several times, "how much longer before my treatment?"

Patience often involves waiting — waiting for people to undress or dress, to give you information, or to pay their bill. You may want to hurry them, interrupt their sentences, or speed things up so you can move on to the next task. When you feel yourself becoming impatient, you must maintain your self-control, breathe deeply, smile, and look for realistic ways in which you can remedy the problem. Consider the following case scenario.

Case Scenario #7:
The reception area of the office is crowded because an emergency patient required 20 minutes of the physical therapist's time. Although waiting patients were understanding and gracious about the emergency when it occurred, they are now complaining to one another about the delay, and several have become irritable. One patient asks if he can be placed ahead of others because he has planned to go to a baseball game after his treatment.

"Mr. Adams, I'm sorry you have been delayed, but I know you understand how important it is for the therapist to see emergency patients at once. Only two people remain ahead of you, and they, too, want to leave. Your wait will not

be much longer, at most 30 minutes. You may reschedule the appointment if you like."

Important Points:
a) The physical therapy aide recognizes that the patient's point is valid and that the wait has been long.
b) The physical therapy aide tries to give the patient a time frame for any additional wait and offers an alternative to waiting.
c) The physical therapy aide does not place this patient ahead of others.

◆ TYPES OF COMMUNICATION

There are two basic types of communication. They include the use of words that we form into sentences, known as oral or verbal communication, and messages that do not use spoken words, called nonverbal communication. Expressions such as "a look that would kill," "red-faced in anger," or "love written all over her face," are examples of messages delivered without words. It is important to remember that when you work with patients, you must be careful that your verbal and nonverbal communication sends the same message; otherwise, you may confuse, hurt, or offend someone. Consider the following case scenario. Do you think the physical therapy aide's verbal and nonverbal messages agree?

Case Scenario #8:
A physical therapy aide who is engaged in a telephone conversa-

tion ignores a patient who stands at the reception desk and waits several minutes. After finishing the call, the physical therapy aide looks at the patient, picks up a medical record, and reviews it while talking to the patient. The physical therapy aide then leaves the room while talking over her shoulder to the patient who remains standing. "Good morning, Mr. Brown. How are you this morning. Are you feeling better? I'll be right back."

Oral Communication

Oral communication, as we already stated, refers to oral messages and includes face-to-face encounters, announcements, questions, off-hand remarks, telephone conversations, gossip, and other forms of communication. Successful communication depends on correct word choices and on the listener's understanding of what is being said.

There are many factors that influence the communication process and affect understanding between communicators. These include one's level of education, economic status, prior experiences, and cultural heritage. Since there is no absolute universal meaning for words existing in the minds of people, each defines words based upon his or her own influencing factors. The greater the difference in one's background, the more difficulty he or she may encounter in understanding another person.

An area in which many health care professionals get into trouble involves using medical or technical terms beyond the scope of the patient's understanding or background. Some people use technical words to impress the listener or to prove their superior knowledge. New employees or recent graduates often feel important by using big words to show how smart they are. If you are confident in your education, you will recognize that use of medical words does not necessarily demonstrate knowledge, and you should not display a wide vocabulary at the expense of another's understanding or comfort. Consider the following case scenario.

Case Scenario #9:
"Mrs. White, here is a pamphlet on living with low back pain that the physical therapist asked me to give to you. It will help you to understand your illness. You will notice from the pamphlet that weakness of the leg muscles is an early symptom."

This physical therapy aide knows that the patient will not undersand medical language and uses laymen's language to discuss the medical condition. A less informed physical therapy aide might have communicated in the following manner:
"Mrs. White, here is a pamphlet on rheumatoid arthritis of the lumbosacral region that the physical therapist asked me to give to you. The etiology of this disease is unknown, however, the pamphlet will help you to understand your illness. You will notice from the pamphlet that the atrophy of the leg muscles is an early symptom."

Nonverbal Communication

Nonverbal communication, as we have already discussed, refers to messages sent without words or in addition to words. It includes facial expressions, touch, tone of voice, listening, eye contact, gestures, appearance, manner, time, body language, silence, and other nonverbal behavior. Every individual person sends and receives hundreds of nonverbal messages daily. They enhance the communication process and should be used by both the sender and the receiver in order to confirm verbal messages.

Nonverbal communication is important to any relationship, and this is especially true with people who are sick, uncomfortable, or anxious. When we hear the statement, "What is not said may be more important than what is said," we should understand that this makes reference to the significance to nonverbal behavior. As a physical therapy aide, your competence in using and interpreting nonverbal behavior will oftentimes determine the degree of success you enjoy in your relationship with others.

◆ COMMUNICATION IN THE PHYSICAL THERAPY SETTING

Now that we have spent some time discussing the components of communication and how the process of effective communication occurs, let's talk about how and when communication occurs in the physical therapy setting.

Using the Telephone

In any clinical or administrative setting, the telephone is generally considered the most important line of public relations. Because you create an impression each and every time you

talk on the telephone, it is extremely important that the techniques you use are correct.

Proper use of the telephone usually depends upon many different skills. since the impression you create on it, for the most part, tends to influence a patient or any other caller, it is most important that you always remember to be tactful, diplomatic, courteous, professional, and firm, but flexible. You should also be capable of making decisions, as well as willing to accept responsibility for making those decisions.

In addition to developing such essential skills as using a correct tone of voice, being pleasant, clear and distinct, and using correct grammar, there are very specific abilities which you must acquire which are necessary for proper telephone techniques.

To begin with, you should always answer the telephone promptly. In addition, try to answer with a smile. This helps the caller to feel secure in your response, as well as helping you to create a pleasant voice. Even though the caller may not be able to see this gesture, he or she will be able to detect it in your voice.

Another important skill necessary in correct telephone usage is identifying both yourself and the office or department in which you are working. And never use slang when you answer the telephone. A "Good morning, this is Ms. Jones," or "Dr.Smith's office, can I help you," generally goes a lot farther than being rude or short with the caller (see Figure 3-1).

Whenever you are talking on the telephone, it is also important to keep the receiver firmly against your ear and put the mouthpiece approximately one inch away from the center of your lips.

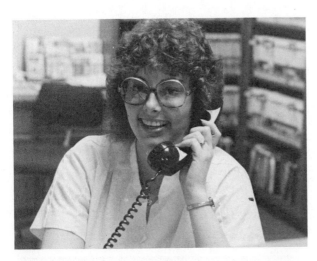

Figure 3-1 Answer the telephone with a smile. (From Simmers, *Diversified Health Occupations*, 2nd edition, copyright 1988 by Delmar Publishers Inc.)

This usually helps the caller receive the best transmission of your voice.

Screening Telephone Calls

In some hospitals or physical therapy agencies, you may be responsible for screening telephone calls. This has to do with determining which calls should be transferred to the physical therapist or the appropriate person and which can be handled by you or another worker in the department. You will find that most departments or agencies have their own or policy regarding the screening of telephone calls.

In order to properly screen calls, it is important for you to determine the purpose of the call. Many patients simply ask to talk with a particular person. By asking the caller, "May I help you?" or "May I tell Ms. Smith why you are calling?" generally helps in determining the nature of the call.

Screening telephone calls may also involve evaluating emergency situations and then dealing with them appropriately. In some cases, for example, a patient may be upset even though there is no real emergency. By asking pertinent questions and remaining calm, you may be able to determine what is a real emergency and what is not. Most emergencies are referred to the appropriate person if she is available. If that individual is not available, you should obtain important information regarding the nature of the call, so that you can help the caller obtain help from the correct source. In most cases, hospitals and medical facilities usually have a procedure to follow for emergency situations that might occur when an appropriate person is not available.

Procedure #1: Using the Telephone

1. Assemble your equipment. This includes a telephone message pad, a pen or pencil, and a telephone setup.
2. Answer the telephone promptly and with a "smile."
3. Identify yourself and the facility to the caller.
4. Ask the caller his or her name and the purpose of the call.
5. Watch your tone of voice, manners, grammer, and responses.
6. Deal with the call or refer it to the appropriate person.
7. Close the conversation with saying "Thank you for calling."
8. Gently replace the receiver in its cradle.
9. Immediately record the message, noting the time and date of the call, the caller's name, a brief message and your initials.

Procedure #2: Screening Calls

When required to screen telephone calls, consider the following procedure:

1. Ask the person's name and the reason for the call.
2. Ask questions that clarify the reason for the call.
3. Handle the call personally if you can.
4. Transfer the call to another staff member when appropriate.
5. Get the details for a callback message if the physical therapist should return the call.

Typical Telephone Screening Situations

When screening incoming telephone calls, consider the following scenarios. At the completion of each scenario, ask yourself, as the person answering the call, would you have responded in the same or similar manner.

Scenario #10: Incoming Call to Make an Appointment

Physical Therapy Aide: "Valley Physical Therapy Center. May I help you?"
Caller: "I'd like to talk to the head physical therapist."
Physical Therapy Aide: "I'm sorry, the head therapist, Ms. Smith, is with a patient at the moment. May I ask who is calling?"
Caller: "This is John Jones."
Physical Therapy Aide: "Are you a patient of Ms. Smith's?"
Caller: "Yes."
Physical Therapy Aide: "Would you like to make an appointment with Ms. Smith?"
Caller: "Yes, I would."
Physical Therapy Aide: "What is your medical problem, Mr. Jones?"
(Continue with conversation by scheduling an appointment.)

Scenario #11: Incoming Call for Billing and Insurance

Physical Therapy Aide: "Ms. Jones office. May I help you?"
Caller: "This is Jose Garcia with AAA Insurance Company. I would like information about the charges for your patient, Robert Brown."
Physical Therapy Aide: "Mr. Garcia, I will transfer your call to Ms. Short, who is in charge of insurance payments for our office."

Scenario #12: Incoming Call for "Personal" Business

Physical Therapy Aide: "Good morning, physical therapy department. May I help you?"
Caller: "Mr. Black, please."
Physical Therapy Aide: "I'm sorry, Mr. Black is with a patient. May I ask who is calling?"
Caller: "This is a personal call. I'm a friend of his."
Physical Therapy Aide: "Mr. Black usually returns his calls just before lunch. If you leave your name and number, I will ask him to return your call."
Caller: "It's Jane Good at (818) 555-1234."

Telephone Etiquette

It is always important to use discretion whenever you are required to use the telephone. You would never say "The physical therapist is out to breakfast," or "The therapist isn't in yet and I don't know when she'll be in." Statements such as "The therapist is not available at present," or "I expect Ms. Smith to return at 4:30 p.m., may I take a message," are more appropriate.

Whenever you are about to end a telephone conversation, it is always appropriate to close with "Thank you for calling," and then say good-bye. This should be followed by your gently replacing the receiver in the telephone cradle and, if possible, allowing the caller to hang up first.

If your facility requires that messages be taken for persons not available, you should always make sure that the message is taken accurately and that the time and date of the call is recorded appropriately. Telephone messages should always contain the name of the caller; his or her telephone number, with the area code; a brief summary of the reason for the call; the action taken, if any; and the initials of the person taking the call. Remember too, that it is important to always keep a memo pad and a pen or pencil close to the telephone in order to record messages. If a copy of the telephone call is necessary for the patient's record, you may also use carbon paper and a ballpoint pen in order to record the information.

Procedure #3: Taking Call-back Messages

Since physical therapists do not routinely answer telephone calls, you will generally be required to take call-back messages. To take such a message, consider the following procedure:

1. Write the date and time of the call.
2. Write the name of the person called.
3. Ask the caller's name and telephone number.
4. Ask whether the caller will telephone again.
5. Write down the complete message.

Always remember to ask for specifics if the message is unclear. Complete the task by adding your initials as the person who took the call (see Figure 3-2).

To:_____
Date:_____
Time:_____

While you were away:
Mr./Mrs./Miss:_____
Of_____
Phone:(___)_____
                              ext.

❏ Telephoned   ❏ Please call
❏ Called to see you ❏ Will call again
❏ Wants to see you   ❏ Urgent
❏ Returned your call

Message:_____
_____
_____
_____
_____
_____ Operator

Figure 3-2 The telephone message pad.

Dealing with Problem Calls

Problem calls may occur in any health agency. Some people may refuse to give their name or discuss the purpose of their call. At times, they may even try to intimidate you or make threats toward you or your co-workers. Always try to remain calm and control your temper and attitude, and never hesitate to tell the caller that the person he or she is asking for is unable to answer the telephone. While it may be difficult, try to remain polite yet firm in dealing with this type of situation. If a patient does give his or her name but refuses to state the purpose of the call, remember that this type of situation also requires tact. If ever in doubt, you can always put the patient on "hold" and check with the individual the caller wants. It is then up to that person whether or not to take the call.

Putting the Caller on Hold

The term **holding,** refers to the telephone's capability of keeping a call waiting on one line while a second call is on another line. The two callers do not hear one another's conversations. When a call is placed on hold, the telephone line is blocked, making the line unavailable to incoming and outgoing calls. Asking a person to hold is necessary at times, however, the hold function can be abused if it is used too frequently or if callers are kept waiting too long. You should use the "hold" function when the person being called cannot come to the telephone immediately or when the person answering the telephone is busy with another call.

If you find that you have to put the caller on hold or if you know there will be a slight delay before the appropriate person answers the call, always make sure you inform the caller of this fact. Never leave a caller on hold for long periods of time, and if there is a delay, offer to take the caller's number and have the individual return the call.

♦ APPOINTMENT SCHEDULING

Another important administrative task that you might be responsible for completing and that generally goes along with using the telephone, has do to with scheduling appointments for patients who are to receive physical therapy treatments. Such appointments may either be for treatments that the patient will receive at the bedside, if he is confined to the hospital, or may be for outpatient visits, either in the physical therapy department of the facility or in a private physical therapy office or center.

The most important point to remember when scheduling appointments is that efficient operation of the department or office depends on the correct scheduling of appointments, an activity that requires clear thinking and good judgment. Whether appointments are scheduled by hand in a daybook or with the help of a computer using scheduling software, the entire staff depends on a smooth flow of patient traffic in order to maintain a workable schedule. Appointments must be made so that they allow sufficient time for each patient's treatment, yet without wasteful time gaps.

Generally speaking, one of the most frequent complaints heard from patients who are required to come into the department or the office has to do with them having to spend a great deal of time sitting in a waiting room before they are scheduled for their treatment. In order to avoid this as much as possible, a carefully planned appointment book can be used.

Appointment books vary from facility to facility (see Figure 3-3). However, most of them contain one-half page for each day. Time is usually blocked off in quarter hour periods in order to ensure that all time can be used wisely. Try to become familiar with the type of book or log your facility uses, and get to know what block of time each line represents.

Since you will always want to make sure that appointments are not scheduled with individuals who are not available, try to take an organized approach to appointment scheduling. Before scheduling any appointments, make sure you block out periods of time when the individual is not available. Such time may include lunch, meetings, or even afternoons in which the person may be off or out of the office. The easiest way to block out the period of time is to place a big "X" through those times so that no errors of scheduling can occur.

Another important point to using the appointment book is to always make the appointments in pencil. In this way, if an appointment must be canceled, names can be erased and the time can be rescheduled for another patient. Since not all facilities may follow this policy, you should always follow your individual facility's procedure for this particular practice.

When you are required to schedule appointments for patients, you should also have a pretty good understanding of how long specific therapies might take. If, for example, you know a patient is coming in for an ultrasound of the lower back, followed by hot packs to

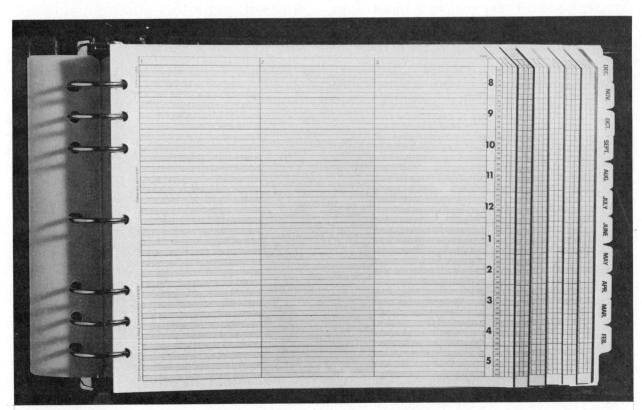

Figure 3-3 A sample appointment book. (From Simmers, *Diversified Health Occupations*, 2nd edition, copyright 1988 by Delmar Publishers Inc.)

the area, you should check with the therapist or the posted schedule, if one exists, about how long such a procedure takes prior to making the appointment. If you discover that this procedure takes approximately 45 minutes to an hour, you would not want to schedule another patient during that time.

Even though most facilities or physical therapy departments generally have a posted schedule that indicates which patients are coming in for specific therapies, always try to get the patient to tell you why he is coming in. By doing this, you can double-check your schedule and if necessary, make any corrections to the appointment book prior to the patient's coming in. In order to do this, however, you should also make sure that when the patient calls you get her telephone number, which is then written in pencil next to her name under the scheduled appointment time.

Since appointment scheduling on the telephone with the patient is more often done in a private physical therapy facility than in a hospital physical therapy department, when the patient does call for an appointment, you should make sure that you have the necessary information before closing your conversation. This includes obtaining the patient's full name, as well as the name of the physician ordering the treatment; the reason for coming into the office, that is, what type of treatment is to be given; and the patient's telephone number. As we have already discussed, by securing the patient's telephone number and putting it directly into the appointment book, it may save time, later, if the patient's appointment has to be canceled or rescheduled.

After you have obtained all the required information from the patient, make sure you repeat the date, day of the week, and the exact time of the appointment. By repeating both the date and day of the week, you provide the patient with a doublecheck and thereby prevent needless errors in the long run. Once you have completed your conversation with the patient, make sure that you mark the full amount of time in the appointment book.

If a patient calls to cancel an appointment, always try to be polite and understanding. Ask the patient if he or she would like to reschedule the appointment. Since the original appointment was written in pencil, you may then erase it and record all the new information in the correct day and block of time.

Chronic problems of scheduling generally occur in all health care agencies. If a specific patient becomes a chronic offender, there are several methods of dealing with the problem. One method involves scheduling this patient at the end of the day. If he does not appear, this will not affect other patients or schedules as much. Some offices send bills for time scheduled. In these facilities, patients must be told in advance that if they cannot keep the appointment, they must notify the office within a specified period of time, usually 24 hours prior to their appointment, or they will be charged for the missed appointment. Some departments or private offices, also note broken appointments as "no shows" on the patient's chart. Usually, the final decision as to how to deal with these situations rests upon the individual in charge.

The proper scheduling of appointments takes time and practice. If you find that your position requires that you schedule appointments, always make sure that you review your facility's individual policy regarding their system, and once reviewed, make sure you follow the facility's method appropriately.

♦♦♦

Procedure #4: Scheduling an Appointment

If required to schedule appointments, the following procedure should be considered:

1. Assemble your equipment. This includes the appointment book and a pen or pencil.
2. Check the appointment book or log and note how much time each line represents.
3. Place the day of the week and date on the top of each of the daily columns.
4. Block off those periods of time when the person for whom the appointments are being scheduled will not be in. Cross through the block with a large "X."
5. Schedule the appointment in the correct time slot. Include the patient's correct name, his or her physician's name, and the telephone number. Include the reason for the appointment.
6. Doublecheck your entry.

♦♦♦

♦ ♦ ♦
SUMMARY OUTLINE

Communicating Effectively
- Parts to effective communication
- Empathy
- Tactfulness
- Patience

Types of Communication
- Oral or verbal communication
- Nonverbal communication

Communication in the Physical Therapy Setting
- Using the telephone
- Screening telephone calls
- Telephone etiquette
- Taking call-back messages
- Dealing with problem calls
- Putting the caller on "hold"

Appointment Scheduling
- Purpose and importance of appointment scheduling
- The appointment book
- Cancelled appointments
- Procedure for appointment scheduling

CHAPTER REVIEW QUESTIONS

1. Define oral and nonverbal communication and explain why each is valuable.
2. Why do you think a physical therapy aide should choose his words carefully when interacting with patients?
3. Define empathy and explain how it differs from sympathy.
4. Define tactfulness.
5. Define patience.
6. Explain the circumstances in which putting a caller on "hold" would be acceptable.
7. Briefly explain the procedures for screening telephone calls.
8. List at least five pieces of information needed for a call-back message:

   a._____   d._____

   b._____   e._____

   c._____

9. Explain how you handle the following calls:

   a. A patient asks to speak to the bookkeeper who is on another line.

   b. Another physical therapy aide, who is busy, receives a personal call.

   c. A patient asks to talk with the physical therapist.

10. What would you do if the following situations occurred during regular office hours?

    a. A patient who has an 11:00 A.M. appointment does not appear.

    b. The physical therapist is behind schedule by 45 minutes.

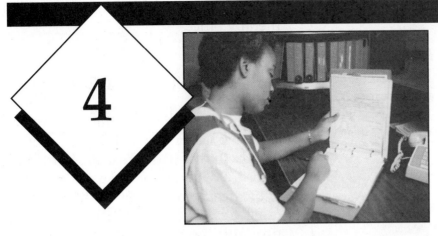

4

Administrative Skills

Objectives

After studying this chapter, you will be able to:

1. Identify clerical and administrative tasks that may be required of the physical therapy aide.

2. Describe what constitutes a patient's medical record.

3. Identify five forms found in a patient's medical chart.

4. Describe how to complete a medical record form.

5. Describe the procedure for correcting a medical record.

6. Explain how fees may be collected from patients.

7. Define professional courtesy.

8. Briefly explain how a Superbill system works.

9. Identify three common methods of bookkeeping used in a medical or physical therapy office.

10. Discuss the purpose of insurance and briefly describe how to fill out an insurance form.

11. Identify two common methods of filing in the physical therapy office.

12. List at least five different types of letters a physical therapy aide might be required to type.

In Chapter 3, we discussed some of the basic clerical or administrative skills the physical therapy aide might be required to perform as part of her daily workload. According to your previous reading, we discovered that effective communication was the most basic skill of all, particularly as it related to greeting patients, answering the telephone, and setting up appointments in the office or department. However, when we discuss the role of the physical therapy aide as it relates to administrative tasks, we must also be concerned with other areas such as working with and maintaining the patient's chart, billing and record-keeping, and many of the skills involved in running the physical therapy office.

◆ THE MEDICAL RECORD

As in all medical facilities, there may be times when you will be required to work with the patient's chart or medical record. While there are a wide variety of medical records kept on the patient in most health care facilities, you will probably be most involved with his physical therapy record sheet.

Understanding the Medical Record

A patient's **medical record** is information set down in writing that documents facts and events during the administration of patient care. The **medical report** is part of the medical record and is a permanent legal document that formally states the consequences of the patient's examination or treatment in letter or report form. There are three important reasons for keeping the patient's medical records.

The first reason is that it may be used by the physician to aid in the diagnosis and treatment of a patient. The second reason medical records are used is that they are able to assist in the research of diseases and injuries so that other patients may benefit from previous patient care. Finally, a patient's record is kept, because of the legal ramifications involved in health care. The record may be used to avoid legal problems, comply with laws, and to defend the physician or other health care provider in the event of a lawsuit.

Patient records may also be used to complete various reports required by law such as reports on communicable diseases; child abuse; injuries, such as gunshot wounds and stabbings which result from criminal actions; and diseases and illnesses of newborns and infants. They are also helpful in completing insurance claims for government and state programs so that proof is available to show specific services charged to the patient.

The patient record may consist of a variety of documents such as a patient registration form, which might consist of identifying information as well a as medical history questionnaire; progress or chart notes; laboratory reports; x-ray and other medical reports, such as those used in a specific treatment involving physical therapy. The patient's ledger card, which is used specifically for billing and insurance information, is also considered part of the record but is generally filed in a separate file. Generally speaking, the specialty of a physician or the type of office in which the record is kept most influences the kind of records maintained.

All entries in the patient's record must be as legible as possible because hospitals and physicians and specialty offices have been held liable when a medication or treatment has been given to a patient in error as a result of handwritten notes incorrectly read. Although some physicians and physical therapists prefer to handwrite their notes, it is common today for these professionals to dictate their notes if their handwriting is illegible so that they can be typed to avoid errors that might result in an expensive lawsuit. Typed entries made during the continuing care or treatment of the patient should always be signed or initialed by the attending physician or therapist. For a chart to be admissible as evidence in a court of law, the individual dictating or writing the entries should be able to attest that the entries were true and correct at the time of writing. A signature or initials after the typed notes indicates this fact.

Since medical forms may vary according to individual facilities, let's take a look at the ones used most frequently and which you will be more apt to encounter in the physical therapy office.

Statistical Data Sheet

The statistical data sheet, sometimes referred to as the **patient's registration form,** (see Figure 4-1), is generally filled out during the patient's first visit to the office. It usually includes such information as the patient's full name, address and telephone number, marital status, sex, date of birth, place of employment, insurance company, if any, and the name of the referring physician.

Medical History Record

The medical history record is used in most agencies and its purpose is to provide information that may assist the department or office in caring for the patient. It usually includes such vital information as the patient's name, address, age, and sex; a past medical history, including any treatments, operations, allergies, and childhood diseases; a *family history*, which provides information on the patient's immediate family members; a *personal history* such as the patient's marital history, personal habits like smoking and the use of alcohol, and, if the patient is a female, their menstrual history and history of pregnancy. The medical history form also includes information pertaining to the patient's present illness, including a description of the signs and symptoms for which the patient is seeking treat-

STATISTICAL DATA SHEET

Case Number __12345__   Date __MAY 18, 19--__

Mr.
Mrs.
(Miss) __BROWN__   __BARBARA__   __B__   _____
        Last   First   Middle   Maiden

Address __50 FOX DRIVE__

City __ALBANY__   State __N.Y.__   Zip __12205__

Telephone __(518) 469-8550__   Birthdate __10__ / __2__ / __62__
                               Mo.   Day   Yr.

(S.) M. W. D.   Age __31__   Social Security __117-22-1949__

Spouse's Name in full __NONE__

Occupation __RECEPTIONIST__

Place of Employment __WRGB RADIO STATION__

Business Address __4 NISKAYUNA ROAD__

City __ALBANY__   State __N.Y.__   Zip __12206__

Business Telephone (Include ext.) __(518) 469-7234 (EXT. 24)__

Person Responsible for Account __JOHN BROWN__

Relationship __FATHER__   Address __50 FOX DRIVE__

City __ALBANY__   State __N.Y.__ Zip __12205__ Telephone __(518) 469-8550__

Insurance Company __METROPOLITAN LIFE__

Address __74 WEST 89TH STREET__

City __NEW YORK__   State __N.Y.__   Zip __18900__

Group Number (if any) __01210__   Policy Number __4673__

Other Health Insurance __NONE__

Referred by: __DR. SEBASTIAN WARD__

Figure 4-1 A sample statistical data sheet. (From Simmers, *Diversified Health Occupations*, 2nd edition, copyright 1988 by Delmar Publishers Inc.)

ment; a *physical examination form*, always completed by a physician, in which notations are made showing the different areas of the body where treatment may be necessary; and finally, a *prognosis, diagnosis or treatment record form*, which are generally used to indicate the final outcome of the disease or treatment being used.

Confidentiality and the Medical Record

All forms that make up the patient's medical record or chart, are considered confidential and should be handled as such. This means that all the information which you may come into contact with on the chart should never be shared with anyone other than those individuals providing care to the patient. Also, whenever you are required to obtain information from the patient, it should be done in complete privacy. Since specific questions regarding the patient's private life may have to be asked, it is essential that all questions be asked in a professional manner.

Correcting the Medical Record

Because of the medicolegal problems that might arise, it is important to know how to properly correct chart notes as well as other records. You must never *erase* or *white out* handwritten or typed entries that require correction on a patient's medical record. Instead, a line is neatly drawn through the incorrect entry so that it remains readable. If there is adequate room above or below the original entry, the correct information is inserted there. The person making the correction writes the abbreviation "Corr.," the date, and his or her initials in the margin of the chart sheet (see Figure 4-2). If there is no space above or below the correct entry, the correction must be made below on the next available section on the sheet. There, the person making the correction enters the date, writes or types "correction to chart

---

♦♦♦

Procedure #5: Completing a Medical Record or Form

If required to complete a medical record or report form, the following procedure should be considered:

1. Assemble all of your equipment. This includes the physical therapy treatment form, a pen, or a typewriter.
2. Use a private area for questioning the patient.
3. Complete the form as required by your facility. Make sure the form has the patient's correct name, address, and telephone number; the referring physician, diagnosis, if any, and other pertinent information.
4. Recheck all information provided by the patient.
5. Complete the form as required by your facility. This may include a statistical data sheet, medical history, family history and history of the present illness.
6. Prepare the patient for treatment as indicated by your facility.
7. If you are required to type the information from a written record, recheck all parts to be sure the information is accurate.
8. Replace all your equipment.

♦♦♦

							Treatment or Medication	Nourishment	Remarks
Date	Time	Temp.	Pulse	Resp.	Urine	Stool			
4-1-	7 30 A.M.	99	84	20					65 yr. old male adm. to rm.
									602-B via wheelchair
							B/P 128/72		c/o "Cramp like abd. pains"
							wt. 146 lbs.		abd. distended
	8				150 ml				to lab.
	8 15						C B C)		ordered
							Hinten)		Dr. Darin notified
									J. Mathews, Ass't
	9 30						Darvon Comp. 65 mg.		P.O.
	11 30							tea and dry toast	appetite good
	11 30							tea and dry toast	refused
	12	99.4	88	18					c/o increased pain and
									abd. disten.
	1						Harris Flush		given c̄ tap H₂O- 105°
									lg. amt. flatus expelled
									J. Mathews, Ass't
	4	99.4	88	22	150 ml		B/P 128/70		Coughing—had some diffi-
									culty holding thermometer
									in mouth
									R. Jones, Ass't

Figure 4-2 Making an entry correction. (From Hegner and Caldwell, *Nursing Assistant: A Nursing Process Approach,* 6th edition, copyright 1992 by Delmar Publishers Inc.)

note of (date)," and follows that with the correct entry and his or her initials or signature at the end of the notation.

It is acceptable when typing a chart note or medical report, to use correction fluid or tape on typographical errors at the time of typing, but you should *never* obscure, erase, or put self-adhesive typing strips over an original entry to correct the chart at a later time. If the physician or the physical therapist has discovered she has neglected to enter a notation or needs to make a correction after the chart has been typed, it must be added as an addendum or corrected in the specified manner.

♦ BILLING, BANKING, AND INSURANCE

While most large hospitals and private physical therapy facilities generally have a separate department or individual responsible for the financial record keeping, billing, and insurance intake,

you may encounter a situation in which the physical therapy aide is responsible for such tasks.

Although the practice of medicine and physical therapy has its primary aim at providing health care and treatment to those that require it, it would be quite foolish and unrealistic to ignore the fact that another motive for providing this care and treatment is the production of a livelihood for the physician or physical therapist and his family. The production of this livelihood depends upon the good credit of those the individual practitioner serves. When we speak of the word credit, meaning "to believe" or "to trust," we also speak of one's trust in others. In today's financial world, however, credit also means a trust in a person's business integrity and her financial ability to meet all obligations when they become due.

Since physicians and physical therapists generally prefer not to discuss financial matters with patients, it usually becomes the job of the physical therapy aide or the individual responsible for running the front office of the physical therapy center. Because financial matters are personal, it is important that any discussion of fees be private so that the patient can feel free to talk about any problems he or she might have. A mature, courteous, tactful, firm, and businesslike approach is vital. It has been proven that stating the amount of the fee for the service actually improves public relations and reduces patient complaints, business office turnover problems, accounts receivable, and financial charge-offs.

Fees

As with anything else, there is a right time and a wrong time for the discus-

sion of fees for services provided. Most patients who arrive at the office to obtain treatment are more concerned with their health problem than with the expense incurred as a result of their office visit. You should always begin by listening to the patient's medical problem; however, you must also be prepared to discuss the expense should the patient be inquisitive about costs. After the patient has explained his medical problem or the reason for the visit, the physical therapy aide should tactfully inquire whether he has health insurance coverage because the initial office visit usually begins the credit process and establishes the credit relationship. Generally speaking, a patient who has health insurance will have coverage that will offset some of the office or hospital expenses.

Fees for services rendered should always be clearly and accurately stated. A misquoted price may make a patient angry. Also, never try to hedge by stating the approximate amount nor apologize for the fee. If a patient is having difficulties, this may come out during the initial interview. If this is indeed the case, you may then discuss a payment plan or a discount if warranted.

In some instances, a patient may be emotionally unable to handle a discussion of fees; that is why it may be wise to ask, "Would you like to know something about the expense?" If a patient is elderly and someone in the family is responsible for the bill, the fee discussion should take place with both the paying party and the patient present.

Professional Courtesy

The term *professional courtesy* refers to a discount or no-charge exemption extended to certain people authorized by the physical therapist or administrator of the office or department. It is important to know the office policy on this issue so as not to bill an individual in error. Professional courtesy is usually extended to physicians, nurses, medical assistants, clergy, pharmacists, and dentists, and any other individual deemed appropriate by the physical therapist or administrator in charge.

Billing

If you are working in a private physical therapy office, you will discover that each office has its own fee collection system based on the individual discretion of the therapist or administrator in charge. Such a system also takes into account the amount of the average bill and the number of patients seen on a daily basis.

In most offices, there are several methods of billing and fee collection. The following are a few of the most frequently used methods:

1. **Fee for Service:** This type of service involves the collection of fees for office visits when the service is rendered. For most offices it is an attractive method of billing, since it usually includes an increase in cash flow and collection ratio, reduction of collection costs, reduced billing chores, settlement by insurance companies directly to the patient, and quick identification of nonpayers.
2. **Cycle Billing:** In this method, certain portions of the accounts receivable are billed at specific times during the month on the basis of alphabetical breakdown, thus allowing for continuous cash flow throughout the month and prevention of having to send a heavy load of statements out at one time.

3. **Monthly Itemized Statement:** This type of billing involves sending the patient a bill for the office visit after the service has been rendered. The greatest disadvantage to this method, is that it often increases collection costs and delays cash flow.
4. **Credit-card Billing:** Putting a bill on a credit card so that the payment is received by the office directly from the credit card company is a method often used in large group practices and in some specialties such as dental care, plastic surgery procedures, and contact lens and vision centers because of the major expenditures resulting from these practices. Usually the credit card company requests a five percent service fee, and if a bill becomes delinquent, the office cannot collect it because that is the responsibility of the credit card company. This method, while not used by all practices, does reduce office overhead and collection costs.

The Superbill System

Another type of billing system that many offices have adopted is called the **Superbill.** The major advantage of this system is that it combines a bill and an insurance claim in one statement rendered to the patient at the time of the office visit (see Figure 4-3). The superbill two-or three-part form can be printed for use with a pegboard, computer, or charge-slip system. Each superbill contains the patient's name, date, services rendered, treatment codes, diagnostic information appearing as an ICD-9CM code number (*International Classification of Diseases*, 9th revision, *Clinical Modification*), insurance require-

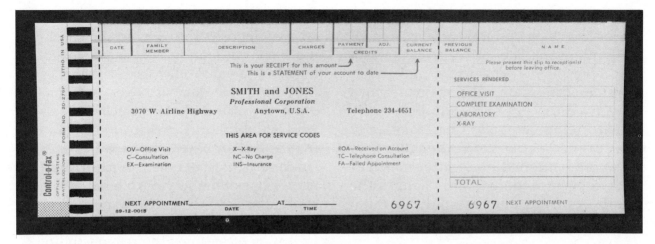

A

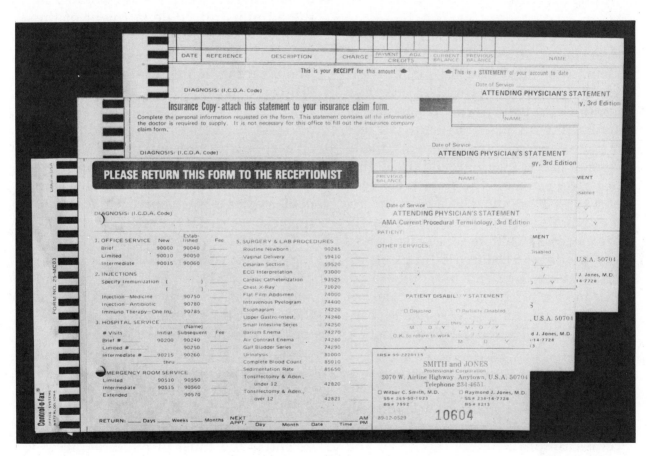

B

Figure 4-3 (A) A statement receipt provides information on past balance due, charges, payment received, and current balance; (B) The communication form is a three-layer version of the statement-receipt form that also lists treatments and insurance codes. (From Simmers, *Diversified Health Occupations*, 2nd edition, copyright 1988 by Delmar Publishers Inc.)

ments, assignment of benefits, and the physician's or physical therapist's identifying data. The form also includes a section for the patient to complete her indentifying data. The major reasons many offices uses the superbill system is that it eliminates the vast majority of insurance paperwork, it encourages payment immediately after services have been rendered, and changes the habits of patients by making them financially responsible for themselves.

Billing Services

When patient ledgers are used as a financial record as well as a billing statement, some offices employ a billing service. A good billing service can improve the patient's understanding of statements because they show all fees incurred and previous payments, thereby eliminating questions and promoting faster collections. The service can also ensure prompt billing because it can get statements out on time, more easily because it is free from office disruptions while billing. Using a billing service often saves time and money because expensive billing equipment is not required in the office and valuable space need not be allocated to billing supplies.

Banking

Every financial transaction in a medical or physical therapy practice concerns cash or the use of checks. If you work in an office where banking is the responsibility of the physical therapy aide, it is essential that you understand fundamental banking procedures and common banking terms. Banking transactions involve privileged information, and the physical therapy aide must be aware of the importance of confidentiality in such matters.

Banks are financial institutions that receive deposits into savings or checking accounts, loan money, make collections, and render other services such as providing safe deposit boxes and handling trust funds. Many such services are also offered by credit unions, savings and loan associations, and other financial institutions. A thorough knowledge of the services offered by the banks and how to make the most effective use of them as they relate to your facility is oftentimes the responsibility of the physical therapy aide working in the administrative department of the facility.

Bookkeeping in the Physical Therapy Office

When discussing billing and banking as each relates to the physical therapy office, it is also important that we spend a few moments discussing the role bookkeeping plays as part of the overall financial picture of the office.

The main purpose of any bookkeeping system is to record the financial affairs of the business. Most medical and physical therapy practices rely on the administrative personnel to manage the bookkeeping transactions so that the physician or physical therapist has a clear daily picture of the income derived from patient accounts as well as detailed information on office expenditures. Accurate financial records are essential and must provide the necessary figures for income tax purposes.

Most medical or physical therapy practices will employ one of three bookkeeping systems. These include a single-entry, double-entry, or pegboard system.

A **single-entry bookkeeping** system is neither self-balancing nor is it articulated. It does not rely on equal debits or credits and is relatively easy to learn and use. It is also acceptable to both federal and state authorities as a basis for filing tax returns.

The **double-entry bookkeeping** system is more an art than it is a system. It involves keeping books that balance and utilizes assets, capital, and liabilities. Because of its complexity, most physical therapy offices do not use this system, since it most often must be kept up to date by a full-charge bookkeeper or accountant.

The use of **pegboard bookkeeping** is probably the most popular bookkeeping method employed by most physician's and physical therapy offices around the country because it is an accurate system, it is easy to learn, and it uses a write-it-once process for recording daily office transactions, thereby minimizing errors and saving clerical writing time. The system uses a lightweight board with pegs on the right and/or left side and forms with holes for the pegs. The forms may be layered one on top of the other and held in place on the board by the pegs (see Figure 4-4). Usually the layered forms are printed on NCR paper, but if not, carbon paper may be used to carry the entries onto the various layered sheets.

When using the pegboard system, the day's transactions, which are kept on a daily journal sheet, are placed on the pegboard. Then a series of prenumbered, perforated charge receipts or service or transaction slips are added. Each slip acts as a receipt in the event of payment and a portion of the slip can be removed and given to the patient to show the next appointment date. Each patient's ledger card is slipped between the daily journal sheet and his transaction slip as the patient is seen. When an entry is written, it then registers simultaneously on all three items — the daily journal sheet, the patient's ledger card, and the charge slip. After each patient has left the office, his other ledger card is removed and the next patient's card is inserted.

◆ COMPLETING INSURANCE FORMS

One of the more common tasks the physical therapy aide assigned to work in the front or administrative office may be required to perform involves the completion of insurance forms. Since many patients rely heavily on insurance companies to pay their medical expenses, completing insurance forms accurately is one of the most important administrative practices in the office. In order to obtain prompt payment from the companies, these forms should be completed correctly and in a timely manner.

Since there are many insurance companies that provide different types of coverage for patients, many forms exist and are currently in use. Generally speaking, most insurance companies provide the patient with booklets that outline the type of coverage available.

All information regarding the patient's insurance coverage is essential, and it is usually obtained at the time of the patient's first visit to the facility. Always make sure that all names, addresses, and contract numbers are correct since any errors could result in nonpayment or slow payment from the insurance company.

If it is the policy of your department to allow patients to file an insurance claim, as opposed to paying for the visit at the time of treatment, make sure that you have the correct forms available.

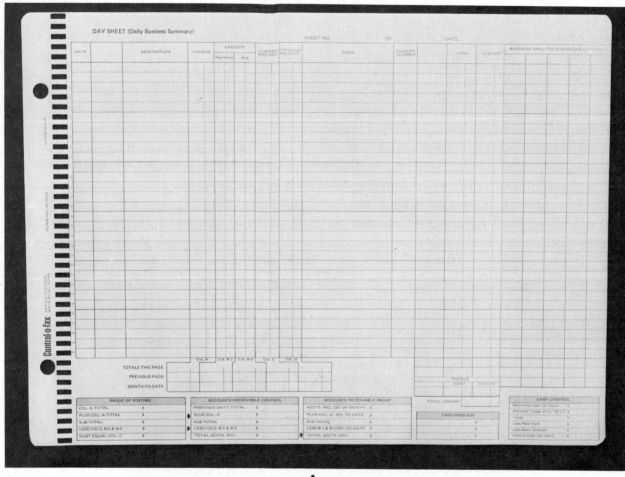

A

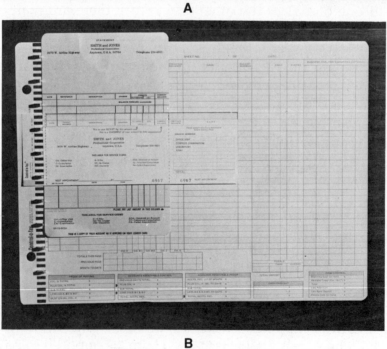

B

Figure 4-4 (A) The day sheet provides a daily record of patients seen, charges incurred, and payments received; (B) The ledger card is inserted between the statement-receipt record and the day sheet on the pegboard. (From Simmers, *Diversified Health Occupations*, 2nd edition, copyright 1988 by Delmar Publishers Inc.)

Many facilities keep a supply of standard insurance forms such as those used by most major insurance companies and those used by the state for State Disability Insurance claims. In other cases, the patient may have to obtain the forms from his insurance company and bring them to the office. Whether or not the patient brings in his own form, or uses one of your standard forms, always make sure that the patient has completed his section of the form. It is also important to make sure that the form has been properly signed. If the patient is a dependent, such as a spouse or a child, it is also necessary to obtain the signature of the person to whom the insurance contract has been issued. This person is referred to as the "insured."

If you are required to assist in the completion of insurance forms, there are some general guidelines that you should always follow. First, always make sure that you are using the correct form. Read it thoroughly and make sure that you understand what information is required. Always check to be sure that the patient has completed the proper sections on the form. This includes making sure that the appropriate signatures have also been obtained.

Secondly, always make sure that the correct names, addresses, and contract numbers have been listed on the form. If necessary, use correct codes for properly identifying the treatment being offered, as well as codes that relate to the office or department. Make sure that all questions on the form are correctly answered.

The final and most important guideline to remember is that you must always make sure that the doctor, therapist, or authorized person has signed the form in the required area. Many forms require the physician's or therapist's identification or licensing number. Make sure it is entered correctly. Also, you should note the boxed area for *assignment of benefits*. If the physician, therapist, or facility will accept the payment amount from the insurance company, this section must be checked or marked "yes." If the amount will not be accepted, make sure that either the box is not checked or that "no" is marked. After you have completed the form, a good practice is to make a copy of it and place it into the patient's chart.

♦ ADDITIONAL ADMINISTRATIVE DUTIES

Depending upon the size of the facility or department in which the physical therapy aide is employed, she may be called upon to complete any number of administrative tasks. In addition to those areas already discussed in this chapter, there may be other clerical tasks required of the aide. Some of these may include filing, typing, working on the office computer system (see Figure 4-5), and letter writing.

Filing

Because medical records constitute the collective memory of any physician's or physical therapist's practice, the physical therapy aide required to file must exercise good judgment in maintaining the office's filing system.

There are two basic types of filing systems that most facilities use. These include the alphabetical system and the numerical system.

Alphabetical filing deals with filing information according to where it fits in the alphabet. It is the system used for

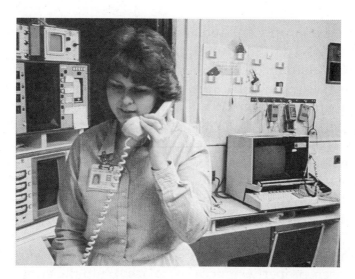

Figure 4-5 Computers are used in physical therapy departments to maintain records and serve as a valuable source of information. (From Hegner and Caldwell, *Nursing Assistant: A Nursing Process Approach,* 6th edition, copyright 1992 by Delmar Publishers Inc.)

listing names in a telephone book, and it is generally used most often because of its simplicity. This type of system involves following some basic rules, including:

1. Indexing names before putting them into alphabetical order.
2. Filing names of organizations and businesses in alphabetical order.
3. Never including such words as *of, and, at, the, on,* or *a* as part of the indexing unit when filing in alphabetical order.
4. When filing a name or a company, always follow strict alphabetical rules.
5. Including prefixes as part of names.
6. Including hyphenated names as part of one unit.
7. Treating familiar abbreviations, such as St., as though the word was spelled out.
8. Using titles or degrees as the last indexing unit.
9. Using notations such as Jr., Sr., II, etc., as final indexing units.
10. If a woman is married, indexing her name with her husband's surname as the first unit.
11. Indexing numbers as though the number were spelled out in letters.

The second most common method of filing in the physical therapy office is called numerical filing. If this system is used, a cross index or reference is generally required. Patient's names are usually indexed as they are in alphabetical filing, with the name placed on a card and a number assigned.

Numbers used in a facility are usually run in order, and a record is kept as to which numbers have been assigned. The card with the name and number is then kept in an alphabetical file. When a patient comes to the department or office, the alphabetical card is located in order to determine the patient's number. The number file is then located. Remember, in this system, numbers always go in order from small to large.

Letter Writing

One basic procedure the physical therapy aide may encounter as part of his responsibility in the administrative office, is assisting in letter writing or typing business letters for the facility. However, the type of letter and the procedure that is followed will almost always depend upon the facility in which the physical therapy aide is employed.

There are five basic types of letters that you may be requested to type. These include collection letters, appointment letters, recall and consultation letters, and inquiry letters. It's important to note, that no matter which type you may be asked to complete, you should always remember that all letters must be typed accurately and neatly and never be altered to change their original content or meaning.

◆ ◆ ◆
SUMMARY OUTLINE

The Medical Record
- Understanding the medical record
- Understanding the medical report
- Statistical data sheet
- Medical history record
- Confidentiality and the medical record
- Correcting the medical record
- Completing a medical record form

Billing, Banking, and Insurance
- Fees
- Professional courtesy
- Billing
- The Superbill system
- Billing services
- Banking and bookkeeping
- Completing insurance forms

Additional Administrative Duties
- Filing
- Letter writing

CHAPTER REVIEW QUESTIONS

1. Briefly explain the purpose and function of a medical record.
2. Briefly explain the purpose and function of a medical report.
3. All records and forms that make up the patient's medical record are considered _____.
4. The term _____ _____ refers to a discount or no-charge exemption extended to certain people.
5. List four frequently used methods of billing in the physical therapy office:

   a._____   c._____
   b._____   d._____

6. What is the major advantage of using a "Superbill" billing system?
7. List three methods of bookkeeping used in most medical offices:

   a._____
   b._____
   c._____

8. What does the phrase "assignment of benefits" mean?
9. List the two basic types of filing systems used by most medical or physical therapy offices:

   a._____
   b._____

10. _____ for services rendered should always be clearly and accurately stated.
11. A _____ _____ _____ usually includes such information as the patient's name, address, and telephone number.

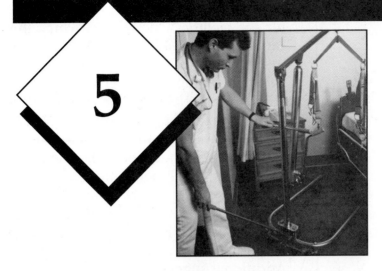

Maintaining the Facility

Objectives
After studying this chapter, you will be able to:

1. Describe the purpose of maintaining the physical therapy facility.

2. Discuss the physical therapy aide's role in maintaining the physical therapy facility.

3. Explain how maintaining the physical therapy facility helps to increase office productivity.

4. Define the function of office procedure manuals.

5. Discuss what is involved in office housekeeping and maintenance.

6. Describe how office supplies and equipment control is maintained.

7. Explain the purpose of inventory control and discuss at least two different methods for a good inventory control system.

8. Discuss the importance of the proper control and storage of drugs in the physical therapy facility.

VOCABULARY

Learn the meaning and the correct spelling of the following words and abbreviations:

Maintenance
Productivity
Housekeeping
Inventory control
Supply control card
Running inventory card
Guarantee

The physical therapy aide assigned to administrative responsibilities must be able to take initiative and exercise independent judgment. This is especially true when such tasks and responsibilities include the maintenance and smooth and effective running of the entire office or department. As the person in charge of maintaining the office, the physical therapy aide must be able to develop an effective management plan that will foster a cooperative effort, provide for an equitable division of the work load by assigning each member of the staff well-defined tasks with a minimum of overlapping duties, and efficiently maintain equipment and supplies necessary to reduce delays and keep the office or facility operating efficiently.

◆ INCREASING OFFICE PRODUCTIVITY

The key role of the physical therapy aide responsible for the administrative department is to continuously strive to boost office productivity which is neces-sary to improve both output and income for the facility. One way in which this can be accomplished includes encouraging specialization of office members such as assigning one person to handle all insurance claims while another handles cash payments. Another way is to encourage continuing education for employees by suggesting that the facility pay a specific percentage toward it. Adopting flexible work hours, allowing some personnel to arrive before normal office hours while others start later also helps to improve office productivity. Additional suggestions, such as varying job assignments, installing productive office equipment, and scheduling regular staff meetings, are all ways in which office productivity can be increased.

Office Procedure Manuals

Some facilities use office procedure manuals to assist them in maintaining an effective workplace. The purpose of these manuals are to spell out specific job descriptions which can guide each staff member in performing his work assignments. It also provides all the employees with a compilation of sample forms for office tasks. A procedure manual can also foster cooperative spirit by making clear to all employees exactly what their jobs entail. In addition, it may be used for orienting new employees and as a handbook for people who may have to substitute for absent personnel.

Housekeeping and Maintenance

If your facility is to project an orderly, hospital-like image, patients must be able to associate its cleanliness with good medical practices. This can easily be accomplished if housekeeping duties are divided among all office personnel,

making it less likely that any one person will feel imposed on. The result will be an accident-free, sanitary office for both the patients and the staff.

Many offices contract with private cleaning agencies or janitorial services to clean their facilities thoroughly on weekends and sometimes at periods during the week when there are no scheduled patient appointments. Before a contract can be negotiated, however, it is best to obtain several bids from different companies for comparison of prices. If during the contract period, work proves inadequate and discussion fails to solve the problem, new bids should be sought and a new service obtained. Most janitorial services will generally include vacuuming rugs, washing woodwork, damp-mopping floors, scrubbing sinks and toilets, emptying wastepaper baskets, washing countertops, and refilling containers.

Most housekeeping tasks assigned to the physical therapy aide will be in the outer-office complex. An uncluttered secretarial workstation with personal items out of sight and office work stored upon completion of each task is most desirable. Other than replenishing secretarial supplies, the physical therapy aide will probably not be concerned with tidying the physical therapist's desk. Additional housekeeping tasks may also include emptying wastebaskets in the front and back offices, replenishing paper supplies, removing fingerprints from work station windows, and checking restrooms.

Nonflowering indoor plants, ferns and terrariums are usually desirable in a medical or physical therapy office because they add decorative accents to the reception area and make it a pleasant place for patients to wait. Therefore, part of your responsibility may be to make sure that all plants are watered and occasionally fertilized as needed.

Depending on the size of your facility, additional housekeeping and maintenance tasks may also be necessary. These may include making sure fire extinguishers are checked and up to date, x-ray rooms are properly cleaned and stocked, and all equipment and supplies are properly cleaned, restocked, and stored in their proper location after use.

♦ MAINTAINING CONTROL OF OFFICE SUPPLIES AND EQUIPMENT

Ordering supplies and equipment and maintaining an adequate inventory is usually delegated to the aides or assistants who use the supplies on a daily basis. The physical therapy aide assigned to work in the clinical area is primarily concerned with keeping on hand medical supplies and equipment for patient care, whereas the aide assigned to work in the administrative or clerical office is more often responsible for ordering business stock and equipment necessary to maintain office efficiency.

Inventory Control of Office Supplies

A continuing stock of office supplies depends on an effective inventory control system, one that provides an up-to-date list of all supplies, the amount of each on hand, the reorder point, and the time required to fill an order. The best way to keep an inventory controlled is to either list each inventory item on an individual sheet of notebook paper, kept in a separate inventory control notebook, or to use file cards arranged in alphabetical order. Entries, written in pencil because some data may have to be changed, should record the name of the item, the identification or catalog number, the supplier's or manufacturer's name, address, and telephone number, the quantity ordered, the reorder point, the price of the item, and the dates when each order was placed, received, and paid for.

If you are required to keep the facility's inventory control, you may find that using *supply control cards* or a *running inventory card* helps maintain better control of your stock. A supply control card provides space for a typed heading and is preprinted with the appropriate columnar headings, thereby providing an efficient method for managing inventory and for facilitating reorders (see Figure 5-1). The amount of an item to purchase can be determined by evaluating information dealing with the consumption rate, cost, and the amount of storage space available.

A running inventory card provides preprinted columnar headings for listing quantity, reorder point, and the location of supplies (see Figure 5-2). Each time an item is removed from the shelf or storage area, the amount listed as "on hand" is corrected downward, providing sufficient warning of a need to reorder. Running inventory cards should always be kept near the supply cabinets.

Another method for maintaining an adequate amount of office supplies is to label each inventory item with a strip of plastic adhesive tape on which is written the name of the item and the minimum number of units constituting a safe reserve. Each time stock is removed, the units remaining are checked against the reorder point. When the reserve supply matches the number on the label, an order can then be placed.

♦ MAINTAINING OFFICE EQUIPMENT

An inoperative or broken piece of equipment can cause a loss of time and money. Repairs may be facilitated by keeping a service file folder containing maintenance instructions on all office and medical equipment. Major equipment repairs should always be handled by qualified repairmen. Leased equipment, such as many of the instruments used in a physical therapy office, often includes a servicing guarantee. Written guarantees, instruction manuals, information pamphlets, and service contracts for reference should all be kept in the service file folder, and guarantee cards should be mailed as soon as equipment has been delivered. To manage equipment maintenance in the office, the physical therapy aide should follow the guidelines listed below:

1. Always assign one person to request repairs on all equipment, thereby eliminating the potential of everyone or no one calling for service.
2. Arrange for equipment to be serviced immediately when a failure occurs.
3. Keep an up-to-date list of all equipment and note repair costs. This helps to both determine when the cost of maintaining a piece of equipment might justify its replacement and having costs readily available for the office operating budget.
4. Before purchasing any new equip-

ment, understand the agreements made for service. A service agreement is a type of "insurance policy" against future repair costs and, as such, contains certain specifications that should be thoroughly understood by the person maintaining the equipment.

5. Only deal with service companies that can respond quickly to requests for service.

Date	Item	Quantity Ordered	Vendor	Price

Figure 5-1 The supply control card.

If the physical therapy aide carries out a well-organized approach to equipment repairs, delays due to downtime will be minimized and many of the problems that can destroy operating efficiency will be relieved.

♦ CONTROL AND STORAGE OF DRUGS

While the vast majority of physical therapy offices and departments would normally have very little or nothing to

Date	Item	Quantity Ordered	Vendor	Price	Quantity On Hand	Last Date Ordered

Figure 5-2 The running inventory card.

do with the dispensing of drugs, some facilities, particularly those that include a physician on staff, may require that specific medications be kept in the facility. If this indeed is the case, the physical therapy aide can help the physician to avoid potential liability by setting up a systematic plan for the management and storage of all drugs. The nurse or medical assistant who handles the medications daily, is usually the individual delegated to the task of keeping an inventory, that is, evaluating the needs and writing down in a notebook the names of drugs that are running low. Then the administrative aide follows through by contacting the pharmacy or sales representative to place the order. Some physicians who have offices near pharmacies prefer to keep a low drug inventory or to rely on free samples dispensed by suppliers, whereas physicians in rural areas oftentimes maintain a large supply of medications. Some system for the control and storage of all drugs kept on the premises is required no matter how small the supply.

◆ ◆ ◆
SUMMARY OUTLINE

Maintaining the Facility
- Increasing office productivity
- Office procedure manuals

Housekeeping and Maintenance

Maintaining Control of Office Supplies and Equipment
- Inventory control of office supplies
- Maintaining office equipment

Control and Storage of Drugs

CHAPTER REVIEW QUESTIONS

1. Briefly explain the key role of the physical therapy aide who is responsible for the administrative department.
2. What is the purpose of an office procedure manual?
3. Why is it important to maintain control of office supplies and equipment?
4. If an office dispenses drugs or medication, who is the person generally responsible for keeping the inventory?
5. Who determines which supply agencies to use for the physical therapy facility?
6. What is the purpose of a supply control card?
7. List at least four items that should appear on any type of inventory control card.
8. Why should the physical therapy aide consult the physical therapist or office supervisor before ordering expensive items or equipment?

9. List at least three responsibilities of an office janitorial staff:
   a._____
   b._____
   c._____
10. Using _____ _____ _____ or a _____ helps maintain better control of office stock.
11. Leased equipment usually includes a _____ _____ and an instruction manual.
12. Describe how the physical therapy aide can help the physician in the control and storage of drugs.
13. Why is a service file folder recommended for equipment maintenance?

SECTION III

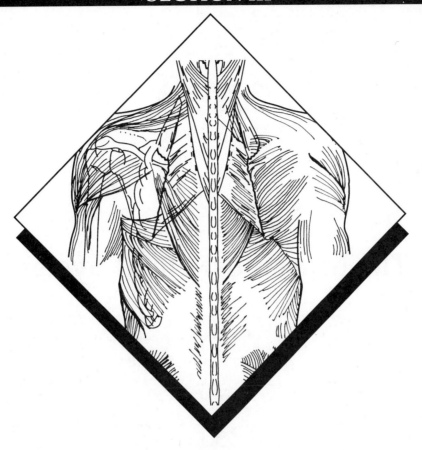

SCIENTIFIC PRINCIPLES

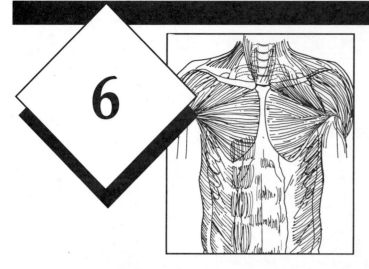

The Musculoskeletal System

Objectives

After studying this chapter, you will be able to:

1. Define the term *anatomy*.

2. Define the term *physiology*.

3. Describe the role the musculoskeletal system plays in the overall function of the human body.

4. Describe the anatomical position of the human body.

5. List the main bones of the skull.

6. Describe the vertebral column and list each of its parts.

7. List and describe which bones make up the shoulder girdle and the pelvic girdle.

8. Define joint movement and explain each of the four types.

9. List the main muscles of the body and briefly describe the function of each.

VOCABULARY

Learn the meaning and the correct spelling of the following words and abbreviations:

Anatomy
Physiology
Skeletal
Anatomical position
Abduction
Adduction
Rotation
Flexion
Extension
Humerus
Olecranon
Acetabulum
Phalanges
Atrophy
Sternocleidomastoid
Extensors
Proximal
Distal
Anterior
Posterior
Maxillary
Mandibular
Frontal
Parietal
Temporal
Radius
Ilium
Ischium
Joint
Masseter
Diaphragm
Flexors
Occipital
Vertebrae
CNS
Atlas
Axis
Thorax

Sternum
Clavicle
Scapula
Ulna
Femur
Tibia
Muscle
Trapezius
Intercostal
Energy

The human body is made up of various structures such as cells, tissues, membranes, muscles, and organs. Each of these very unique entities is responsible for performing a specific task that is important for the body's proper function. While there are many structures and organs which make up the human body, the physical therapy aide, who is most concerned with how the "physical" body parts move, will need to understand the bony structures, including the joints and ligaments, and the muscles. In addition to those concepts which make up the study of the musculoskeletal system, the aide should also have a basic understanding of the theories related to the cardiovascular system, the nervous system, and the integumentary system. However, before we can discuss these concepts, it is important that you first have an understanding of the two basic components which allow each body part to function.

Every minute, intricate parts of the human body hve both a function and a structure. In health care, when we refer to the science of the structure of the body and the relationship of its parts to each other, we call it **anatomy.** If we are discussing the science that deals with the activities or dynamics, that is, the functions, of the body and its individual parts, it is called **physiology.** While there are many different functions of each structure in the human body, for our purposes, we will only address those areas that relate to the physical therapy aide's involvement in caring for the patient.

♦ THE SKELETAL SYSTEM

The framework which makes up the bones of the body is called the skeleton. Its main function is to provide body support, protection for underlying organs, and to serve as levers for body motions and movements.

Whenever bones come together, they form a structure called a joint. The bones of the joint are held together by structures called ligaments, which look like strong, nonelastic bands of dense tissue. The main function of a ligament is to provide stability and thus limit the joint to a very specific range of motion.

Structures that are responsible for producing movement are called muscles. They have the ability to contract (shorten) and to relax (lengthen). Muscles are attached to bones and run across joints. Either muscle contraction or gravity can cause motion in the joint. A muscle must also have a nerve and blood supply. The nerve is responsible for stimulating the muscle to contract, while the blood brings nourishment and oxygen to the muscle and carries away waste products.

The Anatomical Position

When the skeleton assumes the anatomical position, we say that this refers to the point of reference in which motions of the various body parts are being described. In this position, the

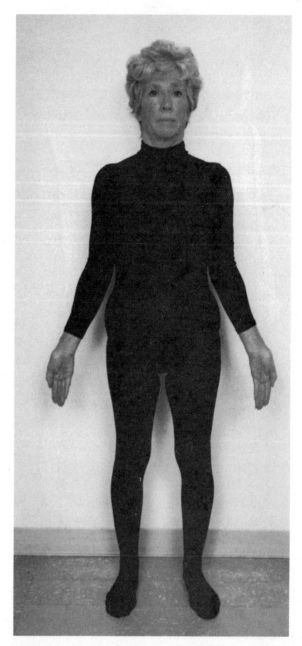

Figure 6–1 The anatomical position. (From Hegner and Caldwell, *Nursing Assistant: A Nursing Process Approach,* 6th edition, copyright 1992 by Delmar Publishers Inc.)

body is erect, with the palms of the hands facing forward (see Figure 6-1). Other postures or positions, have to be taken up, in order to provide the body with the ability to perform various physical tasks and movements.

When an extremity, or part of it, deviates, or departs from the anatomical position in a direction away from the body's midline, we refer to it as *abduction*, meaning to lead away. If this same extremity moves toward the midline, we call it *adduction*. When an extremity turns around on its longitudinal axis, we call the motion *rotation*, meaning to turn. When the joint angle becomes smaller by motion of the corresponding bones, the motion is said to be *flexion*,

meaning "not to bend." When the joint angle becomes larger, this is called *extension* or a stretching out or stretching further (see Figure 6-2).

The part of a body structure nearest the trunk is called the *proximal end*, while the part farthest away is called the *distal end*. The front of the body, that is, the side of the abdomen and the face is called the *anterior* side, while the back is

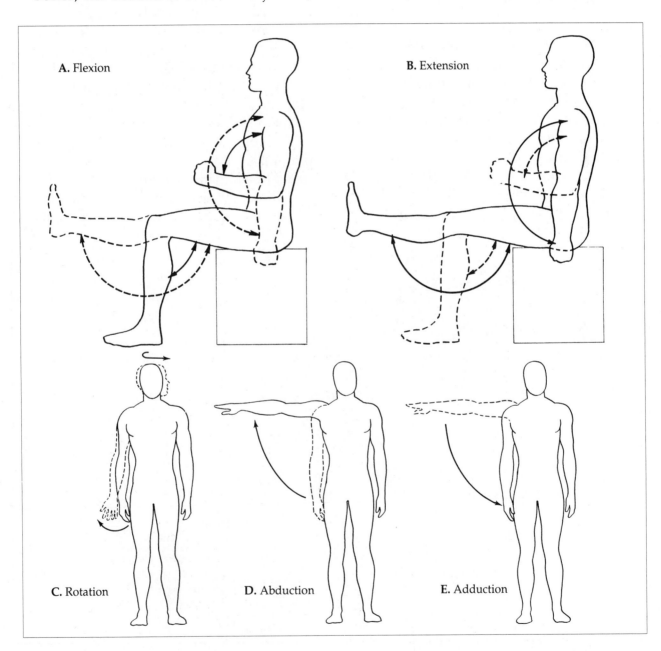

Figure 6-2 Examples of limb motions (abduction, adduction, rotation, flexion, and extension). (From Hegner and Caldwell, *Nursing Assistant: A Nursing Process Approach*, 6th edition, copyright 1992 by Delmar Publishers Inc.)

referred to as the *posterior* side.

Groups of bones form specific skeletal units. These units, or sections, include the skull, the vertebral column, the shoulder girdle with the bones of the upper extremities, the thorax, and the pelvic girdle with the bones of the lower extremities.

The Skull

The skull is divided into two sections, the cranial and facial parts. The cranial part contains the brain, which is part of the central nervous system. The bones of this section include the *frontal, parietal, temporal,* and *occipital* bones. The facial part of the skull is composed of the *maxillary* bone (cheekbone), the *mandibular* bone (chin), the *nasal* bones (nose), and the *palatine* bone (gum).

The Vertebral (Spinal) Column

The entire vertebral column consists of a total of 33 **vertebrae.** A vertebrae is made up of a *body,* the solid round bone in the anterior part of the vertebrae. Attached to each side of the body and joining in the back is a structure called the *arch;* the main part of the arch on each side is called the *lamina.* A projection located on the lamina is called the *transverse process.* Posteriorly, there is a slender bony plate, called the *spinous process* (see Figure 6-3). This is the structure we feel when we palpate the vertebral column with the patient bending forward.

The space enclosed by the body and the arches of the vertebrae is called the *spinal canal.* This structure contains the spinal cord, which, along with the brain, forms the **central nervous system.**

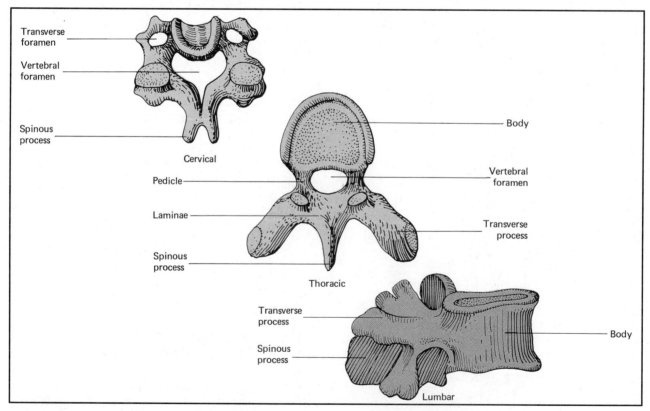

Figure 6-3 Vertebrae: (A) Cervical; (B) Thoracic; (C) Lumbar. (From Burke, *Human Anatomy and Physiology for the Health Sciences,* 2nd edition, copyright 1985 by Delmar Publishers Inc.)

Between the bodies of each vertebrae lies a thick pad called the *intervertebral disc*, whose main function is to act as a shock absorber.

The weight of the upper body is transmitted to the lower body through the vertebral column. This column consists of five sections (see Figure 6-4). The first seven vertebrae are called *cervical vertebrae*. These primarily make up the neck. The first two cervical vertebrae have a strikingly different shape from the remaining ones. The first one, called the **atlas,** is the one on which the skull rests. The second vertebrae is called the **axis;** it is at this structure where most of the head motions occur.

The remaining sections of the spine consist of 12 *thoracic* vertebrae, referred to as the chest region; five *lumbar* vertebrae, located in the lumbar region, called the lower back; the *sacrum*, a bony plate made up out of five vertebrae rigidly fixed to one another; and the four vertebrae of the *coccyx,* or tailbone. The sacrum and the hip bones together form the bony structure, called the **pelvic girdle.**

Each individual vertebrae of the spinal column is designated by the first letter of the name of the section in which it is located. For example, the ninth thoracic vertebrae is designated, *T-9* and the second lumbar vertebrae is

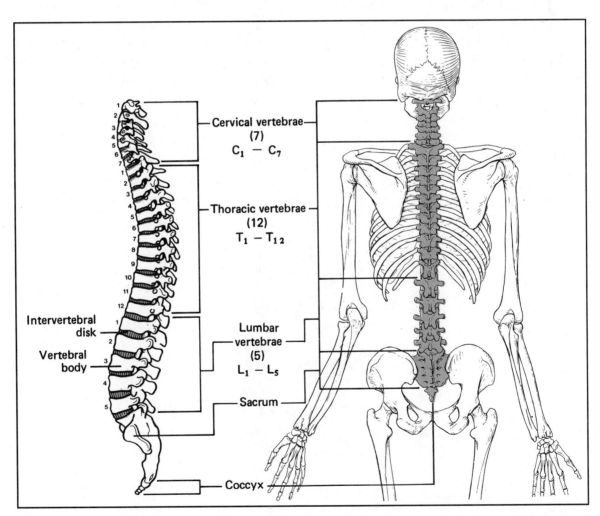

Figure 6-4 The spinal column (two views). (From Kinn, *Medical Terminology: Building Blocks for Health Careers,* copyright 1990 by Delmar Publishers Inc.)

called *L-2.* There are two exceptions. The first two cervical vertebrae, as previously noted, are called the atlas and the axis, respectively. The seventh cervical vertebrae has the most prominent spinous process. Hence, it can be easily felt, or palpated, through the skin.

The Thorax

The bones of the thoracic cage are referred to as the **sternum,** or breastbone, and the 12 pairs of ribs, which are attached posteriorly to the 12 thoracic vertebrae. Anteriorly, the upper 10 pairs of **ribs** are connected to the sternum by cartilage. The lower two pairs, called floating ribs, are free at their anterior ends (see Figure 6-5). The function of the thorax is to provide a rigid cage for the lungs. Furthermore, the rigid cage is able to increase and decrease the volume of the thoracic cavity, which is necessary for maintaining pressure difference within the thoracic cavity and the outside atmosphere.

The Shoulder Girdle and Upper Extremities

The main structures that make up the shoulder girdle include the scapula, with a joint base for the upper arm, and the collarbone (see Figure 6-6).

The collarbone, or **clavicle,** is an S-shaped bone, located in the anterior part of the chest. The proximal end is connected with the sternum and the distal part with the scapula. The function of the clavicle is to serve as a stabilizer for the shoulder girdle.

The shoulder blade, or **scapula,** is a flat, triangular-shaped bone, located in the posterior part of the upper body. A ridge, called the *scapular spine,* extends behind and across the upper part of the scapula. The lateral end of this spine extends over the shoulder joint and is called the *acromion,* or the highest point of the shoulder girdle, which denotes its relationship to an extremity's top or to an extreme. Below the acromion, on the side border of the scapula, is a hollowed

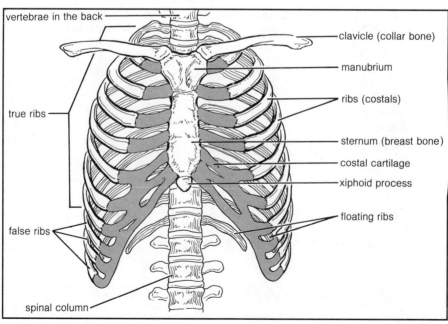

Figure 6-5 The thorax (rib cage). (From Burke, *Human Anatomy and Physiology for the Health Sciences,* 2nd edition, copyright 1985 by Delmar Publishers Inc.)

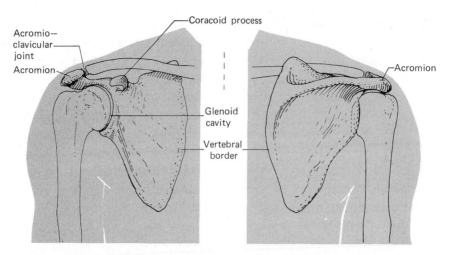

Figure 6-6 The shoulder girdle. (From Burke, *Human Anatomy and Physiology for the Health Sciences*, 2nd edition, copyright 1985 by Delmar Publishers Inc.)

area called the *glenoid cavity.* This provides the joint for the *humerus* or upper arm. The scapula is held to the thoracic cage mostly by muscles and serves as a base for insertion of the trunk and the upper arm muscles.

The **humerus** is the bone of the upper arm. The upper, or proximal end, consists of a rounded head and a narrow part, the neck, and the two prominences, called the *greater* and *lesser tubercles.* The distal part flares out to form two rounded

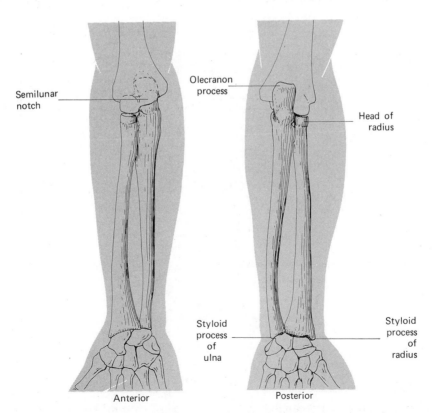

Figure 6-7 The radius and ulna. (From Burke, *Human Anatomy and Physiology for the Health Sciences*, 2nd edition, copyright 1985 by Delmar Publishers Inc.)

parts called the *medial* and *lateral condyles.*

The **radius** is the long bone of the forearm, which is located on the side or thumb side. Its proximal end is called the *head.*

The **ulna** is also a long bone of the forearm located at the medial or little finger side. The proximal end of the ulna is the sharp protrusion of the elbow, called the **olecranon,** and the distal end forms a *styloid process* (see Figure 6-7).

The **wrist** is made up of eight small bones, called *carpals,* which are arranged in two rows of four each. The five *metacarpal* bones, which are cylindrical shaped, connect the wrist and the fingers. They are numbered one to five from the thumb to the little finger.

The **fingers** are formed by structures called *phalanges.* There are two phalanges in the thumb and three in each of the other fingers. A single bone of the finger is called a *phalanx,* and it is further designated by its proximal, middle, or distal position. Therefore, the three bones of the little finger are referred to as the *proximal phalanx,* the *middle phalanx,* and the *distal phalanx* (see Figure 6-8).

The Pelvic Girdle and Lower Extremities

The hip bone forms the sides of the pelvic girdle (see Figure 6-9). It has three parts: the **ilium,** which is the winglike part on the side with the bony ridges, called the crest, and on the top, the **ischium,** and the **pubis.** The three parts join together to form the hip socket, which is referred to as the **acetabulum.** At the lower border of the ischium is a structure called the *ischial tuberosity.* When a person is sitting, these bony prominences carry the body weight. The

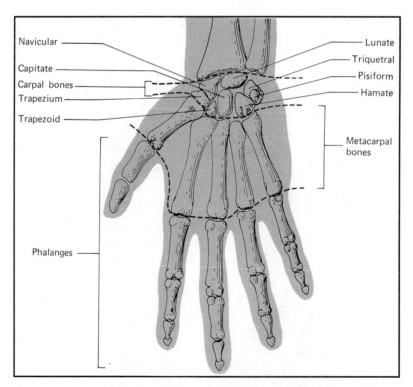

Figure 6-8 (A) The hand, wrist, and fingers. (From Burke, *Human Anatomy and Physiology for the Health Sciences,* 2nd edition, copyright 1985 by Delmar Publishers Inc.)

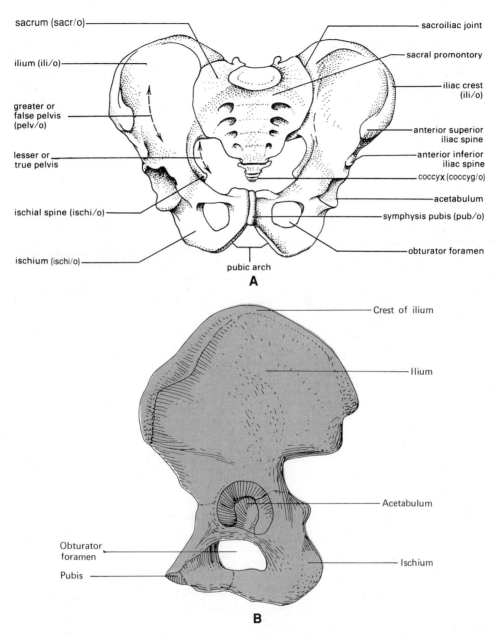

Figure 6-9 (A) The pelvis, (From Smith, Davis & Dennerell, *Medical Terminology: A Programmed Text*, 6th edition, copyright 1991 by Delmar Publishers Inc.; (B) Lateral view of the pelvis, (From Burke, *Human Anatomy and Physiology for the Health Sciences*, 2nd edition, copyright 1985 by Delmar Publishers Inc.); *(Continued)*

bony prominence is also very important for persons who have lost a leg and must wear a prosthesis, or persons who have a weakened leg that has to be supported by a brace. The body weight is transferred onto the prosthesis or the brace through the ischial tuberosity.

The proximal end of the **femur** or thigh bone (see Figure 6-10), together with the acetabulum, forms the hip joint. This proximal end, called the *femoral head*, is connected to the femoral shaft through the femoral neck. Just distal to the neck, there are another two bony prominences, called the *greater and lesser trochanters*. The greater trochanter

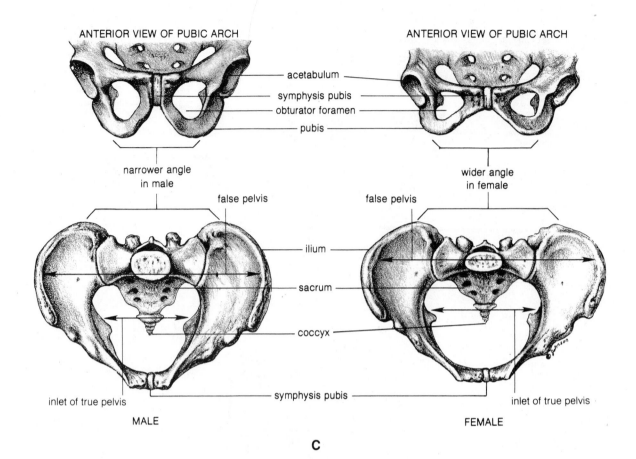

ANTERIOR VIEW OF PUBIC ARCH

ANTERIOR VIEW OF PUBIC ARCH

acetabulum

symphysis pubis

obturator foramen

pubis

narrower angle
in male

wider angle
in female

false pelvis

false pelvis

ilium

sacrum

coccyx

inlet of true pelvis

inlet of true pelvis

symphysis pubis

MALE

FEMALE

C

Figure 6-9 (C) Difference between the male and female pelvis. (From Fong, Ferris & Skelley, *Body Structures and Functions*, 7th edition, copyright 1989 by Delmar Publishers Inc.)

can be felt by deep palpation on the side of the hip. The femoral neck and the trochanters are often the site of fractures in elderly people when they fall.

The distal end of the femur forms the medial and lateral condyles that articulate, or meet with, the *tibial plateu,* which is formed by the proximal end of the tibia. Both bones, together with the **patella,** constitute the knee (see Figure 6-11).

The **tibia,** or shin bone (see Figure 6-12), ends with a prominence proximally and distally; the proximal prominence forms, as we stated above, the tibial plateau. On the proximal anterior surface of the tibia is a bony tubercle, the *tibial tuberosity,* which is used for the attachment of the distal end of the

quadriceps muscle tendon. The distal, or farthest end of the tibia, forms the *medial malleolus,* a part of the ankle joint. Together with the distal end of the fibula, it forms the mortise for the ankle joint.

The **fibula** (see Figure 6-12, page 78) is a long, slender bone located on the lateral aspect of the leg. It is in contact with the tibia at its proximal and distal end. The proximal end is called the *head,* and the distal end is called the lateral *malleolus.*

The **tarsus,** (see Figure 6-13, page 78) or ankle, is made up of seven tarsal bones. The *calcaneus,* or heel bone, is the largest of the tarsal bones and provides a major point of contact with the group for the transmission of body weight. In a normal gait, the stance phase starts with the heel strike. The *talus*, or ankle bone, is the second largest tarsal bone and is the most proximal of the group. It articulates with the distal ends of the tibia and the fibula.

The **metatarsals** are a group of five bones that connect the tarsal bones to the toes. They are similar in shape to those of the metacarpal bones of the hand and are responsible for providing bony support for the toes. They, like the fingers, are numbered from one to five— from the great toe to the little toe.

The toe **phalanges** are much shorter than the finger phalanges. There are two phalanges in the great toe and three in each of the other four toes. Toe phalanges are named in the same manner as are finger phalanges.

♦ **THE JOINTS**

A joint, or *articulation*, is formed wherever two or more bones come together. Moist joints are bound together by *ligaments*, which are tough,

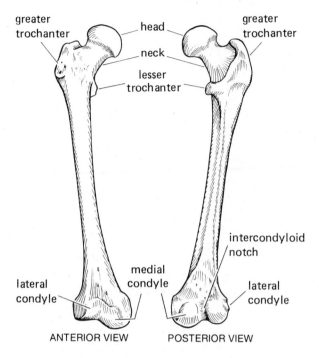

Figure 6-10 The femur. (From Fong, Ferris & Skelley, *Body Structures and Functions*, 7th edition, copyright 1989 by Delmar Publishers Inc.)

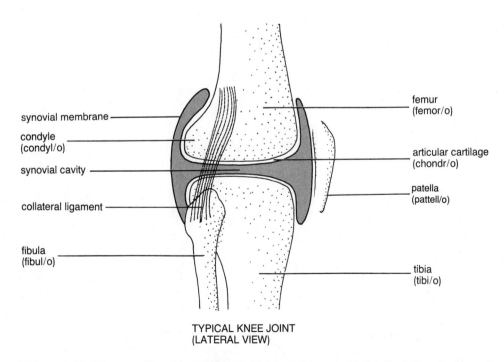

Figure 6-11 The patella. (From Smith, Davis & Dennerell, *Medical Terminology: A Programmed Text*, 6th edition, copyright 1991 by Delmar Publishers Inc.)

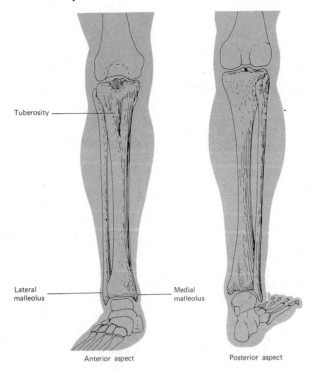

Figure 6-12 The tibia and fibula. (From Burke, *Human Anatomy and Physiology for the Health Sciences*, 2nd edition, copyright 1985 by Delmar Publishers Inc.)

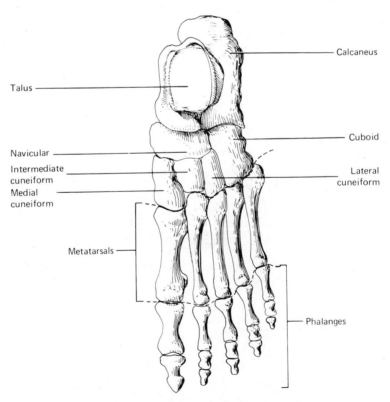

Figure 6-13 The tarsals, metatarsals, and phalanges. (From Burke, *Human Anatomy and Physiology for the Health Sciences*, 2nd edition, copyright 1985 by Delmar Publishers Inc.)

nonelastic fibrous bands, attached to the bones that form the joints. Muscles are secured to the bones by their tendons. Where muscles and their tendons cross a joint, they aid in joint stability.

The joints of the body are capable of various motions according to the structures involved. These include flexion and extension, abduction and adduction, and both internal and external rotation. These are the basic motions of the body parts.

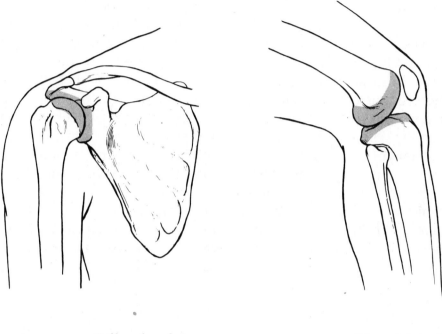

Ball and socket joint—the shoulder

Hinge joint—knee

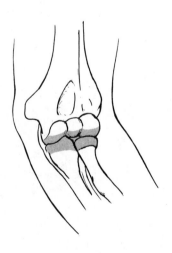

Pivot joint—upper ends of radius and ulna at elbow

Figure 6-14 Types of joints. (From Hegner and Caldwell, *Nursing Assistant: A Nursing Process Approach*, 6th edition, copyright 1992 by Delmar Publishers Inc.)

Throughout the body there are various forms of joints. One of these, called a *hinge joint*, derives its name because the bone is at right angles to the horizontal axis of the joint, thus permitting motion in only one direction. Two examples of hinge joints are the elbow and the finger joints.

In direct contrast to the hinge joint, which only moves on one plane, is the *ball-and-socket joint* such as the hip and the shoulder joints. In these two joints, the ball-shaped head of one bone fits into the cuplike depression of another, permitting rotation around the central axis as well as movement in all ranges.

In addition to the hinge joint, which only moves in one direction, and the ball-and-socket joint, which is capable of moving in all planes, there are other forms of joints with varying degrees of motion within the bony framework (see Figure 6-14).

♦ SPECIFIC JOINT MOTION

The Skull

The only movable skull joint is the one which is formed by the temporal bone and the mandible. Called the *temporomandibular joint* (see Figure 6-15), this joint is capable of flexion, extension, lateral motion, protraction, and retraction. All movements between the skull, the neck, and the trunk are made possible by the intervertebral joints of the vertebral bodies, which are named and numbered for the two adjoining vertebrae that form the joint. For example, the joint between the fourth and fifth vertebrae, is called the *C4-C5* intervertebral joint in the cervical region, *T4-T5* in the thoracic region, and *L4-L5*, in the lumbar region.

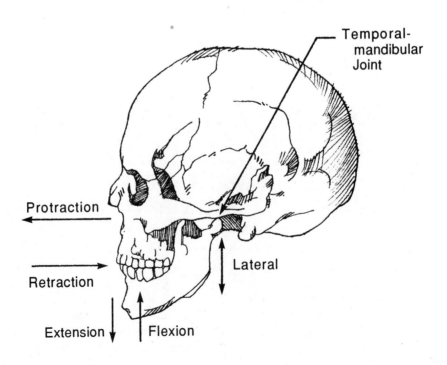

Figure 6-15 The temporomandibular joint.

The Head and Neck

The occipital bone of the skull and the cervical vertebrae form the combination of joints that allows the head and neck motion. These motions are flexion, extension, right and left lateral flexion, and right and left rotation (see Figure 6-16).

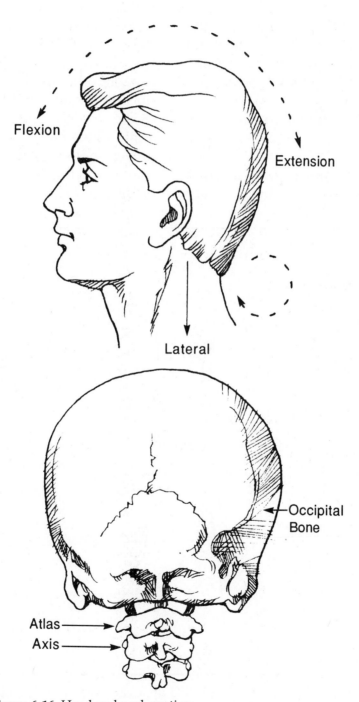

Figure 6-16 Head and neck motion.

The Trunk

The bones of the vertebral column form the joints of the trunk. The trunk is capable of the same motions as the head and neck, that is, flexion and extension, lateral flexion and rotation. Most of the trunk motion is performed in the cervical and lumbar area, and there is no significant difference in the intervertebral joints of the various regions. Motion in the thoracic spine, however, is limited by the rib cage.

The Shoulder Girdle and Upper Extremities

The shoulder girdle furnishes a strong movable base upon which the arms are attached to the trunk. The construction of the shoulder girdle has been especially created for the performance of complex movements, like overhead work. The shoulder girdle (see Figure 6-17) is composed of the two joints, each named for the bones involved. They are the *sternoclavicular joint,* located between the sternum and the clavicle, and the *acromioclavicular joint,* located between the acromial process of the scapula and the clavicle. The shoulder girdle is capable of abduction, adduction, elevation, depression, and rotation.

The *shoulder joint* is a ball-and-socket joint. The glenoid cavity of the scapula is the socket, while the head of the humerus is the ball. This joint is capable of flexion, extension, abduction, adduc-

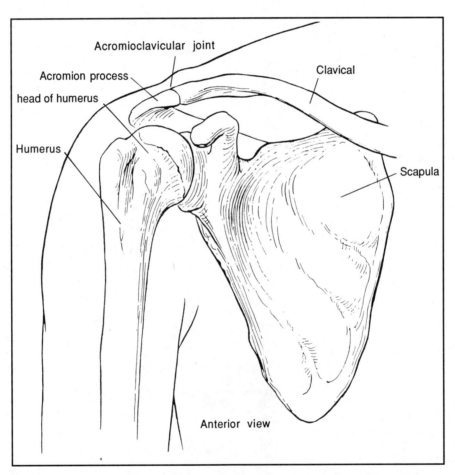

Figure 6-17 The shoulder girdle and upper extremity joints. (From *Medical Art Graphics.* Used with permission.)

tion, and internal and external rotation.

The *elbow* is a hinge joint formed by the distal end of the humerus and the proximal end of the ulna. The elbow is capable of only two motions, flexion and extension.

The *radioulnar joints* are pivot joints located between the radius and the ulna. These joints allow a form of rotation of the forearm called *supination* and *pronation*. In the anatomical position, the radius and ulna are parallel and the palm faces forward. This is called a supinated position. When the palm turns backward, the radius pivots over the ulna and the forearm is *pronated*, or facing downward.

The *wrist* is composed of the distal ends of the radius and the ulna and eight carpal bones. This joint is capable of flexion, extension, radial deviation, and ulnar deviation (see Figure 6-18).

The *metacarpophalangeal* joints are located between the metacarpals and the phalanges. They form the knuckles and are numbered one to five from the thumb to the little finger. They are capable of flexion, extension, and a few degrees of ulnar and radial deviation. Spreading the fingers is called abduction and bringing the fingers together is called adduction.

The *interphalangeal* joints are located between the phalanges of the fingers. Each finger, with the exception of the thumb, has three phalanges and a proximal and distal interphalangeal joint. The thumb has only one interphalangeal joint, which is considered a hinge joint and can therefore only flex and extend.

The Pelvic Girdle and Lower Extremities

The **Pelvic girdle** has been designed for weight bearing and therefore provides a rigid structure through which the weight is transferred from the trunk onto the hips. It has two joints, which are very limited in motion. The first,

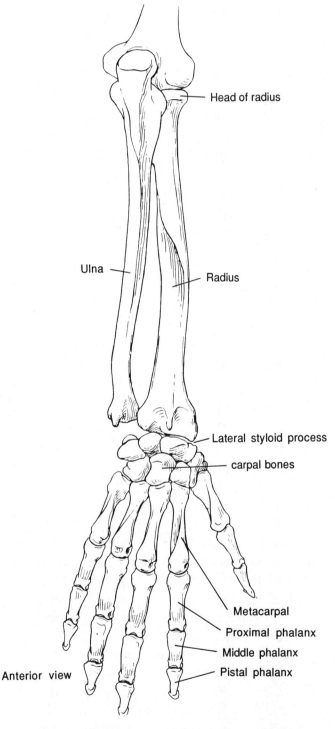

Head of radius

Ulna

Radius

Lateral styloid process

carpal bones

Metacarpal

Proximal phalanx

Middle phalanx

Pistal phalanx

Anterior view

Figure 6-18 Wrist joint. (From *Medical Art Graphics*. Used with permission.)

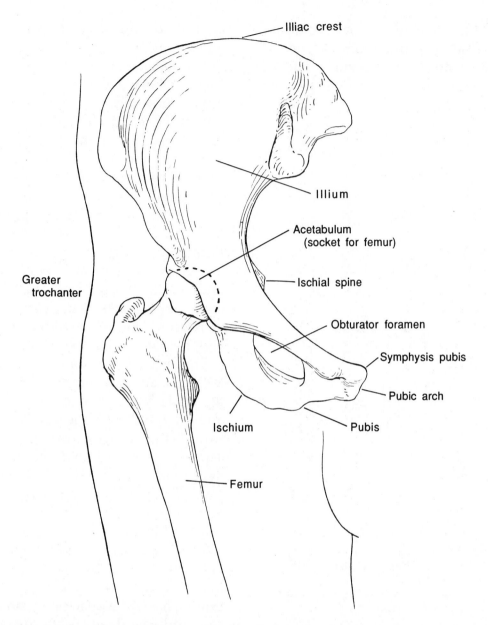

Iliac crest

Illium

Acetabulum
(socket for femur)

Ischial spine

Obturator foramen

Symphysis pubis

Pubic arch

Pubis

Ischium

Femur

Greater
trochanter

Figure 6-19 Pelvic girdle and hip joint. (From *Medical Art Graphics*. Used with permission.)

called the *sacroiliac joint*, is located between the sacrum and the ilium, and the second, called the *symphysis pubis*, is located between the right and left pubic bone (see Figure 6-19).

The **hip**, like the shoulder, is also a ball-and-socket joint, composed of the acetabulum, which is the socket, and the head of the femur, which is the ball (see Figure 6-20). Similar to the shoulder in its motions, the hip is also capable of flexion, extension, adduction, and rotation.

The **knee** is a modified hinge joint composed of the condyles at the distal end of the femur and of the proximal end of the tibia (see Figure 6-21, page 86). It is enveloped in a capsule, formed by its two cartilages, called *menisci*, and is supported by strong ligaments and very strong tendons of the quadriceps muscle. The principal motions of the knee joint are flexion and extension. In addition, a few degrees of rotation are also possible.

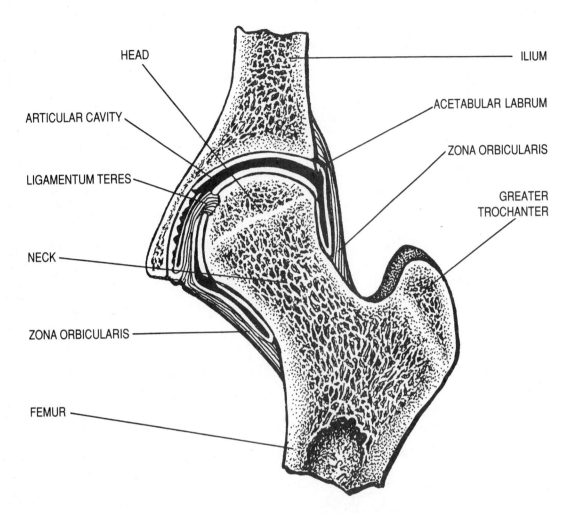

HEAD

ARTICULAR CAVITY

LIGAMENTUM TERES

NECK

ZONA ORBICULARIS

FEMUR

ILIUM

ACETABULAR LABRUM

ZONA ORBICULARIS

GREATER TROCHANTER

Figure 6-20 The hip joint: anterior view, coronal section. (From *Kopy Kit Reproducable Resources*. Used with permission.)

The **ankle** is a combination joint and is similar in composition to that of the wrist (see Figure 6-22, page 87). The distal ends of the tibia and fibula form a mortise for the *talus*, which is one of the seven tarsal bones. The joints between the tarsal bones are sliding joints. The combination of these joints allows flexion, extension, inversion, and eversion.

The **metatarsophalangeal** joints between the metatarsals and the phalanges are similar to the metacarpophalangeal joints. The first metatarsophalangeal joint, which is the one for the great toe, is important in the toe push-off when walking.

◆ THE MUSCLES

The movements of the body are the result of gravity or the contraction of muscles. An unerstanding of the major skeletal muscles of the body, including their location, their relation to skeletal attachment, and the motions they perform, is important for the physical therapy aide. Therefore, the location and action of only those muscles that the physical therapy aide will most likely be concerned with during his or her work will be discussed.

As the name might imply, the skeletal muscles are those muscles attached to

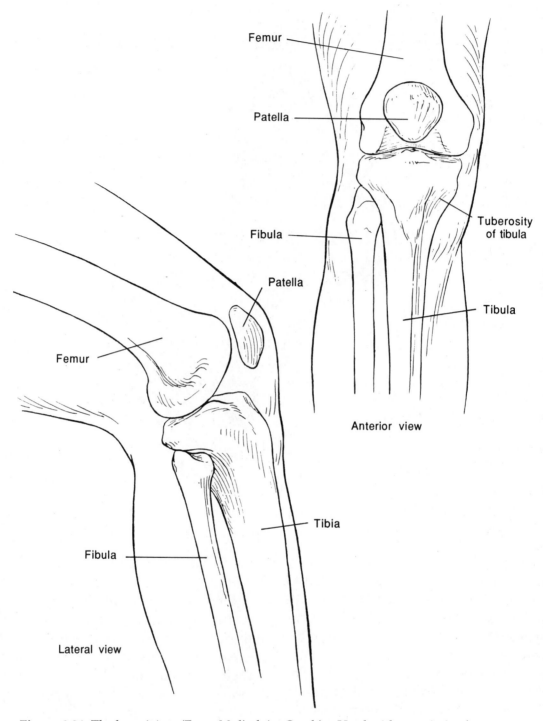

Anterior view

Lateral view

Figure 6-21 The knee joint. (From *Medical Art Graphics.* Used with permission.)

the skeleton and are responsible for the movement of its parts. The muscles and bones together form a system of levers, all of which are capable of producing various motions. A muscle is composed of many muscle fibers. These fibers are grouped and held together by connective tissues in order to form small muscle bundles. These connective tissues also contain blood, lymph, and nerve supplies for the fibers. Groups of muscle bundles held together by sheaths,

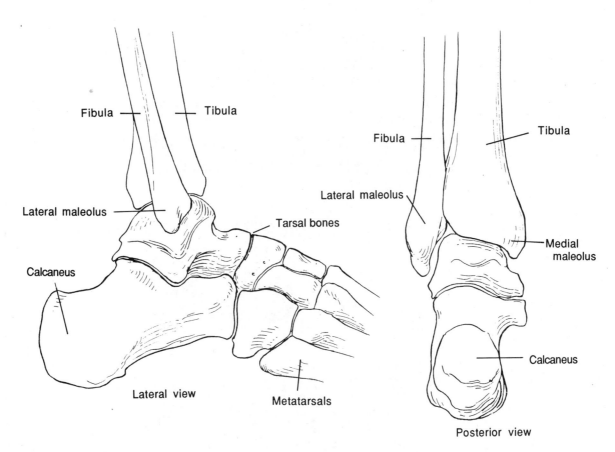

Figure 6-22 The ankle joint. (From *Medical Art Graphics.* Used with permission.)

called *fascia*, comprise the individual muscle. Each muscle is named according to its location, action, or other distinguishing feature. A muscle has a *belly*, or fleshy part, and a *tendon* on each side of the belly. The tendons are attached to the bones and are designated as the muscle's proximal or distal attachment (see Figure 6-23).

A muscle contracts, or shortens, when it receives a stimulus through the motor nerve. If the motor nerves supplying a particular muscle are destroyed by disease or injury, the impulse cannot be transmitted along the nerves, and the muscle cannot be voluntarily contracted. Muscle fibers diminish in size when they are not used. This wasting away or diminution in size is called **atrophy.** A muscle that is overdeveloped due to vigorous activity is called **hypertrophic.**

Muscles seldom act independently. Even a very simple motion is generally the result of an interaction of a group of muscles working together. For each muscle group that produces one motion, there is another group that produces the opposite motion, as, for example, flexion and extension.

Muscles of the Head and Neck

The strongest muscle located in the skull is called the **masseter.** Used for chewing, this muscle can easily be felt when one clenches the teeth together. The facial muscles enable us to wrinkle the forehead, to smile, to close our eyes, to frown, and to perform other similar motions. The more important muscles of the neck are the **sternocleidomastoid** muscle, which turns the neck, and the

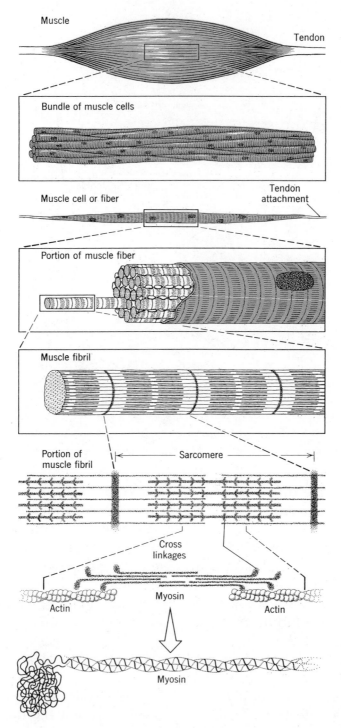

Figure 6-23 Muscle structure. (From Burke, *Human Anatomy and Physiology for the Health Sciences*, 2nd edition, copyright 1985 by Delmar Publishers Inc.)

trapezius muscles, which allow us to shrug our shoulders. The belly of the sternocleidomastoid muscle can be felt on the left when the neck is turned to the right (see Figure 6-24), and it can also be felt on the right when the neck is turned to the left. The belly of the trapezius can be felt when the shoulder is shrugged upward.

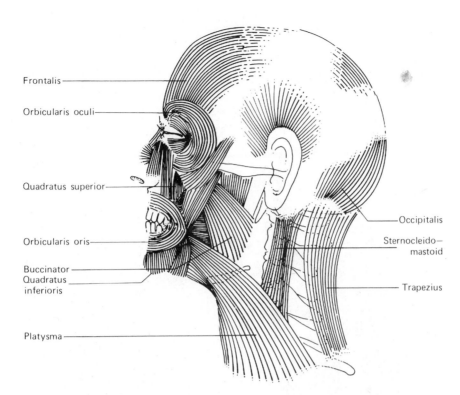

Frontalis

Orbicularis oculi

Quadratus superior

Orbicularis oris

Buccinator
Quadratus
inferioris

Platysma

Occipitalis

Sternocleido-
mastoid

Trapezius

Figure 6-24 Muscles of the head. (From Burke, *Human Anatomy and Physiology for the Health Sciences*, 2nd edition, copyright 1985 by Delmar Publishers Inc.)

Trunk Muscles

Some of the larger muscles of the trunk include the **erector spinae** muscles, which are attached to the vertebrae and help to keep the spine erect, and the **quadratus lumborum** muscles, which are attached to the iliac crest and the vertebrae. The main muscles of the trunk that lift the ribs during inspiration (breathing in) are the **intercostal** muscles, while the muscles of the **diaphragm** flatten during the act of inspiration. When a person becomes very short of breath, other muscles, including the **trapezius, sternocleidal,** and the **latissimus dorsi,** also participate in the act of respiration (see Figures 6-25, 6-26, and 6-27).

Muscles of the Upper Extremities

Muscles of the upper extremities include the trapezius, which helps to shrug the shoulders, the **rhomboid** and **serratus anterior** muscles, which assist in the stabilization of the shoulder and hold it to the rib cage, and the **deltoid** and **supraspinatus** muscles, which help to abduct the upper arm and hold the humeral head in the glenoid fossa.

The **pectoralis** and **teres minor** and major muscles help us to adduct our upper arm to the trunk. The **biceps brachii** helps to flex the elbow and move the upper arm forward, or anterior (see Figure 6-28). The **latissimus dorsi** is a shoulder depressor, and the

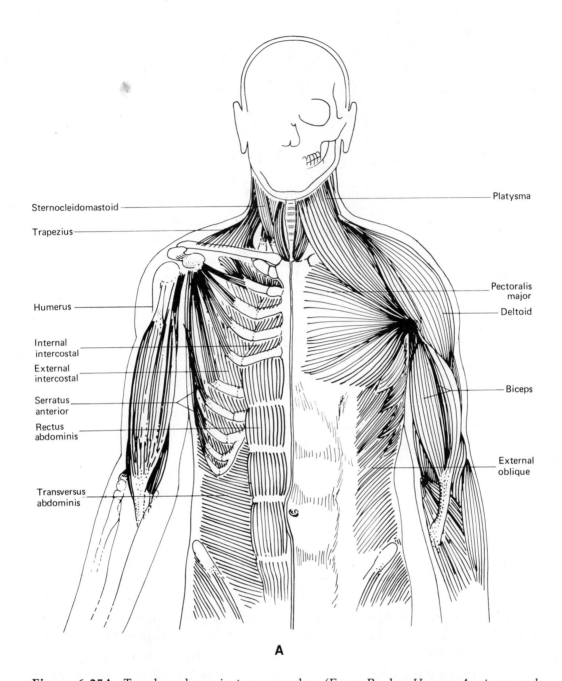

Sternocleidomastoid

Trapezius

Humerus

Internal
intercostal

External
intercostal

Serratus
anterior

Rectus
abdominis

Transversus
abdominis

Platysma

Pectoralis
major

Deltoid

Biceps

External
oblique

A

Figure 6-25A Trunk and respiratory muscles. (From Burke, *Human Anatomy and Physiology for the Health Sciences*, 2nd edition, copyright 1985 by Delmar Publishers Inc.) (*Continued*)

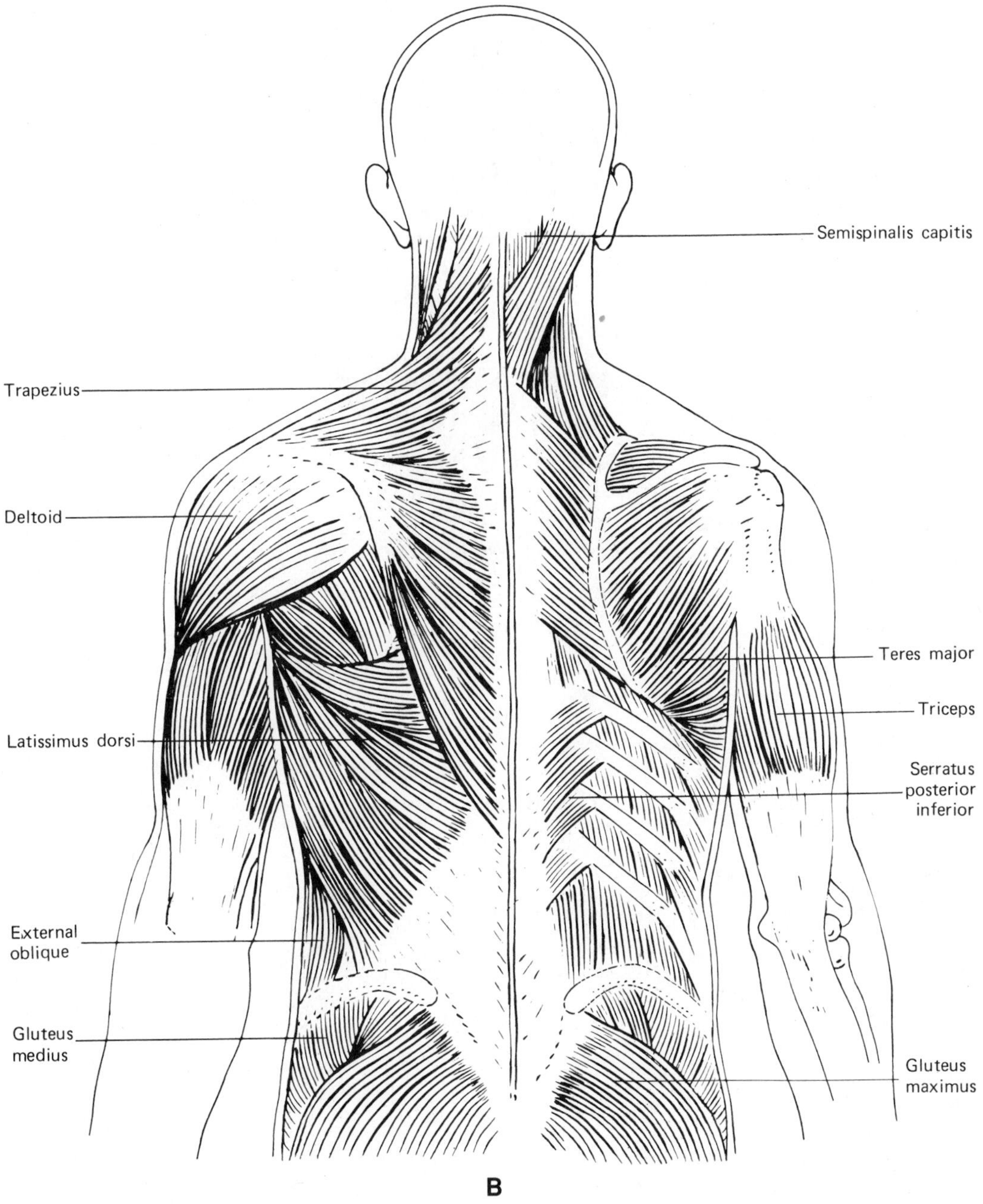

Semispinalis capitis

Trapezius

Deltoid

Teres major

Triceps

Latissimus dorsi

Serratus posterior inferior

External oblique

Gluteus medius

Gluteus maximus

B

Figure 6-25B (From Burke, *Human Anatomy and Physiology for the Health Sciences*, 2nd edition, copyright 1985 by Delmar Publishers Inc.)

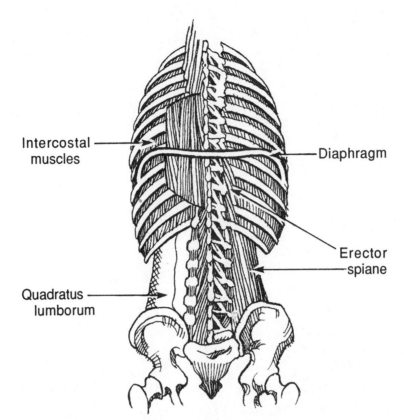

Figure 6-26 Accessory respiratory muscles.

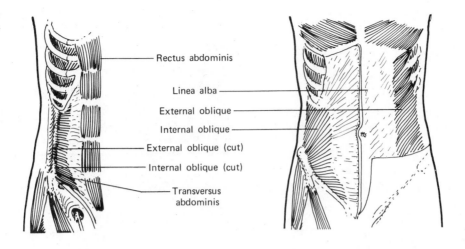

Rectus abdominis

Linea alba

External oblique

Internal oblique

External oblique (cut)

Internal oblique (cut)

Transversus abdominis

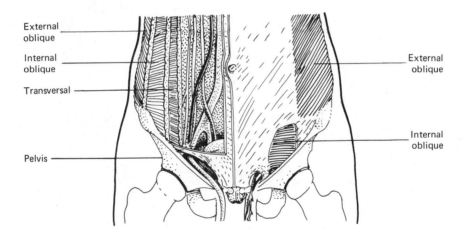

External oblique

Internal oblique

Transversal

Pelvis

External oblique

Internal oblique

Figure 6-27 Abdominal muscles. (From Burke, *Human Anatomy and Physiology for the Health Sciences*, 2nd edition, copyright 1985 by Delmar Publishers Inc.)

ANTERIOR VIEW

POSTERIOR VIEW

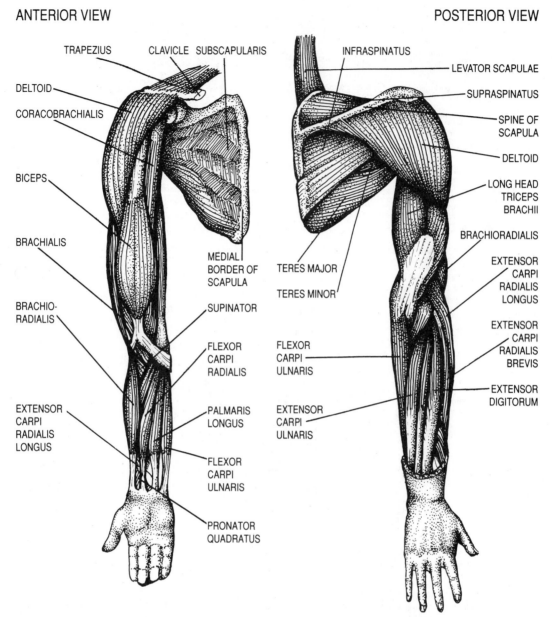

Figure 6-28 Shoulder and upper extremity muscles. (From *Kopy Kit Reproducible Resources.* Used with permission.)

triceps brachii is an elbow extensor. Therefore, the function of these latter two muscles is very important when ambulation aides, such as crutches or walkers, are used. In addition, there are the muscles of the forearm, wrist, and hand. On the dorsal surface of the forearm are located the **wrist** and **finger extensors.** These muscles, in general, have their proximal attachment on the humerus and the radius and are attached distally to the carpal bones

and phalanges. On the volar surface of the forearm, are located the **wrist** and **finger** *flexors.* These muscles, in general, have their proximal attachment on the humerus and ulna and attach distally to the carpal bones and phalanges. In the hand proper, located between the metacarpal bones and making up the fleshy part of the thumb and palm, is a group of muscles called the **intrinsic** muscles of the hand (see Figure 6-29).

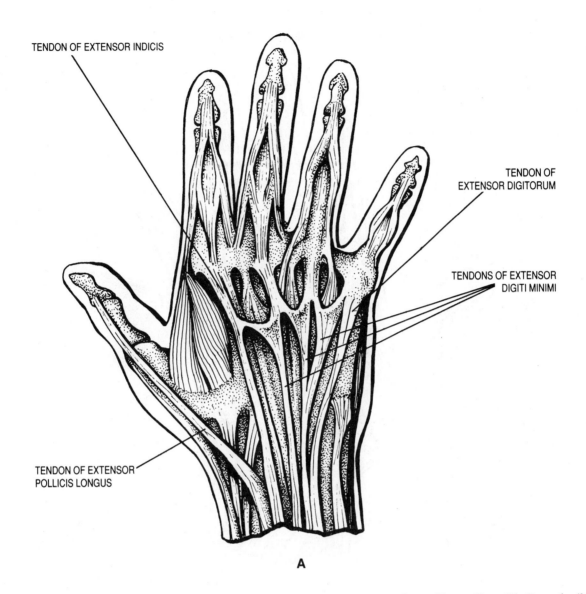

Figure 6-29 Muscles of the hand: (A) Superficial muscles and tendons; (From *Kopy Kit Reproducible Resources*. Used with permission.) *(Continued)*

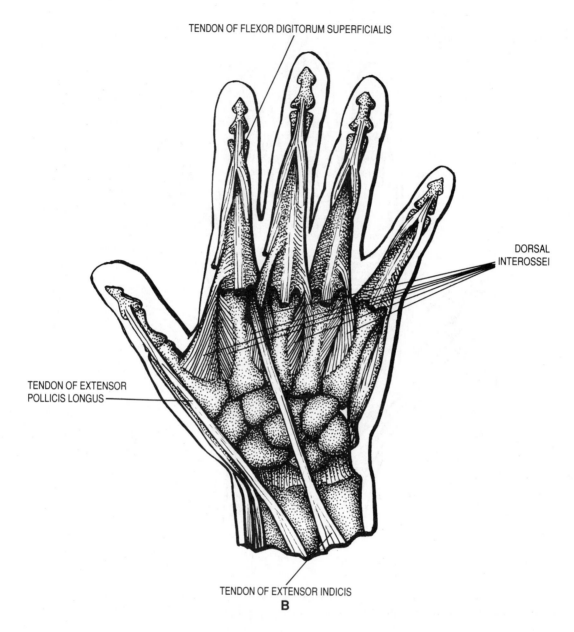

TENDON OF FLEXOR DIGITORUM SUPERFICIALIS

DORSAL INTEROSSEI

TENDON OF EXTENSOR POLLICIS LONGUS

TENDON OF EXTENSOR INDICIS

B

Figure 6-29 Muscles of the hand: (B) Deep muscles and tendons; (From *Kopy Kit Reproducible Resources*. Used with permission.) *(Continued)*

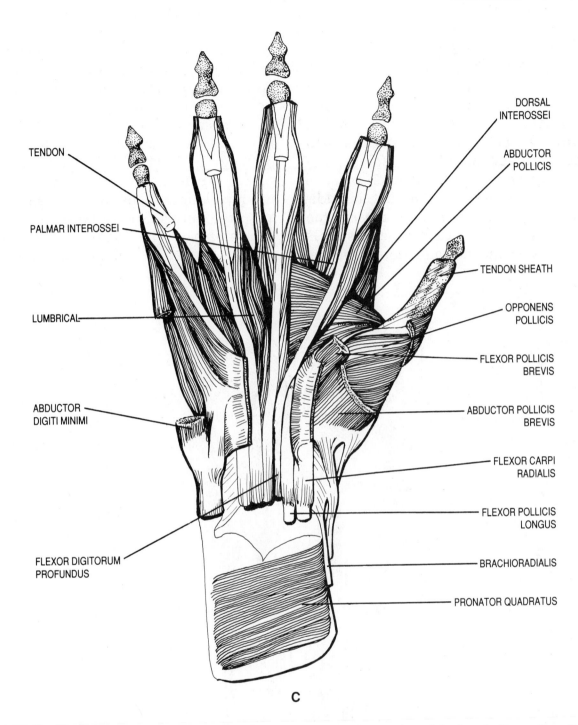

Figure 6-29 Muscles of the hand: (C) Superficial muscles of the palm of the hand. (From *Kopy Kit Reproducible Resources*. Used with permission.)

Muscles of the Pelvic Girdle and the Lower Extremities

Muscles of these structures include the **iliopsoas, gluteii, hamstrings, quadriceps femoris, sartorius, hip adductor, gastrocnemius, soleus, tibialis anterior** and the **peroneli** muscles (see Figure 6-30). In the foot, in addition to the tibialis anterior muscle, the long extensor muscles of the toes cross the ankle joint and cause dorsiflexion as well as toe extension. The iliopsoas muscle, which originates in the lumbar spine and inserts in the thigh bone, helps us to flex our hips. The gluteus maximus and medius, which originate in the iliac bone (a part of the pelvic girdle) and are inset in the femur and its greater trochanter, extend and abduct the hip. The gluteus medius helps to keep the pelvis horizontal when in a stance phase. The quadriceps muscle extends the knee. The gastrocnemius,

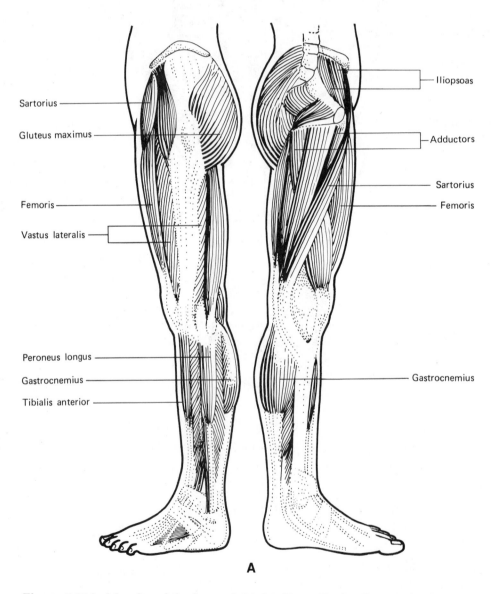

Sartorius — Gluteus maximus — Femoris — Vastus lateralis — Peroneus longus — Gastrocnemius — Tibialis anterior — Iliopsoas — Adductors — Sartorius — Femoris — Gastrocnemius

A

Figure 6-30A Muscles of the leg and thigh. (From Burke, *Human Anatomy and Physiology for the Health Sciences*, 2nd edition, copyright 1985 by Delmar Publishers Inc.) *(Continued)*

which originates in the upper tibia and inserts with the **Achilles tendon** into the calcaneus, is very important in walking. By contraction, it affects plantar flexion of the foot and thereby enables toe push-off at the end of the stance phase. The quadriceps femoris muscle is very important for knee extension and enables us to walk upstairs and downstairs. In the back, the long flexor muscles of the lateral side of the leg, the peroneli muscles, run the tendons behind the lateral malleolus and thereby allow the eversion of the ankle. The tibialis anterior muscles affects dorsiflexion and inversion of the ankle (see Figure 6-31).

♦ PHYSIOLOGY OF THE MUSCLES

Muscular contraction is continuously influenced by a variety of events taking place in the body. Some of the most important considerations will be discussed here.

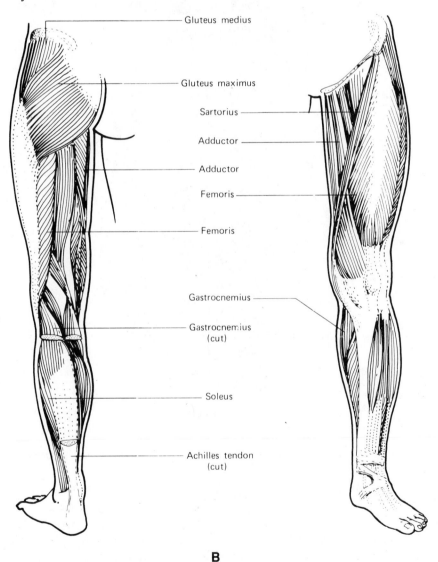

Gluteus medius

Gluteus maximus

Sartorius

Adductor

Adductor

Femoris

Femoris

Gastrocnemius

Gastrocnemius (cut)

Soleus

Achilles tendon (cut)

B

Figure 6-30B Muscles of the leg and thigh. (From Burke, *Human Anatomy and Physiology for the Health Sciences*, 2nd edition, copyright 1985 by Delmar Publishers Inc.)

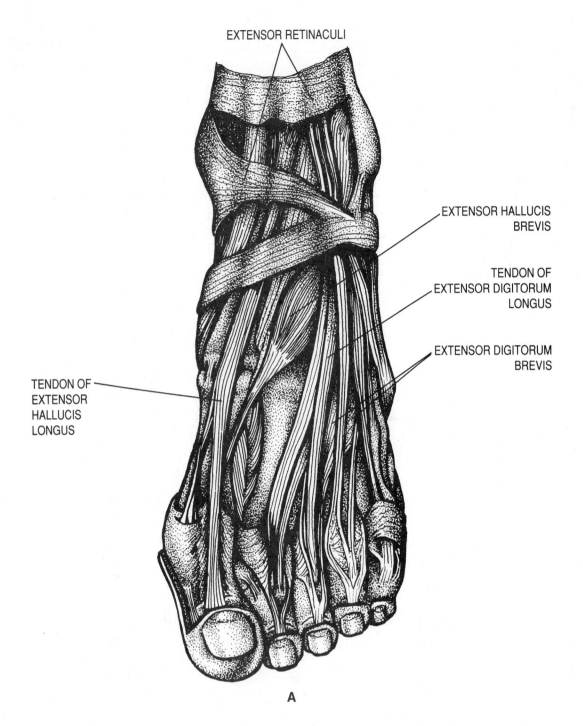

EXTENSOR RETINACULI

EXTENSOR HALLUCIS
BREVIS

TENDON OF
EXTENSOR DIGITORUM
LONGUS

EXTENSOR DIGITORUM
BREVIS

TENDON OF
EXTENSOR
HALLUCIS
LONGUS

A

Figure 6-31 Muscles of the foot: (A) Superior view; (From *Kopy Kit Reproducible Resources*, used with permission.) *(Continued)*

Nerve Supply

Some form of stimulus is necessary in order to initiate muscle contraction. Muscular activity does not actually originate in the motor area of the brain, however, it is associated with sensory inputs. Sensory impulses, such as taste, vision, or touch, are integrated after reaching the brain, and the results of these integrations are responsible for influencing the type of muscular activi-

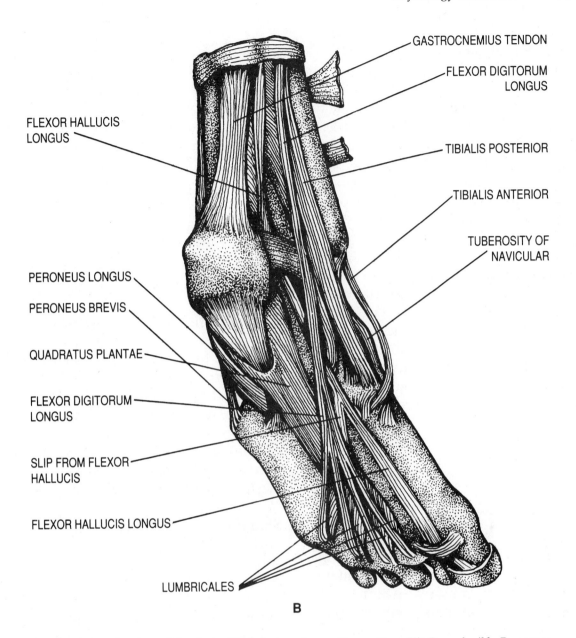

Figure 6-31 Muscles of the foot: (B) Inferior view. (From *Kopy Kit Reproducible Resources*, used with permission.)

ty performed. Previous sensory experiences, such as those experienced at any given time, are stored within the brain and influence patterns of responses. In voluntary contraction of a muscle, the stimulus is provided by the impulse originating in the motor area of the brain. The impulse is conducted by the nervous system to the muscle. Any interruption or impairment of the normal pathway over which the impulse travels can result in an abnormal pattern of motion or in actual failure of the muscle response. Such failure results in paralysis. Similarly, injury or disease of a joint, muscle, or bone can alter the smooth integrated motion normally seen, creating an abnormal pattern of motion and resulting in lack of coordination, imbalance, or weakness.

Energy Supply and End Product Removal

In order to enable the muscle tissue to contract after a stimulus has been received from the motor nerve, an energy supply in the form of glucose and oxygen is needed. This supply is brought to the muscle tissue by the blood flow in the capillaries. At the same time, the end products of the physiologic process, such as carbon dioxide or lactic acid, have to be removed from the muscle tissue as waste products. The venous circulation and the lymph glands are the two structures responsible for accomplishing that task. The frequency of muscle contractions determines the demand for oxygen. In addition, any accumulation of waste products caused by an impairment within the venous or lymph system can also impair muscular activity.

◆ GRAVITY

In all movements, the force of gravity plays a key role. It can either facilitate, impede, or stop muscular action. For example, in a standing position elbow flexion is against gravity since the biceps must lift the weight of the forearm, but extension is achieved with the help of gravity. In a prone position, the effect of gravity reverses this situation.

◆ EXERCISE AND FATIGUE

During exercise, the carbon dioxide and lactic acid that are the end products of metabolism increase within the muscle tissue, eventually causing fatigue. Such a response is partially the result of the body's inability to expel excess amounts of these accumulated end products. Continued exercise will increase the gap between the body's oxygen supply and demand, eventually lessening the fatigue. Physical activity will result in fatigue more readily when the exercising muscles are weakened or otherwise impaired by disease or injury.

◆ MUSCLE ACTION IN SPECIFIC DAILY ACTIVITIES

Many activities are performed without effort by a healthy person. However, they may be a challenge to a person with paralysis, incoordination, or limitation of motion. Therefore, a person who is afflicted with an ailment that causes loss of skilled, well-integrated muscle action or loss of strength may need muscular reeducation in order to master a seemingly simple task.

Standing Erect

Erect posture is maintained by the balance and interplay of specific muscle groups. The extensors of the trunk and the hip are generally the most active muscles because they work against the pull of gravity. They include the extensors of the neck, back, hip, knee, and the plantar flexors of the ankle. Calf muscle interplay is also very important. A paralysis, weakness, or tightness of any muscle used in standing erect, may affect a person's posture or the ability to maintain a standing position.

Walking

In walking, one leg swings forward while the other supports the body. Weakness, paralysis, or tightness of any of the muscles used in walking may cause limping or an alteration in the individual's walking pattern. A patient, for example, who suffers from paralysis of the dorsal flexors of the foot generally has to lift the leg high enough, in order to prevent stubbing his or her toes. Pain is also a cause of abnormal walking patterns.

Specific muscle groups are necessary in order to accomplish walking. These include the extensors of the knees, used to straighten the knees and prevent buckling when your weight is on them as in the case of stair climbing; the extensors of the hips and trunk, used to keep the trunk from falling forward; the abductors of the hips, which are necessary to keep the unsupported side of the pelvis from dropping when the opposite leg is in its swing phase; the flexors of the hips, which are necessary to bring the limb forward in the swing phase; the dorsiflexors of the ankle, which are necessary for the foot and toes to clear the ground, preventing foot slap when the heel strikes the floor at the beginning of the stance phase and, finally, the plantar flexors of the ankle, needed to permit toe push-off at the end of the stance phase.

In cases where there is a permanent or temporary impairment of the weight-bearing structures of the pelvic girdle or the lower extremities, weight bearing must be transferred to body parts that were originally not designed for carrying the body weight and, therefore, have to be adapted to a weight-bearing function. With the aid of crutches, the shoulder girdle and upper extremities may take over this function; therefore, persons who use crutches for years will eventually develop very strong shoulder and upper arm muscles.

◆ ◆ ◆
SUMMARY OUTLINE

The Musculoskeletal System
- Anatomy and physiology

The Skeletal System
- Purpose and function of the skeletal system
- The antomical position
- The skull
- The vertebral (spinal) column
- The thorax
- The shoulder girdle and upper extremities
- The pelvic girdle and lower extremities

The Joints
- Purpose and function of joints
- Specific joint motions

The Muscular System
- Purpose and function of the muscular system
- Muscles of the head and neck
- Trunk muscles
- Muscles of the upper extremities
- Muscles of the pelvic girdle and the lower extremities
- Physiology of muscles
- Energy supply and end product removal
- Gravity and the muscular system
- Exercise and fatigue

Muscle Action in Specific Daily Activities
- Standing erect
- Walking

CHAPTER REVIEW QUESTIONS

1. The framework making up the bones of the body is called the
   _____.

2. Whenever bones come together, they form a structure called
   _____.

3. Structures responsible for producing movement are called
   _____.

4. The _____ _____ is the point of reference in
   which motions of various body parts are described.

5. The two sections of the skull are called the _____ and the
   _____.

6. The vertebral column consists of _____ vertebrae.

7. The main structures making up the shoulder girdle include the
   _____ and the _____.

8. Most joints are bound together by _____.

9. The pelvic girdle has been designed for _____ _____
   and provides a rigid structure for transferring weight from the
   trunk onto the hips.

10. A muscle _____, or shortens, when it receives a stimulus
    through the motor nerve.

11. Match the correct answer in Column A with its correct
    response in Column B:

Column A	Column B
abduction	to bend
anterior	moving toward the body's midline
flexion	to stretch out
posterior	moving away from the body's midline
adduction	toward the back
extension	toward the front

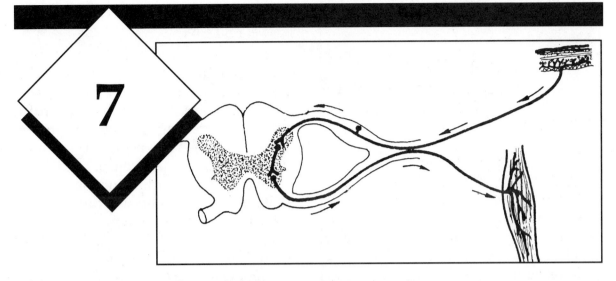

The Nervous System

Objectives
After studying this chapter, you will be able to:

1. Describe the purpose and function of the nervous system.

2. Describe the purpose and function of the central nervous system.

3. Define the term *meninges*.

4. Identify structures of the central nervous system.

5. Explain the function of the brain and identify each of its main parts.

6. Describe the purpose and function of the peripheral nervous system.

7. Identify structures of the peripheral nervous system.

8. Describe the purpose and function of the autonomic nervous system.

9. Describe the difference between sympathetic and para-sympathetic nerve fibers.

VOCABULARY

Learn the meaning and the correct spelling of the following words and abbreviations:

Central nervous system
CNS
Meninges
Optical
Acoustic
Tactile
Cerebrum
Cerebellum
Lobe
Brain stem
Parasympathetic
Frontal
Parietal
Temporal
Occipital
Cerebrospinal fluid
CSF
Peripheral nervous system
Autonomic nervous system
ANS
Sympathetic
Involuntary

The nervous system functions as a highly complex unit that makes it possible for our body to be aware of its surroundings. It also makes it possible for us to coordinate mental and physical activities and to respond as needed to both internal and external stimuli. The nervous system is divided into three distinct systems: *the central nervous system*, the *peripheral nervous system*, and the *autonomic nervous system*. Each part of the nervous system is responsible for carrying out very specific functions.

◆ THE CENTRAL NERVOUS SYSTEM

The central nervous system consists of the brain and the spinal cord. These structures are covered by structures known as **meninges.** The central nervous system is responsible for receiving all incoming optical, acoustic, and tactile stimuli and for coordinating the activities of various body systems. It carries out all activities of learning, thinking, and reasoning, and directs the voluntary actions of the body (see Figure 7-1).

The **brain** is the directional center for the entire nervous system; it is housed in the cranium of the skull. It is divided into two parts: the **cerebrum,** which is the main part of the brain, and a smaller part, called the **cerebellum.** The cerebrum is divided into lobes that are named for the corresponding bones of the skull that protect the individual lobes. The **frontal lobe** is the motor area and the center for all of the body's movement, speech, and writing; the **parietal lobe** is the sensory area that allows us to feel heat, cold, touch, and pressure; the **temporal lobe** is the center for vision (see Figure 7-2).

The cerebellum is located underneath the posterior part of the cerebrum. It is responsible for governing the timing and integration of voluntary muscular movements, coordinating body activity, regulating muscle tone, and it is the center of reflex action and equilibrium.

The **brain stem** is the structure that links the cerebrum to the spinal cord. It contains important tracts that lead to and from the centers of the cerebrum and the cerebellum. Many nerve tracts carry stimuli from the various parts of the brain to the spinal cord, crossing from one side to the other within the brain stem. This crossing over of nerve tracts explains the fact that the impairment of

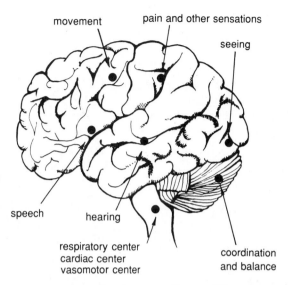

Figure 7-2 The brain. (From Hegner and Caldwell, *Nursing Assistant: A Nursing Process Approach*, 6th edition, copyright 1992 by Delmar Publishers Inc.)

Between the meninges and the structures of the central nervous system is the **cerebrospinal fluid.**

◆ THE PERIPHERAL NERVOUS SYSTEM

The **peripheral nervous system** is composed of nerves located outside the central nervous system. It is frequently designated as the *lower motor neuron system* in contrast to the *upper motor neuron system*, which includes all structures of the central nervous system. The peripheral nervous system contains motor neurons that cause muscles to contract, and sensory neurons that receive stimuli and relay them to the central nervous system.

There are 12 pairs of cranial nerves which supply the organs of special senses and parts of the face, tongue, neck, thorax, and abdomen. There are 31 pairs of spinal nerves which innervate the skeletal muscles and give sensation to both the trunk and the upper and lower extremities. Nerves for the upper

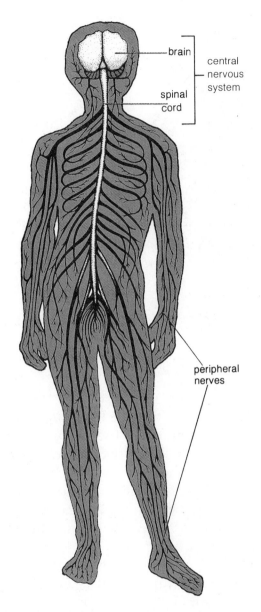

Figure 7-1 The nervous system. (From Hegner and Caldwell, *Nursing Assistant: A Nursing Process Approach*, 6th edition, copyright 1992 by Delmar Publishers Inc.)

the arms and legs of a patient with brain damage is on the side opposite the injury. A respiratory center is also located within the brain stem (see Figure 7-3).

The **spinal cord,** which is protected by the vertebrae, is made up of ascending and descending tracts that connect the brain to the peripheral nerves. It extends from the brain to the level of the second lumbar vertebrae where the spinal cord ends.

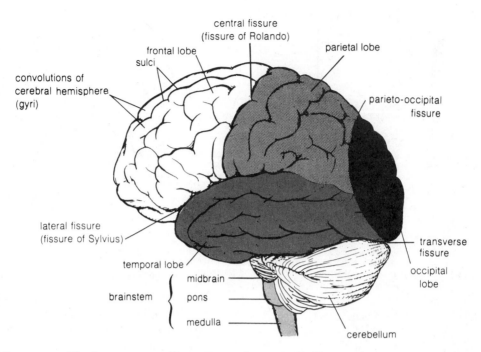

Figure 7-3 The brain stem. (From Fong, Ferris & Skelley, *Body Structures and Functions*, 7th edition, copyright 1989 by Delmar Publishers Inc.)

extremities extend from the spinal cord and eventually form the brachial plexus in the shoulder area.

The **brachial plexus** gives way to five motor nerves from its three cords. These include the short or **axillary** nerve to the deltoid muscle, which abducts the shoulder; the **radial** nerve, which affects extension of the elbow, wrist, and fingers; the **musculocutaneous** nerve, which flexes the elbow; and the **median** and **ulnar** nerves, which run down to the hand. The latter two supply the muscles that flex the wrist and fingers and enable us to have a firm grip and to make a fist.

The nerves that go to the lower extremities form the **lumbosacral plexus**. The three major nerves given off by this plexus include the **femoral obturator** and **sciatic** nerves. The femoral nerve goes to the muscles that flex the hip and extend the knee. The obturator goes to the muscles for hip adduction. The very large sciatic nerves go to the muscles that extend and abduct the hip, flex the knee, and dorsiflex and plantar flex the ankle. At the height of the knee, the nerve divides into the **peroneal** nerve, which goes to the muscles responsible for dorsiflexing the ankle, and the **posterior tibial** nerve, which supplies the plantar flexors of the ankle. From the function of this nerve, one can easily see that a sciatic nerve injury can cause severe impairment in walking.

♦ THE AUTONOMIC NERVOUS SYSTEM

This part of the nervous system cannot be influenced by a person's own will: therefore, it is considered to be an *involuntary* system.

The **autonomic nervous system** (see Figure 7-4), has two types of fibers, the **sympathetic** and the **parasympathetic fibers.** Each of these two forms of fibers causes a very specific effect on the vari-

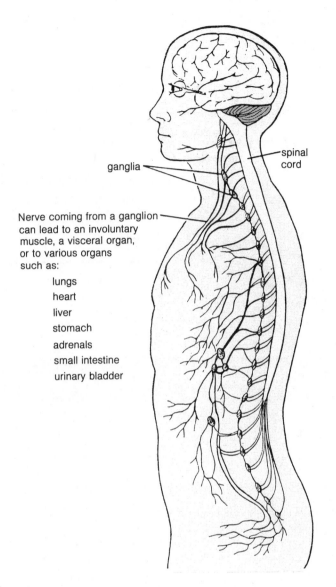

ganglia

spinal cord

Nerve coming from a ganglion can lead to an involuntary muscle, a visceral organ, or to various organs such as:

lungs

heart

liver

stomach

adrenals

small intestine

urinary bladder

Figure 7-4 The autonomic nervous system. (From Hegner and Caldwell, *Nursing Assistant: A Nursing Process Approach*, 6th edition, copyright 1992 by Delmar Publishers Inc.)

ous body organs. For example, a stimulus from the parasympathetic nerves can cause the heartbeat to slow, but a stimulus from the sympathetic fibers will speed up the heartbeat. If a person is nervous and excited, the sympathetic nerves becomes activated and, the heartbeat increases. While an individual is sleeping, or relaxing, the parasympathetic nerves take over, thereby slowing the heartbeat. Many of the essential daily bodily functions, such as digestion, urination, and defecation, all have strong parasympathetic components.

◆ ◆ ◆
SUMMARY OUTLINE

The Nervous System
- Anatomy and physiology of the nervous system
- Purpose and function of the nervous system

The Central Nervous System
- Mieninges
- The brain
- The spinal cord

The Peripheral Nervous System
- Purpose and function
- Structures of the peripheral nervous system

The Autonomic Nervous System
- Purpose and function
- Structures of the autonomic nervous system

CHAPTER REVIEW QUESTIONS

1. Briefly define the function of the nervous system.
2. The _____ _____ _____ consists of the brain and the spinal cord.
3. Where are the activities of learning, thinking, and reasoning carried out.
4. List the three main parts of the brain:
   a._____
   b._____
   c._____
5. The _____ _____ is the motor area of the brain, and thus is the center for all of the body's movement.
6. What is the function of cerebrospinal fluid?
7. The _____ _____ _____ is composed of nerves located outside the CNS.
8. How many pairs of cranial nerves supply the organs of the special senses and part of the face, tongue, neck, thorax, and abdomen?
9. Nerves that go to the lower extremities form the _____ _____.
10. The part of the nervous system that cannot be influenced by a person's own will, is called the _____ _____ _____.

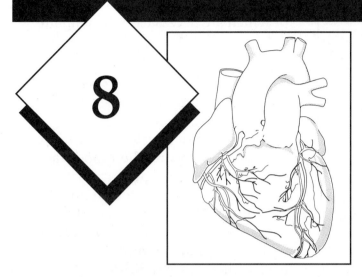

8

The Cardiovascular System

Objectives
After studying this chapter, you will be able to:

1. Describe the purpose and function of the cardiovascular system.

2. Describe the purpose and function of the circulatory system.

3. Identify the structures of the circulatory system.

4. Discuss the structure and function of the heart.

5. Explain how the act of respiration occurs.

6. Discuss the heart-lung cycle and be able to trace the flow of blood through the cardiovascular system.

7. Define the role of the pulse and briefly explain how it occurs.

8. Define blood pressure and briefly explain how it occurs.

9. Discuss the purpose and function of the respiratory system and identify the structures that make it up.

10. Explain how the respiratory process occurs.

VOCABULARY

Learn the meaning and the correct spelling of the following words and abbreviations:

Cardiovascular
Circulatory
Vascular
Plasma
Hemoglobin
Leukocytes
Erythrocytes
Platelets
Artery
Capillaries
Vein
Arterioles
Venuoles
Superior vena cava
Inferior vena cava
Myocardium
Atrium
Ventricle
Aorta
Pulmonary
Repsiration
Aveoli
Oxygenated
Deoxygenated
Systole
Diastole
Pluse
Blood Pressure
Lung
Pharynx
Larynx
Trachea
Dyspnea

The cardiovascular system is made up of two body systems, the circulatory and the respiratory, which work together in order to facilitate the body's ability to circulate and oxygenate blood, both of which are necessary to sustain life.

◆ THE CIRCULATORY SYSTEM

The circulatory system, which is comprised of the heart, the blood vascular system, and the lymphatic system, is responsible for circulating blood throughout the entire body. At the same time, it supplies food and oxygen to the body tissues and removes waste products such as carbon dioxide. Having an understanding of the circulatory system helps the physical therapy aide to recognize important signs and symptoms of failing circulation while physical therapy procedures are being administered.

The **vascular** system, which transports the blood, consists of the blood vessels and the heart. **Blood** is a body fluid, responsible for transporting vital material and circulating it continuously throughout the body. The average person has approximately five to six liters of blood in her body, and approximately 50 percent of it is made up of plasma, the liquid part, while the other 50 percent consists of solid substances or cellular elements.

Plasma is pale yellow in color and is made of water, mineral salts, and proteins. The red blood cells contain a pigment called **hemoglobin,** a form of a protein. It is the hemoglobin that contains globulin and an iron salt, which makes the blood red. Hemoglobin also has the ability to combine with oxygen and carbon dioxide, carrying the former from the lungs to the cells and the latter from the cells to the lungs.

Another solid cellular element found in the blood are the **leukocytes** or white blood cells, which are colorless and whose responsibilities include the penetration of the walls of capillaries in order to enter the surrounding tissues. By penetrating the surrounding tissue, the white blood cells are able to protect, ingest, and eventually destroy any bacteria in the blood and tissues. Another element found in the blood are **platelets.** These round and oval bodies aid in the body's ability to coagulate or clot the blood.

Blood vessels form a network of tubes that allows the blood to circulate to all parts of the body. This network consists of **arteries, capillaries,** and **veins.** Arteries are elastic, muscular tubes that carry blood from the heart to the peripheral body parts. Near the heart, arteries are two to three centimeters in diameter; farther away from the heart, the diameter decreases. They have their own nerve supply, and their diameters vary during contraction and relaxation of the heart. Their terminal branches, called **arterioles,** are connected to the capillaries.

Capillaries are tiny, thin-walled vessels that link arterioles and veins. They form a dense interrelating network within the tissues of all parts of the body. Through their thin walls, the oxygen and food, necessary for the tissues to grow, carbon dioxide, and other waste products can penetrate to be carried away by the veins.

Veins are similar to arteries except that they have thinner and much less elastic walls. They carry carbon dioxide-loaded blood to the heart, and their terminal branches receive oxygenated blood from the capillaries. As the veins approach the heart, they become larger in diameter. The vein responsible for bringing blood from the upper body parts to the heart is called the **superior vena cava,** while the one responsible for bringing blood from the lower body parts is called the **inferior vena cava.**

The heart is a hollow organ with muscular walls called **myocardium.** Its primary purpose is to function as a pump. The interior of the heart is divided into the right and left heart, with each containing two chambers: the upper chamber or **atrium** and the lower chamber or **ventricle.** The right atrium is connected to the largest vein, called the **vena cava,** through which blood with carbon dioxide-loaded red blood cells pass from the body to the heart. The left ventricle is connected to the largest artery, called the **aorta,** which moves the blood being pumped from the heart to the body. The right ventricle is connected to the lungs by the **pulmonary artery,** the only artery in the body responsible for carrying carbon dioxide-rich blood. The left atrium is connected to the **pulmonary veins,** the only veins with oxygen-rich blood; they carry blood from the lungs back to the heart after oxygen has been taken up by the blood in the lungs.

The inner side of the heart has a membranous lining called the **endocardium,** which folds back to form the valves of the heart. These valves include the **tricuspid valve,** made up of three flaps and located between the right atrium and ventricle, and the **mitral** or **bicuspid valve,** made up of two flaps, located between the left atrium and ventricle.

Circulation and blood have several functions within the body. These include their role in both respiration and the heart-lung cycle.

Respiration

Oxygen is carried by the hemoglobin found in the **erythrocytes,** or red blood cells. It is picked up by the red blood cells, which contain hemoglobin, as they pass through the capillaries located along the walls of the **alveoli** in the lungs. Carbon dioxide, the result of the utilization of the oxygen by the tissues, is then carried back by the red blood cells to the alveoli of the lungs and is eventually breathed out of the body. The blood also carries nutrients, such as protein, fat, and carbohydrates, to the tissues of the body after they have been absorbed by the blood from the walls of the intestines. It also carries waste products to the kidneys for excretion in the form of urine. Some waste products are carried to other organs, such as the liver, in order to be less toxic prior to excretion. The blood is also responsible for transporting the water of the body tissues for the proper maintenance of fluid balance. It regulates the body temperature by distributing the heat produced by the body. Because of its water content and mobility, blood also serves as a temperature regulator for the body. It's important to note also that heat applied locally will eventually be distributed into the body by the process of circulation.

♦ THE BLOOD VESSELS

The blood vessels carry blood to the tissues. Since the arteries receive blood from the heart, the arterial stream flows in spurts as the heart beats. The capillaries transmit food and oxygen to the tissues and receive waste products to be excreted from the body. The veins carry the blood from the capillaries back to the heart. Unlike the spurting arterial blood, the flow of blood within the veins is smooth.

Most venous flow is against gravity. The valves of the veins trap the blood so that it cannot flow backward. Active contraction of skeletal muscles helps to propel the blood from the lower body parts to the heart. The heart serves as a pump for the circulatory system; it contracts and forces the blood into the arteries, maintaining pressure in the arteries and controlling the rate of flow.

♦ THE HEART-LUNG CYCLE: TRACING THE FLOW OF BLOOD

Deoxygenated blood flows from the veins via the *superior vena cava* and *inferior vena cava* into the *right atrium*. From there, it passes into the right ventricle and, by way of the *pulmonary artery*, into the *lungs* where the carbon dioxide is removed and oxygen is added. From the lungs, the blood passes through the *pulmonary veins* and enters the *left atrium*. It then goes to the *left ventricle* and, by way of the *aorta*, into the *arteries* (see Figure 8-1). The entire cycle occurs approximately 60 to 80 times a minute. When the heart muscle contracts, the blood is forced from the chamber into the arteries. This phase is called **systole,** or the contraction phase. The time of relaxation, when the chamber fills with blood, is called **diastole,** or a phase in which expansion occurs.

♦ PULSE

The **pulse** of the body is defined as the contraction and relaxation of the arterial walls. A normal pulse is approximately 70 to 80 beats per minute in a healthy adult. The pulse indicates the rate of the heartbeat as well as its rhythm.

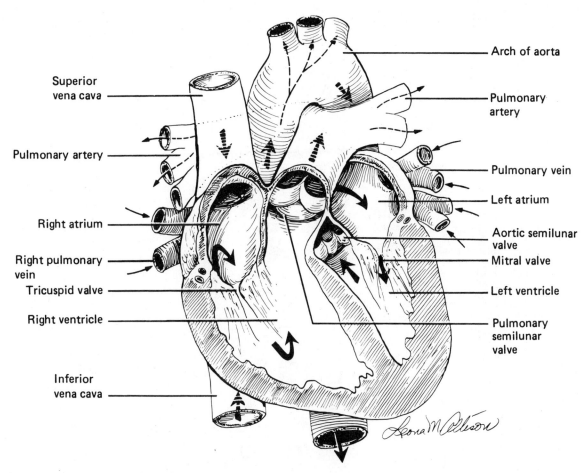

Figure 8-1 Direction blood flows through the heart. (From Hegner and Caldwell, *Nursing Assistant: A Nursing Process Approach,* 6th edition, copyright 1992 by Delmar Publishers Inc.)

♦ BLOOD PRESSURE

Blood pressure refers to the pressure being exerted by the blood against the walls of the artery. It is highest when the left ventricle contracts (systole), and lowest when the left ventricle relaxes (diastole).

♦ THE RESPIRATORY SYSTEM

The metabolic activity of the tissues of the body turns oxygen into carbon dioxide. As a waste product, this must be eliminated. The process of oxygen and carbon dioxide exchange is called **respiration.** And the respiratory system, together with the circulatory system, is responsible for making this exchange possible.

The respiratory system consists of the air passage and the lungs. The air passage allows the air to reach the lungs. It consists of the nose, pharynx, larynx, trachea, and the bronchi (see Figure 8-2).

The Nose

The **nose** is the entrance for the passage of air. It has two openings called the *nostrils.* The nasal cavity is partitioned by a structure called the *septum* and is lined with mucous membrane, that secretes a viscous fluid called

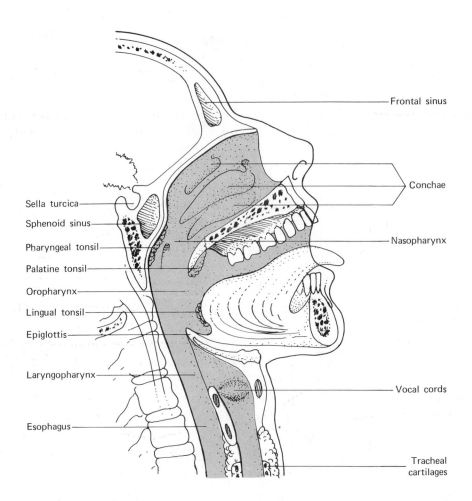

Figure 8-2 The respiratory system: upper airways. (From Burke, *Human Anatomy and Physiology for the Health Sciences*, 2nd edition, copyright 1985 by Delmar Publishers Inc.)

mucus. Air is warmed, moistened, and filtered within the nasal cavity.

The Pharynx

The **pharynx** connects the nose to the larynx. In the walls of the pharynx are masses of lymph nodes called **adenoids** and **tonsils,** that filter bacteria from the outside. The pharynx is also the passage from the mouth to the esophagus.

The Larynx

The **larynx,** or voice box, consists of cartilages. The thyroid cartilage, or *Adam's Apple,* is the largest cartilage and can be palpated and seen through the skin. It moves up and down when an individual speaks or swallows. When food is being swallowed, the **epiglottis,** a cartilage of the larynx, closes its openings so that food is forced into the esophagus and prevented from entering the lungs. The larynx is crossed by two membraneous bands called the **vocal cords.**

The Trachea

The **trachea,** or windpipe, is a tube whose *lumen,* or opening, is held open by cartilaginous rings. It extends from the larynx down to about the level of the second rib where it divides to form two bronchial tubes. The trachea is lined with mucous membranes and *cilia,* which are hairlike projections responsible for filtering the air before it enters the lungs.

The Bronchi

The **bronchi** consist of two bronchial tubes. One bronchus enters each lung, where it branches into many bronchioles.

The Lungs

The **lungs** are the main organs of respiration. They are composed of a light, elastic, spongy tissue. Each lung is divided into sections, or *lobes.* The right lung has three lobes: the upper, middle, and lower lobes. The left lung has two lobes: the upper and the lower. On the left, the place of the middle lobe is largely taken up by the heart and the aorta. The bronchioli connect with the alveoli. Each lobe contains many **alveoli** or air sacs, which are at the end of the bronchioles. The alveoli have elastic walls and thin linings which separate the capillaries of the wall from the air sacs. It is in the alveoli that the actual exchange of oxygen from the outside air to the blood and of carbon dioxide from the blood to the air takes place.

Each lung is covered by a smooth membrane, called the **visceral pleura,** that secretes pleural fluid. In addition, the inner wall of the thorax and diaphragm are covered by the **parietal pleura.** The space between these two pleurae is called the **pleural cavity.** The **diaphragm** separates the respiratory system from the stomach and the intestines.

♦ THE RESPIRATORY PROCESS

The respiratory process begins with the *inspiration* of air. This is an active movement occurring at a time in which the diaphragm lowers its dome in order to increase the capacity of the thoracic cage together with the elevation of the ribs. The pressure decreases in the thoracic cavity and expansion of the lung tissue causes air to flow into the respiratory tract from the outside. *Expiration* is a passive process as the relaxed diaphragm forms a dome upward. The rib cage is lowered by allowing the elastic recall of the structures and forces the air out of the lungs into the outside air. During forced expiration or coughing, additional air is expelled at high velocity by the contraction of the abdominal muscles. Then, the increase of the intraabdominal pressure pushes the diaphragm further upward. Normally, an adult person breathes about 16 times per minute. When the respiration is faster, we define it as being **labored** or difficult. The term given to this type of breathing is **dyspnea.**

◆ ◆ ◆
SUMMARY OUTLINE

The Cardiovascular System
- Purpose and function of the cardiovascular system
- Parts of the cardiovascular system

The Circulatory System
- Purpose and function of the circulatory system
- Blood

- Arteries, veins, capillaries, arterioles, and venuoles
- The heart
- Respiration
- The heart-lung cycle
- The pulse and blood pressure

The Respiratory System
- Purpose and function of the respiration system
- Structures of the respiratory system
- The respiratory process

CHAPTER REVIEW QUESTIONS

1. The circulatory system is composed of the _____, the _____, and the _____ system.
2. The major components of blood are _____, _____, and _____.
3. What structure in the blood helps to destroy bacteria?
4. _____ carry blood from the heart to the peripheral body parts, while _____ carry carbon dioxide-loaded blood to the heart.
5. The two upper chambers of the heart are called _____, while the two lower chambers of the heart are called _____.
6. The inner side of the heart has a membranous lining, called the _____.
7. Which structure in the blood is responsible for carrying oxygen?
8. In the "heart-lung cycle," where does deoxygenated blood originate?
9. _____ _____ refers to the pressure being exerted by the blood against the walls of the artery.
10. List the five major structures of the respiratory system:
    a._____   d._____
    b._____   e._____
    c._____
11. Define the term *dyspnea*.

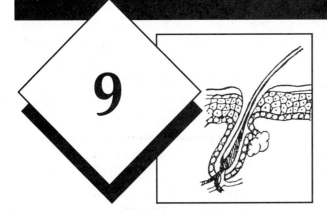

9

The Integumentary System

Objectives

After studying this chapter, you will be able to:

1. Describe the purpose and function of the integumentary system.

2. Identify and describe the structures and functions of the skin.

3. Explain how skin color occurs.

4. Identify the accessory organs of the integumentary system and briefly explain the function of each.

5. Identify the glands of the skin and briefly explain the function of each.

6. Identify the structure of the nail.

7. Describe the role nerves and vitamin D production play in the integumentary system.

VOCABULARY

Learn the meaning and the correct spelling of the following words and abbreviations:

Integumentary
Cyanosis
Subcutaneous
Adipose
Areolar
Dermis
Epidermis
Pigment
Cholecalciferol
Follicle
Bulb
Root
Shaft
Medulla
Cortex
Cuticle
Sebaceous
Melanocyte
Exocrine gland
Endocrine gland
Sweat gland
Matrix
Lunula
Eponchium
Vitamin D
Sebum

organs and systems from infection and injury. It also holds needed fluids inside the body and helps to maintain body temperature. It also acts as a sensory organ for touch and responds to temperature changes in the environment. Finally, the skin is also responsible for excreting some waste products.

The skin also has a social function. We know each other by our outer appearance — the skin of our face, our hands — not by the looks of our livers or our kidneys. Most skin diseases are not physically dangerous, but we are social beings and skin disease tends to be disfiguring. Although a minor skin ailment such as warts, acne, or psoriasis may not threaten a patient's life, it may have an important effect on his confidence and well being.

Finally, the skin reflects symptoms of many different diseases. For example, childhood infectious diseases such as chickenpox and measles can be diagnosed by the characteristic **rash** that appears on the skin. And lack of oxygen in the system appears on the skin as a bluish tinge known as **cyanosis.** In many other instances the appearance of the skin is a crucial element in the diagnosis of diseases that attack organs and systems far beneath the body's outer covering.

The study of the integumentary system, sometimes referred to as dermatology, deals with the anatomy, physiology, and treatment of diseases of the skin, the outer covering of the entire body. It is sometimes called the largest organ in the body because it is more than just a sheet of tissue. It is a complex structure made of several different types of tissue, and it has several functions that are essential to human life.

The skin protects the body's internal

♦ STRUCTURE AND FUNCTION OF THE SKIN

Skin Layers

The skin has three major layers, each made of different kinds of tissues and each responsible for doing a different job. These layers, beginning with the deepest one, are the *subcutaneous* layer, the *dermis,* and the *epidermis.*

Subcutaneous Layer

The subcutaneous layer of the skin is a continuous sheet of **adipose** (fatty) tissue and **areolar** (loose, connective) tissue. The proportions of fatty and connective tissue in this layer depend on the individual and on the part of the body. Subcutaneous tissue attaches the dermis above it to muscles and bones below. The deeper sweat glands and hair follicles that are part of the integumentary system start in the subcutaneous layer of the skin and the nerves and blood vessels that serve the upper layers pass through it.

With age, fat gradually disappears from this layer of the skin. This change, combined with a loss of elasticity in the upper layers of the skin, causes the skin to wrinkle.

Dermis

The dermis is the middle layer of the integumentary system. It has two parts. The area closest to the subcutaneous layer is called the *reticular layer* of the dermis. It consists of connective tissue made up of a combination of collagen fibers and elastic fibers that give the skin its strength and elasticity. When this layer is over-stretched as it is during pregnancy, it causes "stretch marks" such as those that remain after pregnancy.

The upper part of the dermis is arranged in **papillae** or ridges and is called the *papillary layer*. This layer is made of loose connective tissue with some elastic fibers, and is filled with capillaries. These blood vessels nourish the skin cells and also help to regulate body heat.

The papillae show up as regular patterns in the thick skin of the palms of the hands and the soles of the feet, but they are irregular beneath the thin skin of the rest of the body. On the fingertips and toes, the papillae form the unique patterns that produce fingerprints. The lines and creases on the palms can sometimes be linked to genetic disorders. A well-known example is *Down's syndrome*. Children born with this chromosomal abnormality also have a characteristic pattern of creases on their hands.

Epidermis

The epidermis is the outermost layer of the skin. It is divided into either four or five layers, depending on its location. From the inside out, these layers include the basal layer (*stratum germinativum*), the prickle cell layer (*stratum Malpighii*), the granular layer (*stratum granulosum*), the lucid layer (*stratum lucidum*, which is present only on the palms and soles), and the horny layer (*stratum corneum*).

◆ SKIN COLOR: PIGMENT

The lowest layer of the epidermis also contains cells called **melanocytes** that produce the substance melanin, a dark pigment. Every person has some melanin in his or her skin, and the amount of this pigment determines that person's skin color — white, yellow, red, brown, or black. The main factor in the melanin level is inheritance; there are between four and six genes that govern skin color. Environment and hormones also affect skin color. Ultraviolet rays in sunlight stimulate melanin production when they come in contact with the skin, making it darker. This effect is easiest to see in fair-skinned people, but it also occurs in those with darker skin.

♦ ACCESSORY ORGANS AND EPIDERMAL APPENDAGES

A number of accessory organs distributed throughout the skin contribute to its function. These include capillaries, which affect the skin's color, hairs and hair follicles, glands, nails, and nerves.

Hair and Hair Follicles

The skin is covered with hair everywhere except on the thick skin of the soles and palms. The purpose of hair is not known, except that in a few places it serves as a protection against dirt and other pollutants. The major examples of this function are the eyelashes and the nasal hair.

Hair originates in the dermis or in the subcutaneous layer below it. The base of the hair below the surface is called the **root.** It is surrounded by an internal and external sheath of epithelium called the **hair follicle.** The base of the follicle is called the **bulb.** In the follicle, cells multiply in the same way as cells in the basal layer of the epidermis. They move upward, die, and become keratinized

The upper, visible part of the hair is called the **shaft.** It is made up of dead cells arranged in a central **medulla** and surrounded by an outer layer called a **cortex.** The outermost portion of the shaft is the **cuticle,** a single layer of thin, flat, heavily keratinized cells that are arranged like shingles.

Hair follicles are usually set at a slant rather than at right angles to the skin surface. A tiny smooth muscle called the *arrector pili* muscle is attached to each hair follicle. The opposite end of this muscle is attached to the papillae at the top layer of the dermis. Each hair

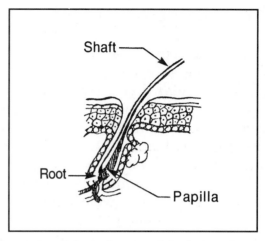

Figure 9-1 Principal parts of the hair and accessory structures.

also has two or more **sebaceous glands** attached to it, which secrete a substance called **sebum** through ducts that open into the hair follicle (see Figure 9-1).

Most hair grows at a rate of about 10 mm per month, and hair is lost and replaced throughout life. Plucking, shaving and cutting hair generally do not damage the root and the rest of the follicle, so the hair continues to grow. To remove a hair permanently, the follicle as well as the shaft must be destroyed.

Hair is generally classified into one of three major categories: straight, wavy, and kinky. These characteristics are inherited and are determined by the shape of the hair shaft. A cross section of a straight hair has a round shaft; wavy has an oval shaft; and kinky has an elliptical or kidney-shaped shaft.

Glands

There are three kinds of glands in the skin. The major ones are the sebaceous glands, which we already stated were responsible for secreting the substance sebum through the ducts that open into the hair follicle, and two types of sweat glands. A fourth type, ceruminous glands, are found only in the outer ear canal. All of these glands are **exocrine glands,** or glands with ducts. Their secretions are conveyed to their destination on the skin's surface through these ducts rather than via the bloodstream as in **endocrine glands.**

Sebaceous glands are located in the dermis alongside hair follicles and just above where the arrector pili muscle is attached to the follicle. They secrete an oily substance called sebum, whose function is to moisturize both hair and skin, to keep them supple, and to prevent dryness.

Sweat glands are coiled glands with their bases in the subcutaneous tissue right where it joins the dermis. Their ducts extend up in a spiral and end at pores, or tiny openings on the skin surface. The ducts of a few sweat glands, known as *apocrine sweat glands*, empty into hair follicles instead of directly onto the skin. The other type, which is far more numerous, is called an *eccrine sweat gland*. It secrets a liquid substance, made of water, sodium chloride, and small amounts of waste materials such as urea. Glands of this type are found all over the body, but they are most concentrated on the palms, soles, of the feet and forehead.

Sweat has two different purposes. The most important one is the regulation of body temperature, and the second is the excretion of waste materials.

Nails

The fingernails and toenails are another specialized form taken on by dead, keratinized epidermal cells. Each nail consists of a nail body, a free edge, and a nail root. Nails are formed in a nail groove on the dorsal surface of the

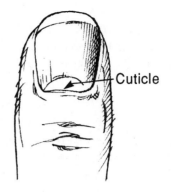

Figure 9-2 Structure of the nail.

terminal end of each finger and toe. The epithelium where the cells multiply, the **matrix** or **root** of the nail, is located in the groove beneath the skin surface. The new cells die and become **nail substance,** a hard, clear form of the protein keratin. These cells are gradually pushed out along the surface of the finger as more and more of them are produced. Nails grow at a rate of about 1 mm per week (see Figure 9-2).

The part of the nail that shows is called the **body** of the nail, or the nail plate. The pale, half-moon-shaped area at the base of the nail is called the **lunula.** This area does not show up on every finger or toe, as it is sometimes covered by the **cuticle** or **eponychium.** The pink color under the nail is from capillaries just beneath the skin surface.

Nerves

Many different types of nerve endings find their way to the skin. Some are wrapped around the hair follicles, some extend to the muscular walls of the small arteries in the capillary beds of the dermis, and others go to the arrector pili muscles and the sweat glands. These nerves send messages to the central nervous system about the immediate surroundings of the body. They detect heat, cold, moisture, contact (touch), and threats such as extreme temperatures and sharp objects. These nerves also allow the body to adjust to the environment by sweating in heat, conserving warmth in cold by rerouting blood away from the skin to the vital organs, and other fine-tuning mechanisms. When the environment threatens, these nerves send pain signals and the nervous system responds with a reflex such as pulling back a hand from a hot stove.

♦ VITAMIN D PRODUCTION

One final job the skin performs in addition to protection, temperature regulation, the sense of touch, and excretion is the the production of vitamin D. This vitamin's function is to aid the body in absorbing calcium from the intestinal tract, making this important mineral available for building and maintaining bone tissue. Vitamin D is available in some foods, but it is also manufactured in the epidermis. Ultraviolet rays from the sun that come in contact with the skin act on a substance in epidermal cells, and transform it to vitamin D, or **cholecalciferol.**

Persons who receive no exposure to sunlight and also have limited diets may develop a deficiency of vitamin D.

♦ ♦ ♦
SUMMARY OUTLINE

The Integumentary System
- Purpose and function of the integumentary system

Structure and Function of the Skin
- Layers of the skin
- Skin color

Accessory Organs and Epidermal Appendages
- Hair and hair follicles
- Glands
- Nails
- Nerves

Vitamin D Production and the Skin

CHAPTER REVIEW QUESTIONS

1. List at least three functions of the skin:
   a._____
   b._____
   c._____
2. What is the deepest layer of the skin called?
3. What is the middle layer of the skin called?
4. What is the outermost layer of the skin called?
5. Define the term adipose.
6. What determines skin color?
7. Circle one: skin glands are endocrine/exocrine glands.
8. The function of sebum is to_____.
9. List the five accessory organs of the skin:
   a._____   d._____
   b._____   e._____
   c._____
10. The function of _____ is to aid the body in absorbing calcium, thus helping in the production and maintenance of bone tissues.

SECTION IV

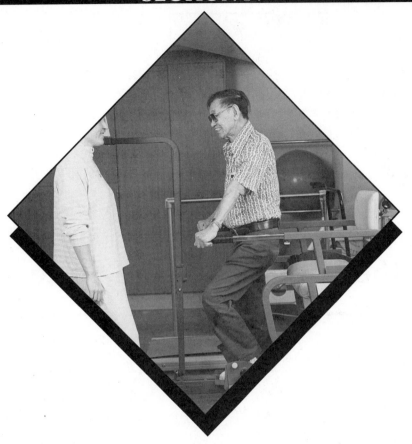

PHYSICAL DYSFUNCTIONS AND DISORDERS AND PHYSICAL THERAPY

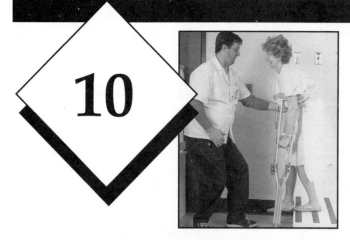

Physical Dysfunction and Disorders of the Musculoskeletal System

VOCABULARY

Learn the meaning and the correct spelling of the following words and abbreviations:

Orthopedic
Fracture
Trauma
Sprain
Strain
Rheumatoid arthritis
Severed tendon
Osteoporosis
Muscular dystrophy
Tenosynovitis
Tendonitis
Joint
Osteoarthritis
Remission
Inguinal
Herniated disc
Vertebrae
Myasthenia gravis
Congenital
Osteomyelitis
Osteomalacia
Biopsy
Chemotherapy
Hernia
Hiatal
Umbilical
Diaphragmatic
Incisional
Collagen

In Chapter 6, we learned about the parts that make up the musculoskeletal system. It is obvious that these parts, that is, the bones, the joints, the muscles, and the connectives tissues that hold them together, depend upon one another and on the rest of the body's systems to function. If any of the parts becomes injured or diseased, the body cannot operate properly. If the problem becomes severe enough, the person involved will have to consult a physician. The physician, in turn, will attempt to determine what is causing the problem. We refer to this process as making a *diagnosis*. Upon completing any tests that might be necessary in diagnosing the problem, the physician will then select a treatment and work with the person, who then becomes a *patient*. The purpose of the treatment is to either cure or alleviate the patient's problem.

If the patient's problem deals with the musculoskeletal system, it is generally referred to as an **orthopedic** condition. Since there are many different types of orthopedic disorders and diseases, for our purposes we will only discuss the more well-known or common problems.

◆ COMMON INJURIES

The skeleton and muscles are susceptible to strains, breaks, and tears for two reasons. First, they tend to be on the outside of the body, and second, they bear the stresses involved in moving the body and holding it together.

Fractures

The term **fracture** refers to any kind of broken bone. There are many different ways of breaking a bone, and each one has a technical name. The most common types of fractures include simple fracture, compound fractures, greenstick fractures, comminuted fractures, incomplete fractures, spiral fractures, impacted fractures, silver fork fractures, a depressed skull fracture, and a complete fracture.

A *simple* fracture occurs when a broken bone does not penetrate the skin and leaves no wound on the outside of the body, while a *compound* fracture occurs when one or more bones penetrates through the skin. This type of fracture is also called an *open* fracture. A *greenstick* fracture, which usually occurs more often in children than in adults, is a result of a break in a bone that has not yet completely ossified. This one splinters on one side only as a green stick does when it is bent.

A break in which the bone has been crushed and/or breaks into several pieces around the injured area is called a *comminuted* fracture. An *incomplete* fracture is one that does not go through the entire bone, unlike a *complete* fracture, which usually breaks all the way across it.

A *spiral* fracture results when a bone is twisted. The fracture makes a spiral-shaped pattern in the bone. And an *impacted* fracture is one in which one piece of the bone is driven into the rest of the bone by the force of the injury. A *silver fork* fracture, which is not often seen, occurs in the lower end of the radius. The name comes from the shape of the bone after such an injury has occurred. Finally, a *depressed skull* fracture is one that results from a fracture of the skull in which the broken piece is pressed into the skull.

♦ OTHER MUSCULOSKELETAL INJURIES

Other injuries, or **traumas,** that may affect the musculoskeletal system without actually breaking a bone include sprains, strains, dislocations, torn cartilage, severed tendons, and inflammation of tendons or joints.

In a **sprain,** the ligaments around a joint are torn but not severed. A severe sprain may cause swelling and pain, and an x-ray may be taken to ensure that no bones have been broken.

A **strain** is a torn or overstretched muscle or tendon in which the tissue is not severed. It is usually quite painful and may also cause swelling, but the pain is generally not at the joint. The term **pulled muscle** is often used to describe a strain, and it is important to note that strains tend to recur in the same place, especially if the muscle is used too much or too soon before healing is complete.

Dislocation occurs most often in the shoulder or the hip, which are *ball-and-socket* joints. The bones of the joint actually move out of their proper places. They sometimes return to the normal position by themselves, or sometimes they must be put back in place.

Torn cartilage is most common in the knee joint. The cartilage at the ends of the long bones in the thigh or lower leg is damaged either by injury or by faulty circulation in the joint area. The symptoms are pain, swelling, and sometimes limited movement of the joint.

A **severed tendon** is often difficult to repair because a tendon is under constant tension. When it is cut, therefore, it snaps back to its origin. Before the injury can heal, the ends of the tendon must be located, stretched back to their normal positions, and stitched together. This may require extensive surgery in order to locate the ends. An injury that involves a severed tendon may take quite a while to heal because of the disruption caused by the search for the severed ends.

Injury or overuse of a limb can cause inflammation of joints or tendons. Inflammation of a joint is called **bursitis** because the bursa, or the sac that holds the joint fluid, is the part of the structure that becomes inflamed. The condition can be caused by a blow to the joint or by irritation from parts of the joint rubbing against each other. Symptoms of this condition generally include pain, swelling, and restricted movement.

Inflammation of the tendon is called **tenosynovitis** or **tendonitis.** Tenosynovitis actually means inflammation of the sheath, or synovium, that encases the tendon. This problem usually is caused by overuse or unaccustomed strain on a tendon. It can also result from a blow or from an infection of the tendon sheath. In severe cases, the tendon's motion may become restricted either because the sheath adheres to the tendon or because the walls of the sheath thicken and reduce the size of the space inside.

♦ JOINT DISEASES

Several diseases or disorders affect the joints of the body. The terms *rheumatism* and *arthritis* have been used interchangeably for a long time to describe these disorders. Many people do not realize that there are several different kinds of problems that may cause pain in the joints. All are uncomfortable but some can be treated and cured while others are very difficult to deal with.

Osteoarthritis

The most common disease affecting the joints is **osteoarthritis,** which is also known as **degenerative joint** disease. Although it can start at almost any age, it is associated more often with the elderly. By the age of 70, 85 percent of the population has some signs of osteoarthritis. The cause of the disease is not known, but apparently in some cases, it occurs in a joint that was previously injured.

The disease begins slowly. It softens the cartilage at the joints, causing severe pain after exercise and stiffness after extended inactivity. In most joints, osteoarthritis is painful but not crippling; however, if it occurs in the hip, knee, or spine, it can be more serious.

Rheumatoid Arthritis

This is a joint disease that is far more severe than osteoarthritis. It usually begins in one or more joints between the ages of 35 and 45, and it eventually spreads to all the active joints in the body. In rheumatoid arthritis, the synovial membranes that surround the joints thicken. This causes inflammation, pain, and stiffness. Nodules or lumps appear beneath the surface of the skin at the joints, and eventually the joints become deformed

This disease cannot be cured, but its spread can be delayed and the pain relieved with medical treatment. Once the initial inflammation has subsided, the patient can return to a somewhat active life, but must take frequent rests to relieve pressure on the joints.

A form of rheumatoid arthritis that affects only children is called **juvenile rheumatoid arthritis.** This form of the disease is accompanied by fever, a rash, and sometimes eye involvement. The treatment is similar to treatment for the adult version of the disease.

Gout

Another joint disease which usually affects the joint of the big toe is called **gout.** This condition is caused by deposits of crystals of uric acid in the affected joint or joints. It flares up suddenly, usually during the night, with a crushing, throbbing pain in the big toe. The toe becomes tender, red, and swollen and remains painful for several days. The attack may be related to an injury, tight shoes, over-eating or drinking, or stress, but it may also have no apparent cause. The problem usually subsides, but it can reoccur at any time. Later attacks may be closer together, last longer, and involve more joints.

Ankylosing Spondylitis

This joint disease affects the spine. It is a chronic or long-term disease that eventually immobilizes the joints between the vertebrae and usually affects men starting between the ages of 20 and 30. The cause is not known.

The first symptoms of ankylosing spondylitis are low back pain and stiffness that is worst in the morning. Pain may also occur in the buttocks, hips, and shoulders. As the joints become "frozen" or immobilized, the pain stops. Treatment is generally aimed at keeping the back as flexible as possible for as long as possible.

Low Back Pain

Another common joint problem that affects the spine, is termed **low back pain.** This is one symptom of ankylosing spondylitis, but it is also a symptom of many other joint problems. It is often difficult to tell what is causing low back pain, so it may be treated for some time as a symptom without a definite diagnosis.

Both osteoarthritis and rheumotoid arthritis are possible causes of low back pain. It may also be the result of muscle strain. In other cases, the cause is a **slipped disc,** also called a *ruptured disc* or *herniated disc.* This condition is sometimes extremely painful. It occurs when the discs of cartilage that serves as a cushion between two vertebrae slips out of place, causing two things to happen.

First, the vertebrae are no longer protected and may rub against each other, causing irritation of the surrounding tissues. Second, the disc itself may come in contact with a nerve, which will cause considerable pain. Treatment is almost always complete bedrest for six or more weeks. Surgery may be necessary to remove the disc and/or fuse the involved vertebrae together so that they no longer rub against each other.

◆ BONE DISEASES

The bones, as well as the joints, can become diseased. There are four major diseases that can affect the bone directly. These include *osteoporosis, osteomyelitis, osteomalacia,* and *bone tumors.*

Osteoporosis

The most common of the major bone diseases is **osteoporosis.** This disorder mainly affects the elderly. As a person ages, the bones are weakened because more bone cells are destroyed than are manufactured to replace them. As a result, the bones become weak and brittle and break easily. This process can reach a point where the bones, especially the back bones, are easily crushed by what was once normal stress. Lifting a heavy object can cause a vertebrae to be crushed. The symptoms of such a break are low back pain and, eventually, abnormal curvature of the spine.

Osteoporosis occurs gradually and is

usually the result of an underlying disease that prevents the renewal of bone, or by a deficiency of calcium or vitamin D. Unless there is a treatable underlying disease, osteoporosis can not be cured.

Osteomyelitis

Another bone disease is **osteomyelitis,** an infection of the bone marrow. This is caused either by an infection in the body as a whole or by an infectious agent that enters the bone directly from an infected fracture or an infected wound near the bone. The problem is usually caused by *Staphylococcus aureus* bacteria and the symptoms include fever and pain, both of which appear suddenly. The disease may be present for some time before these symptoms appear, and if not treated, osteomyelitis can kill the bone cells, leaving a dead and extremely brittle bone in the body.

Osteomalacia

A bone disorder caused by a deficiency of calcium and/or vitamin D is called **osteomalacia.** Both of these elements are necessary for the ossification of bone tissue. The lack of these elements causes the bones to soften and eventually, the skeleton becomes deformed due to the soft bones not being able to hold their shape. Osteomalacia sometimes occurs in children and is called *rickets.*

Bone Tumors

The fourth major bone disease is **bone tumors.** Some bone tumors are benign, or non-cancerous, but others are malignant, or cancerous. There are many types of bone tumors. Some of the most common benign tumors are called *osteo-* *mas* and *chondromas.* Some malignant types are *osteosarcoma,* or osteogenic sarcoma (in the bone), *chondrosarcoma* (in the cartilage), and *myeloma* (in the marrow). The main symptom of a bone tumor is pain in the area of the growth.

If the physician believes a bone tumor may be present, she will generally do a **biopsy** on the bone to find out what kind it is. This procedure involves the removal of a piece of the tumor that will be examined under a microscope to see what kind of cells it contains. Treatment for a benign tumor is surgical removal, however, if the tumor is cancerous, it is removed and either radiation, cancer-killing drugs **(chemotherapy),** or both are necessary as well. Bone cancer can sometimes be cured, but the rate of cure is generally low. It may be a secondary cancer, which means that it has spread from another tumor, often in the lung or the breast. In such cases, the disease is almost always fatal.

♦ MUSCLE DISEASES

Myasthenia Gravis

Muscle tissue is also susceptible to disease. **Myasthenia gravis** is a disease that seems to be caused by abnormal transmission of nerve impulses. Because the nerve impulse is faulty, individual muscle fibers atrophy or shrink, thus inhibiting normal movement. The disease usually starts with the eye and other facial muscles and may then spread to other parts of the body, gradually leading to paralysis. Or the disease may go into **remission** and not return for many years.

This particular disease affects the patient's looks. The eyelids droop, the smile looks unnatural, and choking on food and speech problems may occur. The patient is often tired, and rest helps the muscles to function better.

Muscular Dystrophy

Another muscle disease caused by abnormal muscle function is **muscular dystrophy.** The disease is inherited and almost exclusively affects boys. It is not well understood, but it seems to be caused by an inability of the muscle cells to process some substance that they need. The muscles atrophy, but appear large because the atrophied fibers are replaced by other types of tissue. The symptoms usually appear between the ages of four and seven, after the child has learned to walk. The gait becomes strange, and the child begins to have trouble standing up, because the muscles are weak. The muscles are progressively weaker, so that the child is usually bedridden by the age of 12 and generally dies by the age of 20. There is no effective treatment for muscular dystrophy, but usually the longer the child remains active, the longer he will live.

Tetanus and Trichinosis

There are two muscle diseases that may be caused by outside organisms. The first, called **tetanus,** is rarely seen in the United States because most people are immunized against it. However, it does still occur. Immunization must be renewed at least every five years in order to provide protection against the disease. The organism that causes tetanus, is called *Clostridium tetani.* It enters the body through a deep wound where air does not penetrate. There the organism releases a toxin, or poison,

which causes stiffness and eventually rigidity of the muscles.

Tetanus is painful because of muscle spasms or involuntary contractions. Also, the rigidity of the muscles may make breathing and other body functions difficult. The disease may be of short duration or last for weeks, and recovery is possible if there are no complications. However, complications such as pneumonia are considered quite common. Treatment is generally carried out in the intensive care unit and requires muscle relaxant drugs, breathing aids, complete bed rest, and careful monitoring to prevent complications.

The second disease caused by an outside organism is **trichinosis.** It is from a parasite that may found in insufficiently cooked meat, especially pork. There is no way to test meat to see if the organism is present, so the only way to prevent this disease is to make sure that the meat is cooked well since the heat of cooking kills the organism.

This disease begins with severe diarrhea as the parasite enters the digestive tract. As the larvae or young parasites become embedded in the muscle, they make calcified cysts, or sacs, in the muscle tissue. This causes weakness, fever, and pain. If the nerves or the heart are involved, the disease can be fatal. Treatment includes extra fluids, adequate diet, and drugs to relieve pain and fever and to kill the parasite.

Hernia

A **hernia** is not so much a disease as it is a structural weakness in a muscle. It occurs when an organ such as the stomach or the intestine protrudes through a hole in a muscle wall. It can be dangerous because the section of organ that is on the wrong side of the muscle can become cut off from the rest of the organ and become infected. Severe complications may follow, and function of the organ may be blocked by the hernia.

The least dangerous type of hernia is the hiatal hernia. In this type, a portion of the stomach protrudes through the diaphragm at the point where the esophagus enters the abdominal cavity. A hiatal hernia rarely causes complications and seldom requires surgery. It does, however, cause heartburn.

Other common types of hernia involve the intestines at various weak points in the abdominal wall. They are the **inguinal** hernia, in the groin area, the **umbilical** hernia, located near the naval, the **incisional** hernia, through the site of an imperfectly healed surgical incision, and the **diaphragmatic** hernia, occurring when the abdominal contents protrude into the thorax through the diaphragm wall. In most cases, these are treated surgically to prevent complications.

◆ CONNECTIVE TISSUE DISEASES

Collagen Diseases

There is a group of diseases that affects the connective tissues. They are called **collagen disease**s because they involve the degeneration of the collagen, a protein that is an essential ingredient of the bones, cartilage, and other connective tissues. These diseases are not well understood, and they are usually fatal, either within a short time or over a period of years with occasional remissions. The diseases in this category are called *cutaneous lupus erythematosus, systemic lupus erythematosus (SLE), scleroderma, polymyositis, dermatomyositis,* and *polyarteritis.* Each one affects differ-

ent parts of the body, ranging from the skin to the blood vessels. The symptoms vary according to which part is diseased and treatment is usually aimed at relieving the symptoms, encouraging remissions, and preventing complications.

Congenital Disorders

Finally, there are two disorders, one of bone and the other of cartilage, that are *congenital,* or present at birth. In **osteogenesis imperfecta**, the bones do not develop properly, sometimes starting before birth. As a result of this abnormality, the child's skeleton does not form properly, and the bones fracture easily.

Achondroplasia, the second of these diseases, affects the formation of cartilage. In this condition, the skeleton cannot form properly since bone growth takes place in the cartilage. As a result, a child with this congenital problem will grow up with abnormally short bones in the limbs, normal bones in the torso, and abnormal curavature of the spine *(lordosis).*

Neither of these congenital conditions can be cured, and treatment is designed to make the child's life as normal as possible and, in osteogenesis imperfecta, to try to prevent the breaking of bones.

◆ ◆ ◆
SUMMARY OUTLINE

Understanding Physical Dysfunction and Disorders of the Musculoskeletal System
• Orthopedic conditions

Injuries of the Musculoskeletal System
• Fractures

- Traumas
- Sprains, strains, and pulled muscles
- Dislocation, torn cartilage, and severed tendon
- Bursitis, tendonitis, and tenosynovitis

Joint Diseases
- Osteoarthritis
- Rheumatoid arthritis
- Juvenile rheumatoid arthritis
- Gout
- Ankylosing spondylitis

Low Back Pain
- Causes of low back pain
- Herniated or "slipped" disc

Bone Diseases
- Osteoporosis
- Osteomyelitis
- Osteomalacia
- Bone tumors

Muscle Diseases
- Myasthenia gravis
- Muscular dystrophy
- Tetanus
- Trichinosis

Hernias
- Hiatal hernia
- Inguinal hernia
- Umbilical hernia
- Incisional hernia
- Diaphragmatic hernia

Connective Tissue Diseases
- Collagen diseases

Congenital Disorders
- Osteogenesis imperfecta
- Achondroplasia

CHAPTER REVIEW QUESTIONS

1. If a patient's problem deals with the musculoskeletal system, it is generally referred to as an _____ condition.
2. The term "pulled muscle" is sometimes used to describe a _____.
3. True or false: closed reduction of a fracture is a surgical procedure.
4. True or false: in a strain, a muscle or tendon is torn or overstretched at the joint.
5. A _____ occurs most often in the shoulder or the hip, which are both _____-_____-_____ joints.
6. Inflammation of a joint is called _____.
7. Rheumatoid arthritis usually begins in one or more joints between the ages of ___ and ___.
8. A joint disease that usually affects the joint of the big toe is called _____.

9. What joint disease affects the spine?

10. The disease _____ _____ is a disorder that seems to be caused by abnormal transmission of nerve impulses.

11. A common disorder caused by abnormal muscle function and is inherited, and almost exclusively affects boys, is called

    _____ _____.

12. A structural weakness in a muscle is called a _____.

13. A group of diseases that affect the connective tissue are called _____ diseases.

14. Match the injury with its description:

    | compound fracture | no wound shows |
    | greenstick fracture | bone breaks when twisted |
    | simple fracture | bone splinters on one side |
    | impacted fracture | bone penetrates skin |
    | | bone breaks completely across |
    | | one piece of bone driven into another |

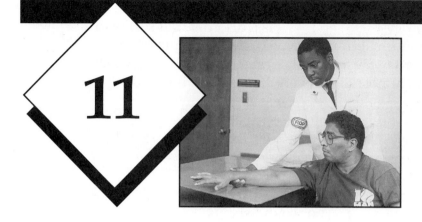

Physical Dysfunction and Disorders of the Nervous System

Objectives
After studying this chapter, you will be able to:

1. Briefly discuss the function of the nervous system.

2. Briefly explain what occurs in the following common neurological disorders: headache, numbness and tingling, pain, photophobia, blurred or double vision, and syncope.

3. Define the following neurological occurances: coma, paralysis, seizure, and confusion.

4. Describe what occurs when a patient suffers from personality changes and mood swings.

5. Define the following disorders: aphasia, ataxia, and apraxia.

6. Describe what occurs when a patient suffers from a cerebral vascular accident.

7. Describe what occurs when a patient suffers from a transient ischemic attack.

8. Describe the difference between a concussion and a contusion.

9. Briefly explain what occurs when the spinal cord is injured.

10. Explain what occurs in the brain when epilepsy is present and identify the types of seizures that might be seen with this disorder.

11. Discuss the following infections of the nervous system: meningitis, encephalitis, poliomyelitis, rabies, and shingles.

12. Briefly explain what occurs to the nervous system in the following structural and functional

disorders: Bell's palsy, cervical spondylosis, carpal tunnel syndrome, peripheral neuropathy, and cerebral palsy.

13. Briefly explain what occurs to the nervous system in the following degenerative diseases: Parkinson's disease, multiple sclerosis, Huntington's chorea, and Friedreich's ataxia.

14. Explain what occurs to the patient's nervous system when Alzheimer's disease is present.

♦ ♦ ♦

VOCABULARY

Learn the meaning and the correct spelling of the following words and abbreviations:

Neurological
Photophobia
Syncope
Convulsion
Seizure
Amnesia
Aphasia
Ataxia
Apraxia
Poliomyelitis
TIA
Concussion
Contusion
Metasticized
Epilepsy

Focal seizure
Grand mal seizure
Meningitis
Encephalitis
Bell's palsy
Neuropathy
CP
Pill-rolling
MS
Chorea
Dementia
CVA

Some nervous system disorders are straightforward and are easily identified as being caused by physical damage, inflammation, or infection. But neurological symptoms are sometimes caused, either partially or completely, by psychological disorders or by stress. A good example of this is the headache. Headaches may be caused by physical problems such as brain hemorrhage, concussion, eyestrain, or meningitis, to name just a few possibilities. Other headaches result from sinusitis or other problems not related to the nervous system. Still others are the result of nervous tension, depression, anxiety, and other problems that may not show up on a CAT scan or a test of cerebrospinal fluid.

In this chapter, we will discuss some of the more common dysfunctions and disorders of the nervous system. Such conditions range from headaches, numbness, tingling, pain, and other dysfunctions that are also considered to be symptoms of neurological diseases to other disorders that may or may not involve the entire body's ability to function and may lead to death.

◆ COMMON NEUROLOGICAL DISORDERS

Some of the most common neurological disorders may also be classified as *symptoms* of other more intense diseases. These include headache, numbness and tingling, pain, photophobia, or extreme sensitivity to light, blurred or double vision, fainting, coma, paralysis, seizures, mental confusion, personality changes, mood disorders, and aphasia, ataxia, and apraxia.

Headache

A headache may vary from a minor complaint to disabling pain. It may be felt as throbbing, stabbing, or a dull ache. In attempting to identify the cause of a headache, the physician will try to get from the patient as detailed a description of the sensation as possible, including the time of day it occurs, how long it lasts, whether it seems to be focused on one place in the skull, and any events that seem to regularly precede or follow it.

Headaches may be caused by pressure on the brain, eyestrain, or pressure on the arteries that lead to the brain. Cutting into brain tissue is not painful, because there are no pain receptors in that tissue; however, there are pain receptors on the surface of the skull and around the blood vessels and other structures of the brain. When brain tissue is injured or infected, it swells like any other injured tissue. This puts pressure on the brain because it is in an enclosed space, the skull. Such swelling causes severe headaches. The same thing happens when a growth occurs on the brain — there is no room for expansion to accommodate the additional tissue.

Numbness and Tingling

Numbness and tingling are often an early indication of damage to the peripheral nervous system or to centers in the brain or spinal cord that govern the area where the sensation is felt. They may be felt down one entire side of the body, in one limb, in the hands or feet, or in the face.

Pain

Pain can have many causes, some of which are merely carried by the nervous system and others which occur because of disease or injury. Some examples of nervous system disorders involving pain include pinched nerves, neuritis, sciatica, and shingles. The usual causes are damage to or pressure on the nerves or inflammation due to infection.

Photophobia

Patients sometimes describe a sensitivity to light that almost amounts to fear. This occurs with infections of the brain such as meningitis. It may also be a symptom of a brain hemorrhage.

Blurred or Double Vision

Several of the cranial nerves are involved with the process of focusing and otherwise adjusting the eyes to see clearly. Many brain disorders, such as stroke, tumors, transient ischemic attacks, and infections can cause vision disorders in one or both eyes.

Syncope or Fainting

Fainting, or brief unconsciousness, is caused by a momentary loss of adequate blood supply to the brain.

Coma

Coma is unconsciousness, or complete lack of responsiveness, that lasts more than two or three minutes. When this condition occurs, the brain is functioning, but the patient cannot be roused into a waking state. Like fainting, it is usually caused by loss of circulation to the brain. If it continues for more than a few hours, brain damage may occur and death may result.

Paralysis

The term *paralysis* means the inability to move some part of the body voluntarily. It may be temporary or permanent. When one side of the brain is damaged by a stroke, tumor, or other injury, the opposite side of the body may become paralyzed.

Seizures

Other terms for this condition include **fit** or **convulsion.** There are many forms of seizures, ranging from the dramatic *grand mal seizure*, in which the patient becomes unconscious, and rigid, falls to the floor, and is shaken by repeated muscle spasms to *petite mal seizures*, or incidents of momentary "absence" that may go completely unnoticed. Seizures are caused by electrical abnormalities in the brain.

Mental Confusion

Disorders of the brain such as tumors and injuries can cause confusion in the patient. This is generally due to disturbances in the memory areas of the brain. Loss of memory of past events is called **amnesia.** In this disorder, the patient may be aware of the problem and very anxious

about it or he may be completely unaware of memory lapses. Another form of mental confusion is **disorientation.** In this dysfunction, the patient does not know where she is or cannot identify the year or the time of day.

Personality Changes and Mood Swings

When the areas of the brain that control mood, emotions, or personality are damaged or bruised, the patient may become anxious, depressed, or elated, have sudden mood changes, known as **mood swings**, or take on a different personality than usual. Often the patient is unaware of such changes, and they are reported by family or friends.

Aphasia

The term **aphasia** means the inability to speak. It is caused by damage to the speech center in the cerebral cortex, usually in the left hemisphere. A person with aphasia may be able to understand verbal communication and to read but may be unable to formulate words either to speak or to write. This dysfunction can be very frustrating for the patient.

Ataxia

A person with **ataxia** cannot control voluntary muscle movements. This dysfunction may be caused by damage to the cerebellum or the motor area of the cerebral cortex.

Apraxia

The term **apraxia** means the inability to carry out learned, voluntary actions such as putting on clothes or eating, even though the patient wants to do them. It is the result of damage to memory centers in the cerebral hemispheres.

Now that we have identified some of the more common dysfunctions of the nervous system, we will look more specifically at some of the frequently seen disorders and diseases that can cause them.

◆ STROKE

The term stroke is a common term used for **cerebrovascular accident** or **CVA.** In a stroke, the circulation of blood to some part of the brain is interrupted. This interruption may be caused by an *embolus* or blocked artery, or by the gradual blockage of a vessel, as a result of *atherosclerosis.* Another cause of stroke may be by an aneurysm or weakness in the blood vessel wall. This condition is called a *cerebral hemorrhage.* Whatever the cause, the result is tissue death in the part of the brain that is no longer receiving a blood supply. The severity of the illness depends upon how much and what part of the brain is damaged.

◆ TRANSIENT ISCHEMIC ATTACKS

Some patients have minor, temporary, symptoms similar to those of a stroke. These include momentary blackouts, temporary blurred vision or confusion, sudden but temporary blindness in one eye, and so forth. These may be warning signs that the circulation to the brain is in danger. Such warnings are called **transient ischemic attacks, or TIAs.** They occur when a cerebral blood vessel becomes blocked but is quickly

reopened or bypassed by the circulatory system.

◆ BRAIN INJURY

Most injuries to the brain that cause lasting damage, occur in traffic accidents, industrial accidents, explosions, or from gunshot wounds. Whether the skull is fractured or not, a severe blow to the head can cause bruising, jolting, or other damage to the brain. The results of a brain injury depend largely on the force of the blow and what part of the brain is involved.

Two dysfunctions that can occur when a brain injury is present include concussion and contusion. A **concussion** is loss of consciousness with possible temporary impairment of brain function. A **contusion,** which is often more serious than a concussion, results from a bruising of brain tissue, which causes loss of consciousness and often is related to a skull fracture.

◆ SPINAL CORD INJURIES

When the spinal cord has been injured, the functions that are controlled by the nerves below that point are affected. However, sometimes an injury will affect only one side of the body.

A spinal cord injury can be fatal if the nerves that control breathing are damaged unless the patient is kept breathing by artificial means. These nerves are in the neck. Injuries lower on the cord often produce permanent disability. The nerves that control the bladder and rectum stem from the spinal cord and are often affected.

If a patient suffers from paralysis from the neck down, including the arms, that person is said to have *quadri-*

plegia. If paralysis is from the waist down, the patient has *paraplegia.* If the paralysis is only on one side of the body, the patient suffers from *hemiplegia.* All of these patients can learn to manage well if they are generally healthy and determined and if they receive the proper help, including physical therapy, and encouragement from medical professionals, family, and friends.

Brain or Spinal Cord Tumors

Tumors of the central nervous system are uncommon. The most common form is secondary cancers that have spread, or *metasticized,* from cancer sites elsewhere in the body, most often from the lungs or breast. A tumor in the brain or spinal cord may be benign or malignant, but both are very serious because they cause pressure on the nerve tissue.

♦ EPILEPSY

Epilepsy is a malfunction of the electrical activity of the brain that causes periodic seizures. Such a seizure occurs more than once and may be in response to a particular stimulus, such as bright light or stress, but more commonly occurs in no particular pattern.

Epileptic seizures may take different forms; however, the most common types include *grand mal,* in which the patient falls down unconscious, goes rigid, and twitches or jerks rhythmically; *petit mal,* in which the patient may go blank for up to 30 seconds and does not know what is happening; *focal seizure,* an uncontrollable twitching that begins in one part of the body and is eventually followed by the twitching of surrounding structures; a *temporal lobe seizure,* occurring after a brief warning or aura, in which, the patient suddenly acts out of character for a few minutes, and *febrile convulsion,* which generally occur during feverish illnesses in childhood and are similar to a grand mal seizure.

Epilepsy can be the result of brain damage caused by disease or injury. It may also be a symptom of a brain tumor, or it may be inherited. In many cases, the cause is not known and no damage is visible in the brain to explain why the seizures occur.

♦ INFECTIONS OF THE NERVOUS SYSTEM

Several infections of the nervous system may lead to further structure and dysfunctional incapacity of the patient. While these disorders are not seen as frequently as those considered to be functional, lack of proper medical diagnosis and attention can lead to death.

Meningitis

This disorder is a viral or bacterial infection of the meninges, the covering of the brain. It often occurs as a complication of a viral illness, such as the flu, or as a complication of sinusitis or a severe ear infection. In severe cases, meningitis can lead to drowsiness, unconsciousness, and, eventually, death or blindness, but it is not always a dangerous condition. It is diagnosed by analysis of cerebrospinal fluid, and treatment is with antibiotics, antipyretics, bedrest, and fluids if the infection is bacterial. Viral forms usually are the less dangerous type and are treated in essentially the same way, except without the use of antibiotics.

Encephalitis

Encephalitis is inflammation of brain tissue, usually due to a viral infection. It may be a complication of mumps or measles, and generally causes a fever, headache, loss of energy, and sometimes irritability, restlessness, drowsiness, and loss of function such as muscle weakness, vision problems, temporary aphasia, and occasionally, coma.

Poliomyelitis

This disease is caused by a viral infection of the anterior horns of the spinal cord. It is commonly known as **polio,** and is not often seen today because a vaccine against it is readily available. In severe cases, polio may cause permanent paralysis or muscular weakness, and the location of the damage in the spinal cord is determined by which muscles have been affected.

Rabies

Rabies is a viral infection of the central nervous system spread by the bite of an infected animal. It is rare today because most domestic animals are vaccinated against it.

Preventive treatment of suspected rabies is based on immunization by a series of vaccine and immune serum injections. When a bite occurs in an area close to the head or in an area with many nerve endings, such as the hands, the virus may reach the brain very quickly. In such cases, treatment should start immediately even though the suspected animal is still being observed.

Shingles

Shingles is a viral infection of the peripheral nerves caused by the same virus that causes chickenpox. It only occurs in patients who have had chickenpox. The virus remains dormant in the body after the patient recovers from the chickenpox and erupts as shingles in some people years later for no known reason. Attacks may be related to stress or injury. Shingles may cause temporary facial paralysis or vision problems if nerves that supply the face and cornea of the eye are involved. This disease cannot be cured, but it may eventually clear on its own.

◆ STRUCTURAL, FUNCTIONAL, AND DEGENERATIVE DISORDERS

Many of the disorders and dysfunctions of the nervous system that may require treatment involving physical therapy, are most often associated with structural, functional, and degenerative problems. The most common of the structural and functional disorders include *Bell's palsy, cervical spondylosis, carpal tunnel syndrome, peripheral neuropathy,* and *cerebral palsy.* Degenerative disorders of the nervous system requiring physical therapy include *Parkinson's Disease, multiple sclerosis, Huntington's chorea, Friedreich's ataxia,* and *Alzheimer's disease.*

Disorders Affecting Structure and Function

Bell's Palsy. In this disorder, the facial nerve on one side swells for no known reason and becomes pinched where it passes through the skull. This causes muscle weakness on that side of the face, resulting in distorted expression, a downward turn to the mouth, and sometimes an inability to close the eye. This condition is almost always temporary.

Cervical Spondylosis. The term **spondylosis** means an immobility of a vertebral joint. In this disorder, the vertebrae in the cervical region develop bony growths. The discs between the vertebrae may harden as well, and the whole structure of the neck may become stiff and misaligned, thus creating an abnormal pressure on the spinal cord and the spinal nerves that supply the arms and hands.

Carpal Tunnel Syndrome. The carpal tunnel is a passageway between the carpal bones of the wrist and the ventral ligaments. Nerves pass through the tunnel on their way from the brain to the hand. The tunnel is rigid. If the tissue in it becomes swollen from accumulated fluid, pressure on the nerves causes carpal tunnel syndrome. Tingling and numbness of the hands and shooting pains that travel from the wrist up the arm may occur. Medication and sometimes surgery may be necessary to free the nerve and create more space in the carpal tunnel.

Peripheral Neuropathy. Peripheral neuropathy means damage to the peripheral nerves. It can be caused by chronic disorders such as diabetes or alcoholism or by a deficiency of vitamin B-12. Symptoms may include tingling in the hands and feet, and numbness or sensitivity of the skin accompanied by nerve pain (neuropathy). Dexterity is sometimes reduced, which can lead to muscle weakness and eventually paralysis.

Cerebral Palsy. Cerebral palsy is caused by brain damage that occurs during fetal development, during birth, or in early childhood. One or more limbs may be immobile or weak, and muscle movements may be poorly controlled or jerky. Accompanying problems may include mental retardation, hearing loss, visual problems, speech problems, and convulsions. This disease is usually not detected until a child is six months old or older, when normal development calls for more coordinated muscle movements.

Degenerative Diseases

Parkinson's Disease. Parkinson's disease occurs because of a deterioration of the basal ganglia and diminished supply of the neurotransmitter chemical dopamine. This imbalance causes shaking and rigidity in the voluntary, skeletal muscles. The patient has characteristic involuntary movements, called *tremors,* such as rhythmic shaking of the head and hands, or a *pill-rolling movement* in which the thumb and fingertips are rubbed together. The tremor goes away when the patient voluntarily moves the limb.

Multiple Sclerosis. In this disease, the myelin sheaths that cover the axons of many nerves become inflamed. The first and, in some cases, the only attack of the disease may cause a number of different symptoms, depending on which nerves are affected. These may include numbness, tingling, or weakness in one or more limbs or in a single spot, ataxia, blurred vision, slurred speech, or urinary incontinence. The disease usually first appears between the ages of 12 and 40 and a period without symptoms, called remission, may follow the first attack. Later attacks may become gradually more frequent and/or more severe over a span of 20 to 40 years.

Huntington's Chorea. Chorea means uncontrollable, jerky body movements. In this rare inherited disease, nerves degenerate in various parts of the body starting in early middle age, causing chorea and mental deterioration. There is no cure and no effective treatment for the symptoms. Genetic counseling is the key to eventual eradication of this disease.

Friedreich's Ataxia. This is another inherited disease, but it affects children beginning between the ages of five and 15. It also causes degeneration of nerve fibers, resulting in ataxia and then problems with speech, movement of the arms, and even standing still. It also causes heart disease. There is no known treatment for the disorder.

Alzheimer's Disease. This disease, also known as **presenile senile dementia,** most often begins in middle age. The symptoms are gradual loss of intellectual ability, memory, and other thought processes due to the death of nerve cells in the frontal and temporal lobes of the cerebrum. The disease eventually causes death and progression is more rapid in younger patients.

There are many possible causes of mental deterioration besides Alzheimer's disease and many of them are treatable. So it is important that any patient who has such symptoms, regardless of age, be tested for other possible causes of the problem. If the patient does in fact have Alzheimer's disease, there is no known treatment. Eventually, close supervision and nursing care will become necessary.

♦ ♦ ♦
SUMMARY OUTLINE

Physical Dysfunctions and Disorders of the Nervous system

Common Neurological Disorders
- Headache
- Numbness
- Pain
- Photophobia
- Blurred or double vision
- Syncope or fainting
- Coma
- Paralysis
- Seizures
- Mental confusion and personality changes and mood swings
- Aphasia, ataxia, and apraxia

Common Neurological Disorders of the Brain
- Cerebral vascular accident
- Transient ischemic attacks
- Brain injury

Spinal Cord Injuries
- Damage that may occur to the nervous system
- Brain or spinal cord tumors

Epilepsy

Infections of the Nervous System
- Meningitis
- Encephalitis
- Poliomyelitis
- Rabies
- Shingles

Structural and Functional Disorders of the Nervous System
- Bell's palsy
- Cervical spondylosis
- Carpal tunnel syndrome
- Peripheral neuropathy
- Cerebral palsy

Degenerative Disorders of the Nervous System
- Parkinson's disease
- Multiple sclerosis
- Huntington's chorea
- Friedreich's ataxia
- Alzheimer's disease

CHAPTER REVIEW QUESTIONS

1. List at least five neurological disorders that may also be classified as symptoms of other more intense diseases:

   a._____   d._____

   b._____   e._____

   c._____

2. What is the medical term for fainting?

3. What is the medical term that means inability to speak?

4. The term is a commonly used word for a _____

   _____ _____.

5. Briefly explain the difference between a concussion and a contusion.

6. A neurological dysfunction which causes minor, temporary symptoms similar to those seen in a stroke, is called

   a _____ _____ _____.

7. _____ is defined as a malfunction of the electrical activity of the brain that causes periodic seizures.

8. What neurological disorder is a result of an inflammation of the brain tissue?

9. In _____ _____, the facial nerve on one side of the face swells for no known reason.

10. The term _____ refers to nerve pain.

11. What neurological disorder is caused by brain damage that occurs during fetal development, during birth, or in early childhood?

12. What neurological disorder is characterized by involuntary tremors and "pill-rolling" movements of the thumb and fingertips?

13. _____ refers to an uncontrollable, jerky body movement.

14. The neurological disease _____ _____ is also known as presenile senile dementia.

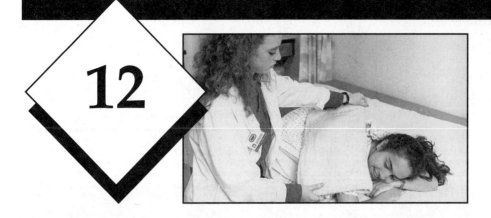

Common Conditions and Disorders and Physical Therapy

Objectives
After studying this chapter, you will be able to:

1. Identify common disorders and conditions generally requiring the treatment of physical therapy.

2. Briefly describe what occurs in Paget's disease.

3. Discuss the role physical therapy plays when a patient has under gone an amputation of an extremity.

4. Describe what occurs when a patient suffers from a decubitus ulcer.

5. Explain what occurs when a patient suffers from contractures and footdrop.

VOCABULARY

Learn the meaning and the correct spelling of the following words and abbreviations:

Paget's disease
Kyphosis
Amputation
Decubitus ulcer
Pressure sore
Contracture
Footdrop

In Chapters 10 and 11, we discussed some of the more commonly seen disorders related to both the musculoskeletal and the nervous system. However, other conditions and disorders, such as those related to amputation, decubitus ulcers, deformities, and other disorders of the body, may necessitate the use of physical therapy as part of their treatment.

♦ PAGET'S DISEASE

Paget's disease (*osteitis deformans*) is a disorder characterized by abnormal bone remodeling. Normally, bone is constantly being formed and resorbed or broken down. In Paget's disease, the resorbed bone is high in mineral content but poorly constructed. The most common areas of involvement are the long bones and the skull, and the cause of the disease is unknown.

Some patients suffering from Paget's disease may be asymptomatic, but may also have some mild skeletal deformity due to the disorder, while others may have marked skeletal deformities, such as enlargement of the skull, bowing of the long bones, and kyphosis (hunch-back). Bone pain and tenderness on pressure may also be present.

♦ AMPUTATION

Amputation of a limb may be the treatment for any one of a number of reasons. It may be necessary due to accidental and extensive trauma to an extremity or as a result of a malignancy. It may be necessary to amputate an extremity because the patient suffers from long standing infections of bone and tissue that prohibit restoration of function or because a deformity of a limb renders it useless and a hindrance. Amputation may also be required when a condition exists that may endanger the life of the patient such as vascular accidents and bacterial infections.

The decision to amputate is made when all other methods of therapy have failed. The physician decides how much of the limb must be amputated to maintain circulation and healthy structures in the remainder of the limb. The procedure can be performed at any level in the lower extremity but there are preferred levels above and below the knee that facilitate fitting with available prostheses.

When the surgeon decides that amputation is inevitable, the first decision made involves the level of amputation. Although a number of tests are available, including arteriography, often the final decision can only be made by observing the vascularity of the tissues while the patient is in surgery.

♦ DECUBITUS ULCERS (PRESSURE SORES)

Whenever nerve impulses to the skin are interrupted, the skin's normal response to injury is diminished. In the normal person, constant movement during waking and even sleeping hours, protects the skin from decubitus ulcers, or pressure sores. People with limited movement or paralysis cannot engage in movement and, therefore, are subject to skin breakdown.

Decubitus ulcers may become infected easily and heal slowly. Skilled nursing management is essential if rehabilitation is to be uncomplicated by decubitus formation.

♦ CONTRACTURES

Contractures occur when a patient undergoes prolonged immobility and his or her extremities are not properly cared for and exercised. It is a condition in which there is an abnormal shortening of muscles that usually results in a deformity of the part and renders it resistant to movement. If preventive measures are not taken, permanent deformity may occur.

♦ FOOTDROP

Footdrop is a frequent complication of patients suffering from contractures, and it occurs as a result of the patient's inability to maintain the foot in a normal position. In essence, it is a dragging of the foot. Since patients suffering from this disorder usually have problems with poor circulation, the physician usually orders that elastic stockings be worn to enhance venous blood return to the major veins. Removing and reapplying the stockings at least twice a day and changing the patient's position at least every two hours generally helps to prevent footdrop, as well as contractures and decubitus ulcers.

♦ ♦ ♦
SUMMARY OUTLINE

Common Conditions and Disorders and Physical Therapy
- The role physical therapy plays in therapeutic treatment of common disorders and conditions
- Paget's disease
- Amputation
- Decubitus ulcers
- Contractures
- Footdrop

CHAPTER REVIEW QUESTIONS

1. What disease of the musculoskeletal system is characterized by abnormal bone remodeling?
2. What does the term "kyphosis" mean?
3. List at least three reasons for which an amputation might be necessary:
    a._____
    b._____
    c._____
4. What is the medical term for a pressure sore?
5. _____ may occur when a patient undergoes prolonged immobility.
6. A patient may suffer from _____ if he is unable to maintain his foot in a normal position.
7. Changing a patient's position at least every ___ hours helps to prevent _____ _____, _____, and _____.

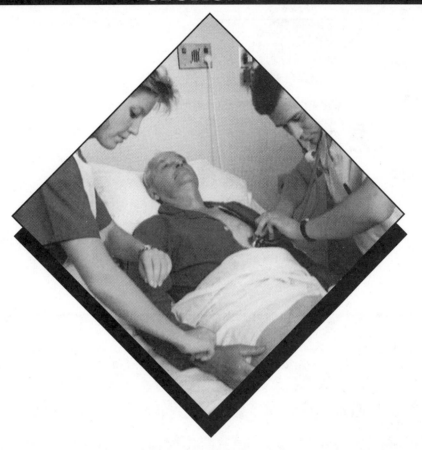

SAFETY AND CHARTING

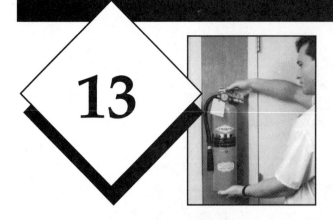

13

Safety in the Working Environment

Objectives
After studying this chapter, you will be able to:

1. Define the term environment as it relates to the medical area.

2. Discuss the purpose for keeping the medical environment safe.

3. Explain how to manage the medical external environment.

4. Discuss the role temperature, humidity, ventilation control, light regulation, color, noise control, neatness and order, control of odors, and providing for the patient's privacy play in managing the health care environment.

5. Discuss the physical therapy aide's role in providing a safe environment.

6. Discuss how to prevent accidents in the health care environment.

7. Identify patients at risk of having accidents.

8. Describe how to prevent falls in the health care environment.

9. Discuss how to prevent burns in the health care environment.

10. Explain the importance of practicing good body alignment and movement in the working environment.

11. Describe how the physical therapy aide can practice good body alignment and movement.

12. Discuss the concept of asepsis and infection control.

13. Explain how medical asepsis is carried out through proper handwashing.

14. Demonstrate correct hand washing technique.

15. Discuss how microorganisms grow and spread.

VOCABULARY

Learn the meaning and the correct spelling of the following words and abbreviations:

Environment
External environment
Temperature
Humidity
Ventilation
Hospital clean
Safety
Body alignment
Body mechanics
Balance
Gravity
Hyperextension
Abduction
Adduction
Asepsis
Medical asepsis
Infection control
Microorganisms

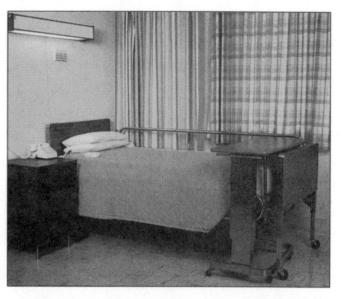

Figure 13-1 The patient's unit becomes his home. (From Hegner and Caldwell, *Nursing Assistant: A Nursing Process Approach*, 6th edition, copyright 1992 by Delmar Publishers Inc.)

All health care workers, including the physical therapy aide, are expected to practice those techniques and skills that provide the patient with a safe and environmentally sound atmosphere (see Figure 13-1).

In the physical therapy area, the aide is concerned with two tasks— carrying out the skills and techniques necessary to assist the patient in achieving a greater degree of health and providing those skills and techniques in a proper and acceptable way. To do so, constitutes providing a safe environment, practicing proper aseptic techniques, and using good body mechanics.

♦ MANAGING THE EXTERNAL ENVIRONMENT

In today's modern health care setting, many people share the responsibility of maintaining and managing the external environment. This includes engineers,

The term environment is a word frequently used to describe any condition that affects the life or development of a person in his surroundings. In health care, we often use the term *therapeutic environment* to describe both those factors that influence the patient's external environment, and those that make up the internal composition of the body.

who maintain temperature through control of heating, cooling, and ventilation; housekeeping personnel, who provide cleanliness and a pleasant appearance; and the health care team, who provides safety, privacy, neatness, and order for the patient's well-being.

There are several specific external environmental factors of concern to the members of physical therapy team. These include the regulation of temperature, humidity control, ventilation, light, use of color, control of noise, neatness and order, elimination of noxious odors, safety, and privacy.

Regulation of Temperature

Temperature affects our comfort and even our disposition. A range between 68 degrees and 72 degrees Fahrenheit is generally maintained in most air-conditioned facilities.

Some air-conditioned facilities have individual controls in treatment rooms to allow for flexibility in temperature control. When this is not available, fans, coolers, and heaters may sometimes be used.

Humidity Control

Humidity is the amount of moisture in the air, and a range of 30 to 50 percent is normally comfortable. Very low humidity dries the respiratory passages. As the temperature increases, air can hold more water. At 50 degrees Fahrenheit, saturated air holds approximately 4.2 grains of water per cubic foot of air. At 90 degrees Fahrenheit, nearly three times as much water is retained.

There is no simple method of decreasing humidity; it has become a technical problem for air-conditioning experts and is accomplished only by modern engineering methods. However, a vaporizer or humidifier can sometimes be used around patients in order to increase the humidity in some respiratory conditions.

Ventilation Control

Ventilation refers to the movement of air; stale air can be oppressive. The use of fans increases comfort because the air is in motion even though the temperature and humidity remain unchanged. In most health care settings, air-conditioning is used for ventilation and temperature control. Windows are not used for these purposes and should not be open.

Light Regulation

Lighting contributes to a patient's well-being; however, some illness, such as those seen in disorders of the nervous system, cause *"photophobia"* in which light is painful to the eyes.

A sunny room is cheerful and can improve a patient's spirits. Therefore, it is important to provide adequate lighting in all patient areas. This means a light that is bright enough to see without *glare* and to avoid eye strain. Good light is *soft* and *diffused*. It does not make sharp shadows. Overhead fluorescent lighting is generally effective (see Figure 13-2).

Use of Color

In the patient environment, some bright colors stimulate while others sooth. The location of the source of light influences color. Decorators are aware of this, and colors in patient treatment rooms are usually subdued pastels.

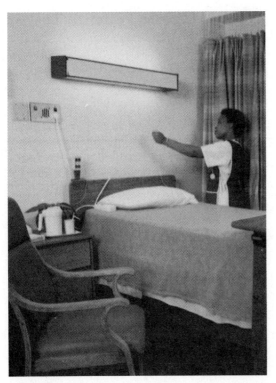

Figure 13-2 The best lighting is indirect lighting; the over–bed light (From Hegner and Caldwell, *Nursing Assistant: A Nursing Process Approach,* 6th edition, copyright 1992 by Delmar Publishers Inc.)

Noise Control

Noise is a negative environmental factor, and it can affect one's health. People who are careless or thoughtless about talking and laughing cause unnecessary noise. Voices carry loudly in corridors, which seldom have drapes or other sound-absorbing materials. Equipment and machinery, such as those that are rolled down hallways, are often noisy. Dropping equipment causes startling noises therefore, many health care facilities and physical therapy offices use carpeting or resilient floor materials and sound-absorbing ceilings in an effort to decrease noise. This still does not reduce the major source of noise — people. Skill in human relations, involving both tolerance and courtesy in dealing with others, is very important for all members of the health care team including the physical therapy aide. By practicing these lifelong skills, you can help reduce "people noise" for all of your patients.

Neatness and Order

Some people seem to thrive on living in clutter while others are offended if a picture hangs even slightly crooked. Therefore, it is important that the office and the individual treatment rooms be kept in sufficient order to be safe. This can easily be accomplished by tidying up and removing used items after every patient, and by doing your part as a member of the health care team in seeing to the office being kept neat and orderly.

Prevention and Control of Odors

Odors can be pleasant or unpleasant. Unfortunately, unpleasant smells have a tendency to permeate in some health care settings. In order to avoid odors from existing in the facility, all members of the staff should follow good prevention techniques. This includes disposing of refuse properly, removing items, such as wilted flowers and stagnant water, from vases, and avoiding being a source of odors yourself.

Good ventilation and cleanliness are far more effective in controlling odors than scented air sprays and other masking devices. "Hospital clean" should be a reality as well as an expression. Prompt and proper disposal and scrupulous cleanliness can decrease odors.

Providing Privacy

Privacy is essential for the patient's well-being. Always remember to knock gently and identify yourself before entering when the door to a treatment room is closed.   Closing the curtain around the patient's cubicle can spare embarrassment to the patient, the physical therapist, and yourself.

Hospital workers, including those working in the physical therapy department, become accustomed to situations and functions that would be embarrassing to the non-medical person. A discreet withdrawal from the room provides privacy for the shy patient to perform such functions as undressing for a treatment.

Remember, lack of privacy, like noise, is a frequent source of patient irritation. The thoughtful aide can do much to decrease these irritations.

♦ PROVIDING A SAFE ENVIRONMENT

Providing a safe environment is everyone's responsibility. Remember that safety is necessary in preventing accidents and in reducing the possibility of lawsuits. Various types of accidents occur in environments where patients are seen. The most common are falls, burns, cuts or bruises, altercations with others, loss of personal possessions, such as money, choking, and electrical shock. The alert physical therapy aide is always on the lookout for safety hazards and corrects them so that accidents can be prevented.

Patients at Risk of Having Accidents

Some patients are more likely to have an accident than others. Those that are more at risk include confused and elderly patients and those taking certain types of medications. Their safety is your concern. Elderly patients often need special

attention. They may be forgetful or have decreased sensory perceptions such as dimmed vision or decreased hearing that deprives them of some of their "danger warning" capabilities.

Another group of patients at risk are children. They have a tendency to climb, touch, taste, and eagerly explore their environments. They need special protection to prevent their curiosity from causing injury.

Preventing Falls

Falls are particularly hazardous in health care settings. Many falls can be prevented by removing foreign objects from the floor that might cause a patient to trip. Handrails and grab bars should also be installed in bathrooms and in corridors to assist weak or debilitated patients.

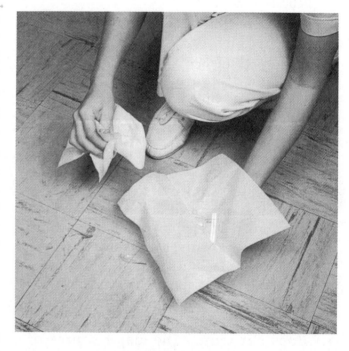

Figure 13-3 Small pieces of glass may be picked up carefully with a folded paper towel or tissue. (From Hegner and Caldwell, *Nursing Assistant: A Nursing Process Approach*, 6th edition, copyright 1992 by Delmar Publishers Inc.)

If you see a spill, mop it up immediately and post a "slippery" sign when it is being mopped. Usually only one side of the floor is mopped at a time, allowing half to remain dry for use (see Figure 13-3).

Another way to prevent falls from occurring is to provide assistance to patients who have poor vision or difficulty seeing. It is especially important that scatter rugs and clutter be removed and that furniture remain in customary locations.

Preventing Burns

The alert aide looks out for safety hazards and corrects them so that burns can be prevented. Testing the temperature of solutions used for soaks or packs and heating devices is necessary to prevent burns. Remember that some patients may have debilitating diseases, such as diabetes, paralysis, or others that cause impaired circulation, and the patient may not even be aware that she has been burned.

Inspection of all electrical plugs, cords, and equipment before use can prevent accidents. Oily rags and other combustible materials usually are stored in metal containers that have tight lids. Oxygen tanks and other gas containers under pressure should be secured with straps or by other means to prevent falling (see Figure 13-4).

Another way in which to prevent fires from occurring is to only allow smoking in designated places. If oxygen is used or kept close by, a "no smoking" sign should be placed in full view for all patients and workers.

Fire in a hospital or health care setting is always a possibility; therefore, it is important to know the rules for fire safety. Generally, the agency's fire regulations will be taught in the first few days of employment. Many local fire departments hold regular fire safety classes for employees in health agencies in their area. These are required in most states if a health agency is to receive its fire safety clearance from the fire department. Know the location of extinguishers and fire doors. Many institutions have occasional fire drills. Always make sure you know what to do in case of a fire or other disaster.

♦ PRACTICING GOOD BODY ALIGNMENT AND MOVEMENT

The practice of good body alignment and using the appropriate movements and proper body mechanics to perform one's work is also part of providing a safe environment. Health care workers

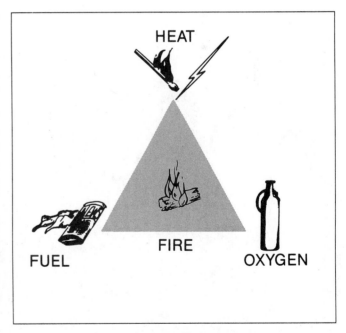

Figure 13-4 (A) The fire triangle–elements needed for combustion (burning). (From Hegner and Caldwell, *Nursing Assistant: A Nursing Process Approach,* 6th edition, copyright 1992 by Delmar Publishers Inc.) (*Continued*)

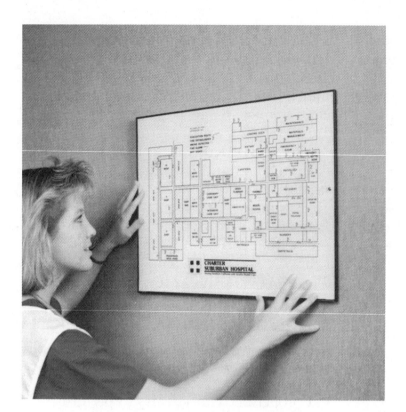
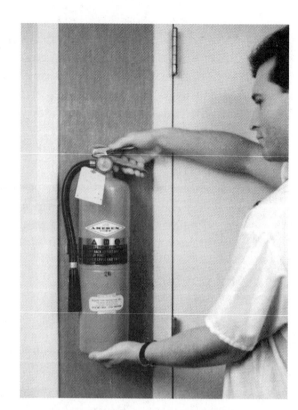

Figure 13-4 (B) All personnel should know the escape plan in the event of a fire and should know where fire extinguishers are located. (From Hegner and Caldwell, *Nursing Assistant: A Nursing Process Approach,* 6th edition, copyright 1992 by Delmar Publishers Inc.) (*Continued*)

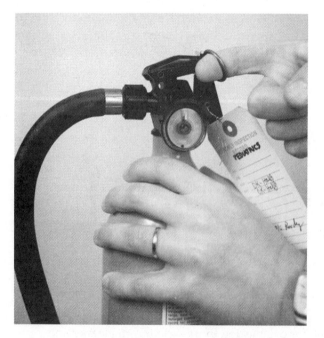
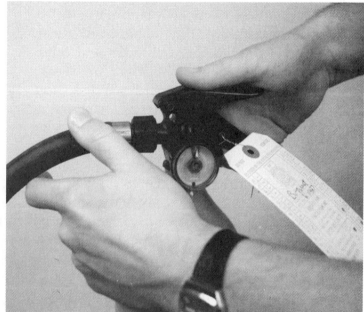

Figure 13-4 (C) Use a fire extinguisher. (From Hegner and Caldwell, *Nursing Assistant: A Nursing Process Approach,* 6th edition, copyright 1992 by Delmar Publishers Inc.)

are very active people. In performing their work, they use a variety of movements as they reach, push, carry, lift, pull, stoop, sit, stand, and walk. Your activities as a physical therapy aide will require that you, too, use these movements as you reach for supplies from a shelf, lift and carry objects, push wheelchairs or stretchers, stoop to pick up objects from the floor, or walk, stand, or assist in ambulating a patient.

All of us have been performing these movements most of our lives, so why do we single them out for consideration now? What is the point? The answer is that with knowledge of proper body alignment and movement your work may be easier, you may prevent injury to yourself and your patient, and you will present a more attractive appearance as you work. You should always be conscious that you are using proper body alignment for yourself and the patient. This includes knowing how to balance yourself correctly in order to avoid strain or injury to yourself (see Figure 13-5).

One of the most common injuries to physical therapy workers is severe muscle strain, usually of the lower back, although it may occur in the shoulders or the abdomen. Low back strain is painful and generally takes a long time to heal. It often requires hospitalization, bed rest, or traction and it is costly in lost salary and medical fees. It is also very preventable. Low back strain and other muscle strains are caused by

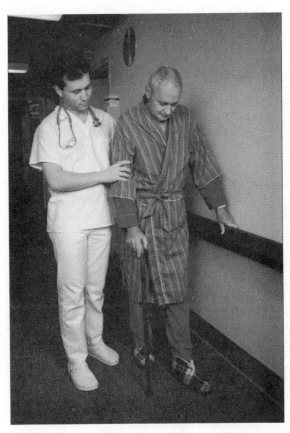
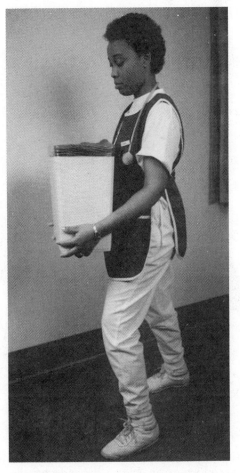

Figure 13-5 (A) The proper standing position allows the physical therapy aide to move safely in any direction as needed; (B) Keeping the feet separated provides a good base of support. (From Hegner and Caldwell, *Nursing Assistant: A Nursing Process Approach*, 6th edition, copyright 1992 by Delmar Publishers Inc.)

improper body alignment, loss of balance, and poor body movements.

Your employer and your co-workers would much rather prefer you to be a healthy worker than a patient with an injury that could have been prevented. The knowledge and use of proper body alignment, balance, and movement will help you to prevent injury to yourself.

Body Alignment and Balance

Alignment is defined as the proper relationship of the body segments to one another. When the segments are properly aligned, it is easier to maintain body balance. Balanced posture means a body that is stable, steady, and not likely to tip or fall.

The main portions of the body, that is

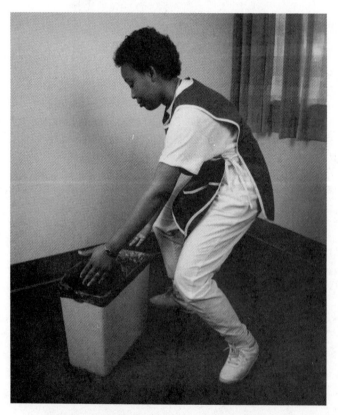

Figure 13-6 The correct way to maintain balance when picking up an object is to bend from the hips and knees. (From Hegner and Caldwell, *Nursing Assistant: A Nursing Process Approach*, 6th edition, copyright 1992 by Delmar Publishers Inc.)

the pelvis, thorax, and the head, are supported by structures below them that are often very small such as the small bones in the feet and in the vertebrae. To maintain the proper relationship and balance of these anatomical parts, the ligaments and muscles must be used effectively (see Figure 13-6).

The force of gravity affects balance because it is constantly pulling the body toward the earth. Therefore, in order for proper balance to exist, there must be a center for the gravity, a base of support, and a line of gravity.

Center of gravity refers to an area located in the pelvis about the level of the second sacral vertebrae. The exact location may vary slightly, depending on body structure. A base of support provides a stable stance for keeping the body from toppling over, as well as stability in movements such as lifting, pushing, or pulling.

Line of gravity pertains to an imaginary line that falls in the frontal plane of the body, that is, one which passes behind the ear downward just behind the center of the hip joint and then downward slightly in front of the knee and ankle joint. Individual variations may occur according to skeletal build and the curvature of a person's spine.

When a person stands in an erect posture so that the line of gravity falls as stated above, body balance is preserved and there is minimal resistance needed to overcome the force of gravity. If the posture is out of alignment, the body weight distribution is shifted, the balance is upset, the muscles no longer work together, and the gravitational pull is increased.

Body Movement

As we discussed in Chapter 6, the joints of our body allow movement when the muscles contract and pull on bones. Various terms are used to describe these movements, they include the movements of flexion, extension, hyperextension, abduction, and adduction.

If you hold your arm out straight, the elbow joint forms a straight line, or a 180-degree angle. By bending the elbow joint, you decrease the angle. This is called *flexion*. *Extension* is the joint movement opposite to flexion. When you straighten the arm that is bent at the elbow, or the leg that is bent at the knee, you are increasing the angle at the joint and extending the arm or leg.

Some joints allow for increasing the angle more than 180-degrees or beyond a straight line. This is called *hyperextension*. You hyperextend your neck each time you raise your chin and tilt your head backward. The knee joint also allows the movement of hyperextension. You can feel this movement if you stand normally with the knee joint nearly straight and then force the knee joint even straighter until the joint is locked or rigid.

Abduction is another term used to describe certain joint movements. Abduct means to move away from the midline of the body. The opposite movement of *abduction* is adduction, the movement to bring the part back toward the midline of the body.

The major body movements are flexion, extension, adduction, and abduction. The muscles that produce these movements are called flexors, extensors, adductors, and abductors.

Checking for Good Body Alignment

Before beginning any body movement, you should always align and balance your body properly in order to prevent strain and injury. To do this, you can use some basic checkpoints. First, always remember to start from a good base of support. Make sure you distribute your weight evenly on both feet, and keep your knees slightly flexed. Remember to tuck in your buttocks and keep the abdomen up and in. Raise your rib cage up, and, finally, always keep your head erect.

When performing a task, always remember to work at a comfortable height, to keep the work close to your body, to use smooth, coordinated movements, and to "set" or prepare the muscles for action. If you are required to reach for an object or to assist a patient, start by checking for good body alignment, stand on a footstool, if needed, with your feet apart. Always advance one foot forward in the direction of the reach, look and reach in front of you rather than overhead, and stabilize your body by "setting" your muscles. Remember to lower the object with smooth, coordinated movements, and, before stepping off the stool, remember to look down.

♦ ASEPSIS AND INFECTION CONTROL

Practicing safety in the working environment includes many factors. As we have already discussed, it includes maintaining the external environment, avoiding accidents, and practicing good body movements. Providing a safe atmosphere for both you and the patient also includes the practice of good medical asepsis and infection control.

It can't be emphasized enough that one of the most important tasks you have in the health care field is providing a healthy environment for both your patients and yourself. A clean, dry, well lit and airy atmosphere goes a long way toward preventing the growth of germs or killing those that already exist.

One of the simplest methods we have to prevent the spread of germs and disease is the use of proper handwashing techniques. It is a safety skill not only for you personally but also for your patient and your co-workers. You will wash your hands before and after doing any procedures that involve direct or indirect contact with a patient, after contact with waste materials, before handling any food or food receptacles, and at any other times when your hands are soiled.

Handwashing for Asepsis: Understanding the Germ Theory

As you enter your career in health care and particularly in the field of physical therapy, you need to develop an understanding of how germs cause disease and how health care workers use principles of medical asepsis to carry out one of the most important patient goals— that of protecting the patient from infection. Medical asepsis includes the techniques and skills used to render any medical setting free of disease-causing microorganisms although nonharmful microorganisms may still be present. The most crucial of these skills, and one of the most effective actions in preventing the spread of infection, is handwashing.

Our everyday world is filled with microorganisms, which are extremely small bits of plant or animal life too small to be seen with the naked eye. They can be seen and studied with the use of a microscope. Only a small number of microorganisms are harmful to the human body and capable of causing diseases. These are referred to as germs,

or *pathogenic* organisms. Bacteria are one-celled microorganisms; some are pathogenic and cause infections, whereas others are *nonpathogenic.*

People come in contact with microorganisms and germs constantly, but the body's defenses are strong enough to protect us from diseases most of the time. Microorganisms consist of protein, have a certain amount of weight, and are unable to move about on their own. Because of their size, they are picked up and carried by the slightest air current, and they settle on any convenient surface. Because they have weight, they drift lower and lower until they settle on a surface, so the heaviest concentration of microorganisms will be present on solid objects.

Microorganisms are found on all skin surfaces. Large numbers are found within the body, especially in the air passages of the respiratory tract, in the mouth, and along the entire length of the digestive tract. Normal, harmless residents of the intestinal tract include *Escherichia coli (E.coli)* (see Figure 13-7). These organisms may cause an infection if introduced into a different part of the body, such as the urinary bladder, or into an open wound. The skin is an effective barrier against pathogenic organisms, and it protects the delicate organs within the body. Vigorous washing removes most of the microorganisms on the surface of the skin that are picked up when we come in contact with objects, but it cannot remove all of those that reside in the grooves and crevices that are present in the outer layers of skin. Additional protection against microorganisms is provided by the immune system of the body.

Infections are caused by germs that invade the tissues of the body and set up a chemical reaction that causes the tissues to react in the symptoms associated with the disease. Generally, an infection can develop if the body is exposed to a large number of pathogenic organisms or if it is attacked by germs that are very strong and virulent. Infections can also be caused if the individual has a low resistance.

Through the use of medical asepsis, health care workers can provide a safe environment for patients who are particularly susceptible to infections. Medical asepsis includes various actions and skills that reduce the number of pathogenic organisms present in the immediate vicinity. It is necessary to reduce the number of all microorganisms in order to lower the number of pathogens; this is done by frequent handwashing, cleaning dirty or soiled surfaces, disposing of highly contaminated items, and using sterile equipment and supplies.

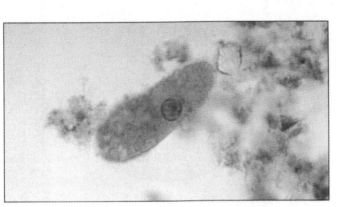

A

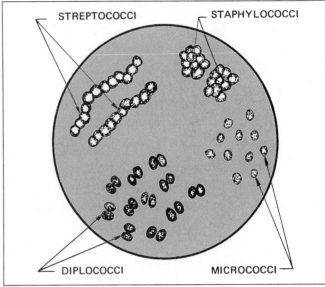

B

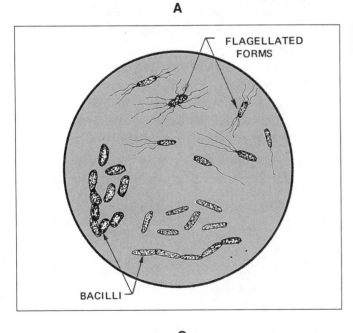

C

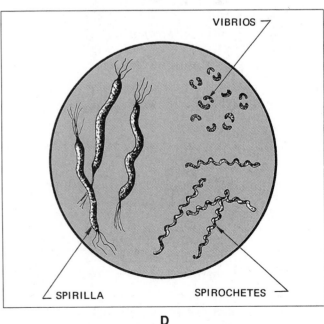

D

Figure 13-7 (A) Intestinal protozoa; (B) Kinds of cocci; (C) Kinds of bacilli; (D) Spirilla forms. (From Hegner and Caldwell, *Nursing Assistant: A Nursing Process Approach*, 6th edition, copyright 1992 by Delmar Publishers Inc.)

How Microorganisms Grow and Spread

Because microorganisms are living organisms, they need certain environmental conditions in order to help them live and grow. These include moisture, food, oxygen, temperature, and darkness.

Microorganisms are incapable of moving by themselves, so they must rely on other vehicles for transportation from one site to another. For an infection to occur, the pathogens have to be able to escape from the reservoir or *host* where they have been allowed to multiply and then be transmitted to another host. They can be carried by human, animal, or insect carriers; on objects, such as furniture, clothing, and medical equipment; by air currents produced by winds, drafts, sneezing, or coughing; and in foods, such as water, milk, and other ingestible materials.

Procedure #6: Completing the Two-Minute Handwash for Medical Asepsis

To complete a two-minute handwash, make sure you have: soap dispenser, waste container, paper towels.

1. Remove all jewelry.
2. Approach the sink; stand in a comfortable position, leaning slightly toward the sink, and maintain good body alignment; avoid contaminating your clothing by touching the sink.
3. Turn on the water with a dry paper towel and keep it running continuously throughout the procedure.
4. Adjust the temperature of the water.
5. Wet your hands with water by holding your hands down toward the sink, lower than your elbows; the water will then drain down the wrists to the fingertips and carry the bacteria away.
6. Apply soap or detergent.
7. Wash your hands. This usually takes about 30 seconds for the palms, 10 seconds for the backs of the hands, and 10 seconds for the fingers. Wash the palms using a rotary or circular motion and friction.
8. Rinse well. Hold your hands with fingers pointing downward and avoid touching any portion of the sink with your hands.
9. Wash your wrists and forearms with soap, spending 10 to 15 seconds per each wrist and forearm.
10. Rinse your arms and hands, remembering to drain in a downward motion.
11. Repeat steps 5 through 9.
12. Inspect your knuckles.
13. Clean your fingernails using an orange stick or a curved end of a flat toothpick.
14. Dry your hands well.
15. Turn off the running water; use a paper towel to turn off the hand faucet; and discard it into the wastebasket after finishing.
16. Apply lotion as desired.
17. Leave the sink area neat and clean.

The most common method of transporting microorganisms is by direct contact with an infected person, contaminated materials, or supplies. They are carried on the hands or skin to another susceptible person. In the health care environment, microorganisms are generally spread from worker to worker, from equipment to patient or worker, from patient to patient, and from worker to patient.

♦ PERFORMING PROPER HANDWASHING

In order to provide a safe environment for the patient and to reduce the number of microorganisms as well as the total number of pathogens, you should wash your hands frequently when providing care. Hands should be washed before and after providing care, after touching contaminated materials or equipment, after going to the bathroom, and before handling food. In addition to washing your hands frequently, you should also follow the appropriate steps for completing a two-minute handwash for medical asepsis.

♦ ♦ ♦
SUMMARY OUTLINE

Safety in the Working Environment
- Defining environment

Managing the External Environment
- Regulation of temperature
- Humidity control
- Ventilation control
- Light regulation
- Use of color
- Noise control
- Neatness and order
- Prevention and control of odors
- Providing privacy

Providing a Safe Environment
- Patients at risk of having accidents
- Preventing falls
- Preventing burns

Practicing Good Body Alignment and Movement
- Understanding the purpose of practicing good body alignment and movement
- Body alignment and balance
- Body movement
- Checking for good body alignment

Asepsis and Infection Control
- Understanding the concept of asepsis and infection control
- Handwashing for asepsis: understanding the germ theory
- How microorganisms grow and spread
- Performing proper handwashing
- Procedure for the two-minute hand wash for medical asepsis

CHAPTER REVIEW QUESTIONS

1. Briefly explain what the term *environment* means.
2. List the 10 environmental factors of concern to the members of the physical therapy team:

   a._____ f._____

   b._____ g._____

   c._____ h._____

   d._____ i._____

   e._____ j._____

3. A range of between ___ degrees and ___ degrees F. is generally mantained in most air-conditioned health care facilities.
4. _____ is defined as the amount of moisture in the air.
5. _____ refers to the movement of air.
6. _____ is a negative environmental factor that can affect one's health.
7. Whose responsibility is it to provide a safe environment?
8. List at least three types of patients who are more at risk of having an accident than others:

   a._____

   b._____

   c._____

9. List at least three ways the physical therapy aide can assist in preventing fires in the office:

   a._____

   b._____

   c._____

10. The practice of good _____ _____ and using good _____ _____ to perform one's work is part of providing a safe environment.
11. _____ is defined as the proper relationship of the body segments to one another.
12. _____ is one of the simplest methods for preventing the spread of diseases and germs.
13. _____ _____ includes the techniques and skills used to render any medical setting free of disease-causing microorganisms.
14. List the five environmental conditions necessary for a microorganism to live and grow:

    a._____ d._____

    b._____ e._____

    c._____

15. To be effective, how long should a medical handwash take?

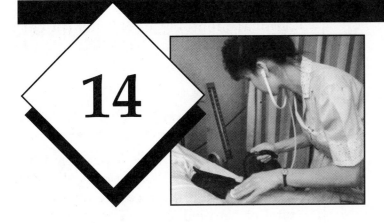

14

Understanding Vital Signs

Objectives

After studying this chapter, you will be able to:

1. Describe the role of the physical therapy aide in understanding and obtaining a patient's vital signs.

2. Describe the purpose of temperature, pulse, respiration, and blood pressure, and the role each plays in the proper function of the body.

3. Describe the variations of temperature, pulse, respiration, and blood pressure.

4. Describe how to obtain a proper reading of the temperature, pulse, respiration, and blood pressure.

VOCABULARY

Learn the meaning and the correct spelling of the following words and abbreviations:

Vital signs
Cardinal signs
Blood pressure
Systole
Diastole
Hypertension
Hypotension
Stethoscope
Pulse
Apical pulse
Respiration
External respiration
Internal respiration
Temperature
Axillary temperature
Rectal temperature
Oral temperature
Sphygmomanometer
Circulation
Radial pulse

As a member of the physical therapy team, you will be most concerned with assisting the physical therapist and the physician in carrying out the treatment for patients in need of therapeutic exercises and care related to the dysfunction of their bodies. There may be times, however, when such regimen may include performing skills which, although they appear unrelated to physical therapy, are just as important, and, in some cases, may contribute to the overall care of the patient and may be helpful to the physician in diagnosing and meeting the patient's needs. Measuring, obtaining, and recording the patient's vital signs are skills that all clinical members of the health care delivery team may be called upon to complete.

◆ VITAL SIGNS

One of the best tools a physician has in evaluating a patient's physical condition is through the measurement of the vital or cardinal signs. They are important signs of one's state of health, and, they include temperature, pulse, respiration, and blood pressure. All are considered measurable, concrete indicators essential for life, and any deviation from what is considered the norm for each individual sign may provide the physician with a clear-cut symptom indicating that one of the body systems may not be functioning properly. It's important to note here that while measuring and recording a patient's vital signs is generally not the responsibility of the physical therapy aide, having a clear understanding of what they represent is important to all health care providers.

◆ BLOOD PRESSURE

When we speak of blood pressure, which is perhaps the body's most significant vital sign, we are defining the amount of force exerted by the heart against its arterial walls as it contracts and relaxes. Two readings, systolic and diastolic, are used to indicate the greatest and least amount of pressure exerted. *Systolic* pressure is created as the force of blood is pushed against the artery walls when the ventricles of the heart are in a state of contraction. It is the upper number in a recorded blood pressure and is measured in millimeters of mercury (mmHg). *Diastolic* pressure occurs when the ventricles of the heart are in a state of relaxation. It is the lower number in the recorded blood pressure and is also measured in millimeters of mercury (mmHg).

Blood Pressure Variations

Blood pressure, like the other vital signs, may vary according to a number of factors, including age, sex, exercise, emotional state, drugs, increased weight or obesity, smoking, heart and renal diseases, and any condition of the blood vessels seen in old age. Additionally, blood pressure is usually higher when standing than when lying down and there is an increase of 3 to 4 mmHg higher in the right arm than in the left.

Normal blood pressure ranges anywhere from 110 to 140 systolic and 70 to 90 diastolic, or 110/70 to 140/90, with the average being 120/80 mmHg for a healthy adult. Because blood pressure increases with age, children usually run lower and older adults generally run higher.

Abnormal Blood Pressure Readings

As we have already stated, many factors can influence blood pressure. In certain instances, these factors become so out of sync with the body's cardiovascular system that the blood pressure either drops or increases to a point where the patient's life may be in danger.

The majority of abnormal blood pressure readings are divided into two major categories. Factors that cause the blood pressure to go below 110/70 mmHg result in a condition known as *hypotension*, while those factors that cause the blood pressure to rise above 140/90 mmHg are said to result in the disorder known as *hypertension*.

Although hypotension is more difficult to detect because there are very few symptoms except for general fatigue associated with this condition, hypertension may be characterized by headaches; irritability; blurred vision; epistaxis, or nosebleed; nausea and vomiting; and vertigo, or dizziness.

Instruments Used for Measuring Blood Pressure

Two instruments are used to measure blood pressure. The first, called a *stethoscope*, consists of earpieces, tubing, and a diaphragm, or bell. It is used to listen to beats of the heart as they are heard through the walls of the artery (see Figure 14-1A).

The second instrument used in the measurement of the blood pressure is the *sphygmomanometer*. It consists of four parts: a manometer, cuff, inflation bulb, and pressure control valve. The manometer is a gauge used to do the actual measurement of the blood pres-

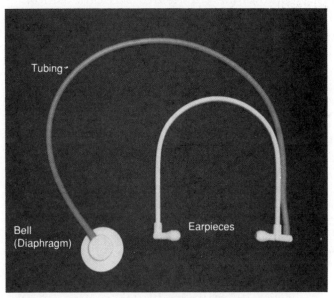

Figure 14-1 (A) The stethoscope. (From Hegner and Caldwell, *Nursing Assistant: A Nursing Process Approach*, 6th edition, copyright 1992 by Delmar Publishers Inc.) *(Continued)*

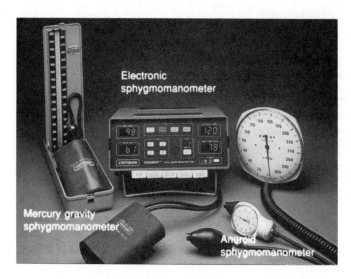

Figure 14-1 (B) Types of sphygmomanometers. (From Hegner and Caldwell, *Nursing Assistant: A Nursing Process Approach,* 6th edition, copyright 1992 by Delmar Publishers Inc.)

sure. There are two types most widely accepted (see Figure 14-1B). The first, called a *mercury manometer,* uses a column of mercury to measure the blood pressure. It is most accurate and reliable because it does not have to be recalibrated and can only be used when the column of mercury is in a vertical position.

The *aneroid manometer* may also be used for measuring blood pressure. It is a portable manometer that uses compressed air in order to measure the blood pressure. It differs from the mercury type in that it requires periodic calibrations.

The cuff of the sphygmomanometer is made of an inflatable rubber bag, covered with a nonstretch material. It is wrapped around the patient's arm and secured with Velcro or clasps. Cuffs come in three sizes: pediatric, for children and thin patients; adult, for normal-sized adults; and large, or obese, cuffs for adults with large arms or for use on a thigh.

The final two parts of the sphygmomanometer are the inflation bulb, which is used to pump air into a cuff through a rubber tube, and the pressure control valve, which is a thumbscrew valve located on the inflation bulb that is used to allow air to escape as it is opened and closed.

♦ MEASURING THE PULSE

Pulse is defined as the beat of the heart as felt through the walls of the arteries. It is the pulsation of the arteries produced by the wave of blood forced through them by the contractions of the heart.

A pulse is measured and recorded according to its individual characteristics. This includes the *rate,* that is, the number of pulsations or beats counted in a given minute; the *rhythm,* defined as the time intervals between each pulse and usually described as regular, irregular, or skipping; and *volume,* or the strength of pulsations, described as full, strong, bounding, weak, or thready. A normal pulse is said to be regular and strong.

Pulse Sites

Since the pulse is the beat of the heart as felt through the walls of the arteries, it stands to reason that a pulse must be taken at a particular location or site — that is, at an artery.

The location of choice for taking a pulse on an average healthy person is at the radial artery, which is located over the inner aspect of the wrist on the thumb side. This site is easily accessible and, therefore, is the most commonly used.

In addition to taking the pulse at the radial artery, pulse measurements may be taken at the brachial artery, located

Procedure #7: Measuring Blood Pressure:

1. Gather the necessary equipment, including the sphygmomanometer, stethoscope, 70 percent isopropyl alcohol, cotton balls or alcohol wipe pads, and the patient's chart.
2. Wash your hands.
3. Clean the earpieces and diaphragm, or bell, of the stethoscope with the alcohol (see Figure 14-2A).
4. Position the patient in a sitting position with the arm supported; make sure the patient is relaxed.
5. Expose the patient's arm by rolling up the sleeve approximately five inches above the elbow or remove the sleeve from the arm if necessary.
6. Place the deflated cuff evenly and snugly around the patient's arm with the lower edge approximately one to two inches above the antecubital space (inside the elbow). Center the cuff over the brachial artery before securing it with clasps or Velcro. If using a mercury manometer, place it on a level surface; if using an aneroid manometer, adjust it so the scale can be easily read.
7. Locate the brachial pulse in the antecubital space by palpating it with your fingertips.
8. Place the earpieces of the stethoscope in your ears, (Figure 14-2B), and place the diaphragm or bell gently, but firmly, over the brachial artery, making sure that the diaphragm or bell is not touching the cuff (Figure 14-2C).
9. With the other hand, close the air valve on the bulb by gently turning the thumbscrew in a clockwise direction; pump the air into the cuff until the level of the mercury is 10 to 20 mmHg above the palpated systolic pressure or about 180 mmHg.
10. Turn the thumbscrew counter-clockwise to release the air at a slow rate so that the pressure falls approximately two to three mmHg per second.
11. Listen carefully for the first tapping sound; this represents the systolic pressure. Note this number on the scale of the aneroid manometer or the exact line on the mercury manometer (Figure 14-2D).
12. Continue to deflate the cuff while listening to the sounds. Read the scale again when the sound becomes dull or muffled; this represents the diastolic pressure.
13. Continue to deflate the cuff at the same speed until you no longer hear the sound.
14. Open the valve completely and rapidly deflate the cuff.
15. Remove the cuff from the patient's arm.
16. Record the results on the patient's chart, noting which arm was used in the appropriate manner.
17. Wash your hands.

over the inner aspect at the bend of the elbow, or at the antecubital space; the temporal artery, located at the side of the forehead at the temple; the carotid artery, located at the right and left sides of the anterior neck and usually reserved for palpitation during cardiopulmonary resuscitation (CPR); the

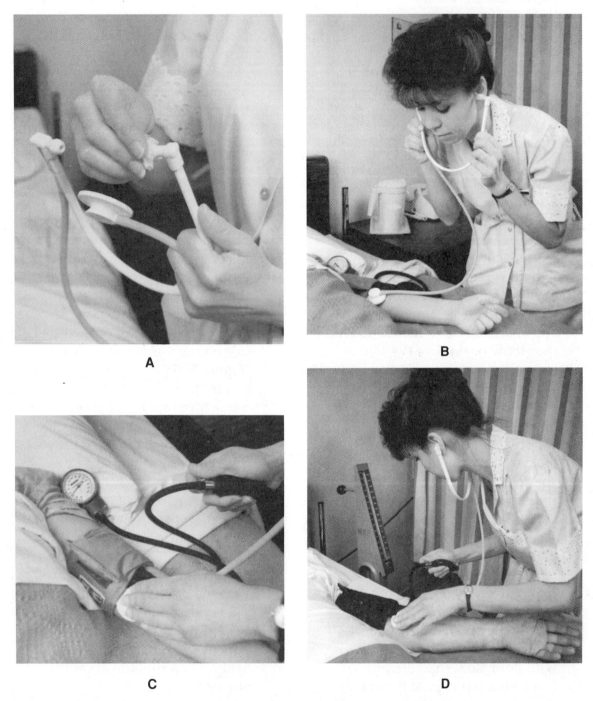

A

B

C

D

Figure 14-2 Measuring the blood pressure: (A) Carefully clean earpieces of the stethoscope before use; (B) Place earpieces of the stethoscope comfortably in your ears; (C) Place stethoscope diaphragm or bell right over the brachial artery; (D) Release the cuff and listen to the first and change sounds; Read the gauge at eye level. (From Hegner and Caldwell, *Nursing Assistant: A Nursing Process Approach*, 6th edition, copyright 1992 by Delmar Publishers Inc.)

femoral artery, located at the anterior lower side of the hip bone in the groin region; the popliteal artery, located at the back of the knee; the dorsalis pedis artery, located on the upper surface of the foot between the ankle and the toes; and the apical site, located between the fifth and sixth ribs and approximately two to three inches to the left of the sternum (see Figure 14-3).

When taking an apical pulse, a stethoscope must be used over the heart to measure the beats being produced (see Figure 14-4).

Pulse Rates and Variations

Pulse rates may vary and are influenced by many factors. These include the patient's age, sex, body size, emotional state, metabolism, whether or not she is involved in exercise, or is taking drugs, is ill, or is feeling pain.

For a normal, healthy adult, the average pulse ranges from 60 to 90 beats per minute, with 80 considered the norm.

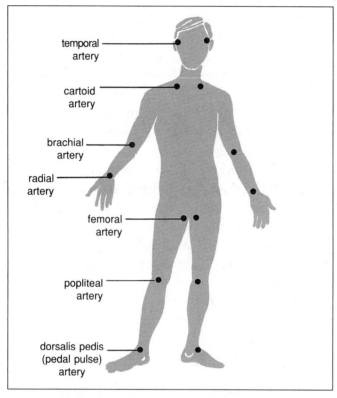

Figure 14-3 Pulse sites. (From Hegner and Caldwell, *Nursing Assistant: A Nursing Process Approach,* 6th edition, copyright 1992 by Delmar Publishers Inc.)

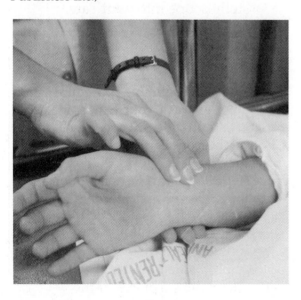

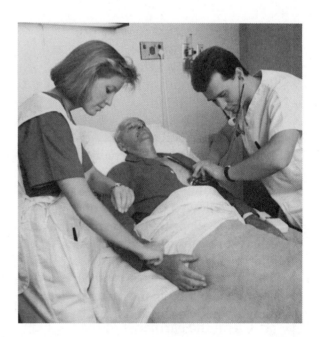

A   B

Figure 14-4 (A) Measuring the radial pulse; (B) Auscultation of an apical pulse. (From Hegner and Caldwell, *Nursing Assistant: A Nursing Process Approach,* 6th edition, copyright 1992 by Delmar Publishers Inc.)

◆◆◆

Procedure #8: Obtaining a Radial Pulse Rate

1. Gather the necessary equipment, including a watch with a sweep second hand, and the patient's chart.
2. Wash your hands.
3. Identify the patient, explain the procedure, and evaluate his medical condition, making sure you do not take the reading immediately after the patient has become emotionally upset or after exertion, unless so ordered by the physician.
4. Position the patient in a sitting or lying position with the arm supported.
5. Hold the patient's wrist and place your first three fingers on his wristbone over the radial artery. Apply light pressure so you can feel the pulsations. *Never* use your thumb to palpate the pulse since it has its own pulse.
6. Count the pulse for 60 seconds.
7. Note the rate, rhythm, and volume of the pulse.
8. Record the pulse rate, rhythm, and volume and note the pulse site used in the appropriate manner.
9. Wash your hands.

◆◆◆

◆◆◆

Procedure #9: Obtaining an Apical Pulse

1. Gather the necessary equipment, including a stethoscope, watch with a sweep second hand, patient's chart, and an antiseptic wipe.
2. Wash your hands.
3. Identify the patient, explain the procedure, and evaluate her medical condition; do not take the reading immediately after the patient has become emotional stressed or after any physical exertion, unless so ordered by the physician.
4. Position the patient in a lying or sitting position.
5. Clean the earpieces of the stethoscope with an antiseptic.
6. Warm the diaphragm of the stethoscope with your hands to provide for the patient's comfort.
7. Place the earpieces of the stethoscope into your ears.
8. Place the diaphragm of the stethoscope over the apex of the heart, located in the fifth intercostal space two to three inches to the left of the sternum (breastbone).
9. Listen for the heartbeat and count the number of beats per minute.
10. Note the rhythm and volume.
11. Record the apical pulse rate, rhythm, and volume, and indicate the site used in the appropriate manner.
12. Clean the earpieces of the stethoscope.
13. Wash your hands.

◆◆◆

Children over seven years of age range from 80 to 90 beats per minute, while children from the age of one to seven, generally range from 80 to 120 beats per minute. Infants and newborns have the highest degree of pulsations, with a newborn ranging from 130 to 160 beats per minute and small infants ranging from 110 to 130 beats per minute.

♦ MEASURING THE RESPIRATIONS

The term respiration refers to the act of breathing in oxygen and breathing out, or expiring, carbon dioxide. As with the other vitals signs, any significant variation in the rate or rhythm of the patient's respirations becomes a clear indication that the body may not be functioning properly.

The process of respiration takes place in the respiratory control center located in the medulla oblongata, or the lower portion of the brain stem. It is an act that occurs both automatically and through voluntary control. That is why an individual may hold his breath, but eventually an involuntary breath must be taken in order to avoid fainting.

Two types of respiration occur at the same time. The first, called *external respiration,* takes place as the exchange of respiratory gases between the alveoli of the lungs and the blood occurs. *Internal respiration* occurs with the exchange of respiratory gases between the body cells and the blood.

Respiration is characterized according to its rate, depth, and rhythm. *Rate* refers to the number of respirations per minute and may be recorded as normal, rapid, or slow. *Depth* depends upon the amount of air being inhaled and exhaled and is recorded as shallow or deep. *Rhythm,* or the intervals of respiration, may be regular or irregular in rate and depth.

Respiration Rates and Variations

Respiratory rates may vary. They are also influenced by a number of factors:

Procedure #10: Obtaining a Respiration Rate

1. Gather the necessary equipment, including a watch with a sweep second hand and the patient's chart.
2. Wash your hands.
3. Identify the patient, explain the procedure, and evaluate the patient's medical condition. Do not take a respiration immediately after the patient has become emotionally upset or after any physical exertion unless otherwise ordered by the physician.
4. Position the patient sitting or lying down.
5. Place three finger on the patient's wrist as if you were taking the pulse.
6. Count each breathing cycle (inhalation and exhalation) as one breath by watching the rise and fall of the chest or upper abdomen.
7. Count for one full minute.
8. In the appropriate manner, record the rate, depth, and rhythm of the respiration as well as the patient's position.
9. Wash your hands.

the patient's emotional state, nervousness, increased muscular activity, the inducement of drugs into the bloodstream, and any diseases of the lungs or circulatory system. In addition to these factors, certain climatic environments may also influence the respiratory rate. High altitudes, for example, tend to affect the rate and depth of the respirations, as do fever, sleep, and any dysfunction or injuries to the brain tissue.

♦   TEMPERATURE

Temperature is defined as the degree of body heat that is a direct result of the balance maintained between heat produced and heat lost by the body.

Many factors affect or influence body temperature. The time of day in which it is taken, for example, may affect the reading on the thermometer. Lowest body temperatures are usually registered in early morning between the hours of 2:00 A.M. and 6:00 A.M. while the highest body temperature generally occurs in the evening hours, predominantly between the hours of 5:00 P.M. and 8:00 P.M.

The sex and age of the patient also have a great deal to do with temperature. Women tend to increase their temperature during ovulation and pregnancy, and infants and children usually register a higher temperature than do adults.

Emotional status, the degree of involvement in physical activities, and environmental changes are all factors tending to influence a patient's temperature. High temperatures usually occur during emotional excitement such as when one is sad or angry, as well as during involvement in strenuous exercise. Emotions, as well as physical activity, will cause muscular contractions to occur in the body. On the other hand, changes in the weather, such as in cold climates, tend to lower body temperature due to the dilation of the blood vessels.

Methods of Measuring Temperature

Three acceptable methods exist for measuring body temperature. These include the most common method taking the temperature orally by placing the thermometer under the tongue; rectally, by placing the thermometer in the rectum (considered the most accurate method), and axillary, by placing the thermometer under the axilla, or armpit (the least accurate of the three). For children, the method of choice is rectal, and for children or adults who have difficulty holding an oral thermometer in place, the axillary method is considered most desirable.

Taking an Oral Temperature

As we have already stated, the most common method of taking a person's temperature is orally, or by mouth. Here the thermometer is held under the tongue and is kept in place for approximately three minutes. Normal readings for an oral temperature range from 97 degrees to 99 degrees Fahrenheit with the average being 98.6 degrees Fahrenheit, or 37.5 degrees Centigrade (see Figure 14-5A-B). When taking a patient's temperature by mouth, it is best to use an oral "security" thermometer. While all glass thermometers are calibrated in Fahrenheit or Centigrade

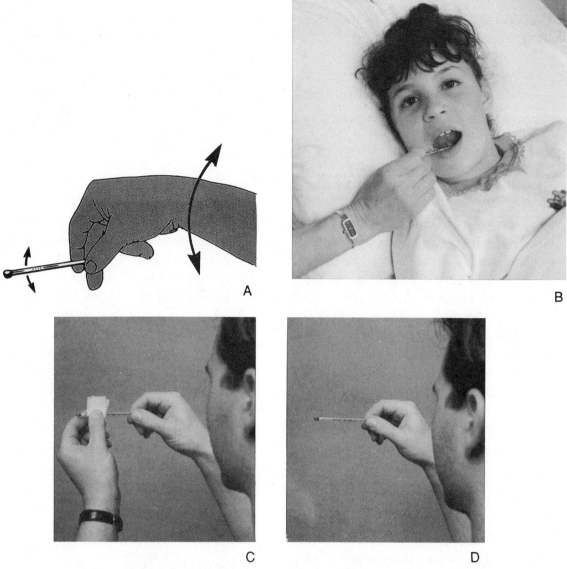

Figure 14-5 Taking an oral temperature: (A) Shake mercury down in the column by holding the thermometer by the stem and snapping the wrist; check the reading and repeat until reading is below 96 degrees Fahrenheit; (B) The bulb end of the thermometer is inserted under the tongue; (C) Wipe thermometer after removing it from patient's mouth; always wipe from stem to bulb; (D) Hold thermometer at eye level; locate the column of mercury and read to the closest line. (From Hegner and Caldwell, *Nursing Assistant: A Nursing Process Approach,* 6th edition, copyright 1992 by Delmar Publishers Inc.)

degrees and consist of two parts — the bulb and the stem — the oral security thermometer has a long, slender bulb and therefore should never be inserted into the rectum. Stubby thermometers have a stubby round bulb that looks very much like a cross between an oral and rectal thermometer and therefore can be used to take either an oral or a rectal temperature.

Procedure #11: Taking an Oral Temperature

1. Wash your hands and gather the necessary equipment. Your thermometer will either be a glass thermometer, a sheath-covered thermometer, a plastic thermometer, or an electronic thermometer. You will also need some tissues, a watch with a second hand, and a pad and pencil.
2. If the thermometer is glass or plastic, remove the thermometer from its container and wipe it with a clean tissue. Check to be sure the thermometer is intact.
3. Read the mercury column. It should register below 96 degrees Fahrenheit. If necessary, shake the thermometer down by standing away from any objects, grasping the stem of the thermometer tightly, and shaking with a downward motion, Figure 14-5A. If used in your facility, place the thermometer in a disposable plastic cover sheath.
4. Insert the bulb end under the patient's tongue, toward the side of the mouth, Figure 14-5B. Tell the patient to hold the thermometer gently with lips closed for three minutes.
5. Remove the thermometer, holding it by the stem. Wipe it from the stem end toward the bulb end, and discard the tissue, Figure 14-5 C.
6. Hold the thermometer at eye level. Locate the column of mercury and read to the closest line, Figure 14-5D. Record your findings on a pad of paper.
7. Wash the thermometer in cold water and soap before returning it to its proper place.
8. Wash your hands.

Taking a Rectal Temperature

The taking of a rectal temperature is usually considered the method of choice for all infants and small children as well as for adults and older children who have difficulty holding an oral thermometer in place. In this method, a rectal thermometer is used. It differs from the oral type in that it has a rounded short bulb that is better held by the rectal muscles. Both the security and stubby thermometers may also be used to take a rectal temperature. Whenever a rectal temperature is taken it is important to remember to leave the thermometer in place for approximately five minutes.

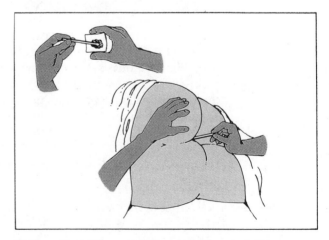

Figure 14-6 The rectal thermometer is lubricated and then inserted 1 and 1/2 inches into the rectum. (From Hegner and Caldwell, *Nursing Assistant: A Nursing Process Approach*, 6th edition, copyright 1992 by Delmar Publishers Inc.)

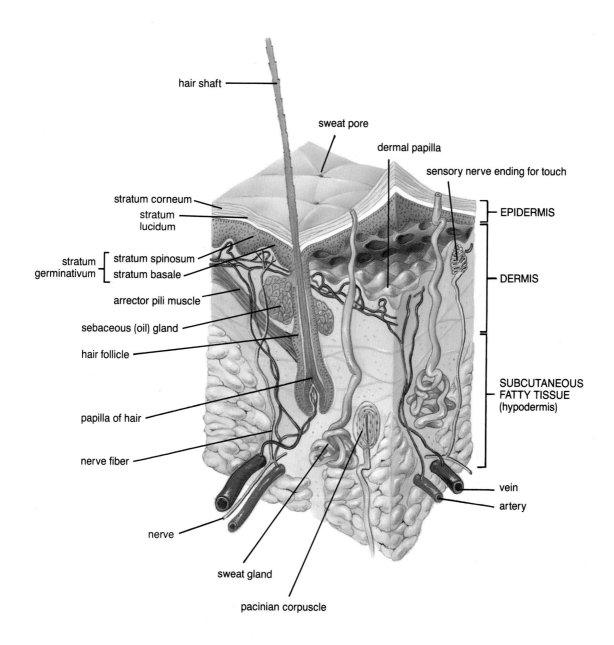

hair shaft

sweat pore

dermal papilla

sensory nerve ending for touch

EPIDERMIS

stratum corneum

stratum
lucidum

stratum
germinativum { stratum spinosum
stratum basale

DERMIS

arrector pili muscle

sebaceous (oil) gland

hair follicle

papilla of hair

SUBCUTANEOUS
FATTY TISSUE
(hypodermis)

nerve fiber

vein

artery

nerve

sweat gland

pacinian corpuscle

Plate 1 Cross Section of Skin

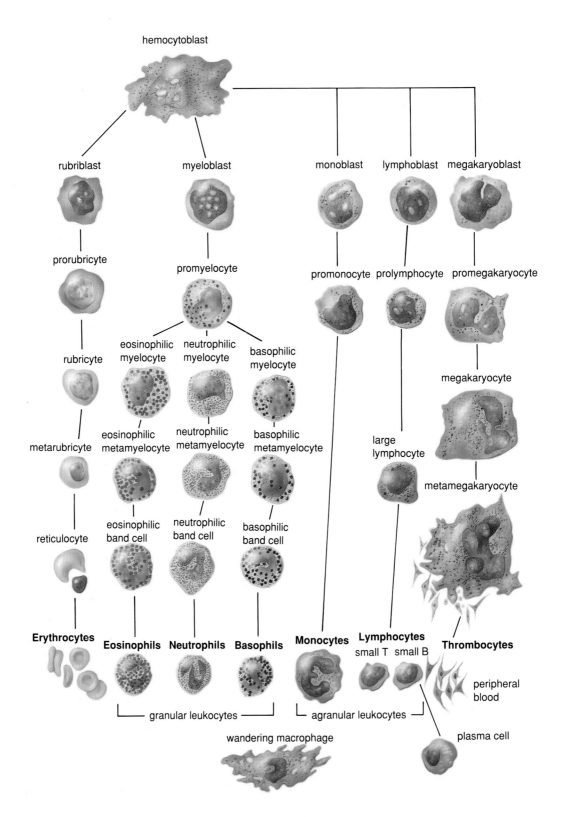

hemocytoblast

rubriblast myeloblast monoblast lymphoblast megakaryoblast

prorubricyte promyelocyte promonocyte prolymphocyte promegakaryocyte

eosinophilic neutrophilic basophilic
myelocyte myelocyte myelocyte

rubricyte

megakaryocyte

metarubricyte eosinophilic neutrophilic basophilic
metamyelocyte metamyelocyte metamyelocyte

large
lymphocyte metamegakaryocyte

reticulocyte eosinophilic neutrophilic basophilic
band cell band cell band cell

Erythrocytes **Eosinophils** **Neutrophils** **Basophils** **Monocytes** **Lymphocytes** **Thrombocytes**

small T small B

peripheral
blood

— granular leukocytes — — agranular leukocytes — plasma cell

wandering macrophage

Plate 2 Blood Cells and Platelets

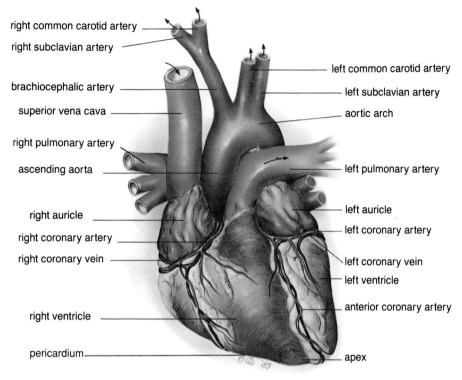

right common carotid artery

right subclavian artery

brachiocephalic artery

superior vena cava

right pulmonary artery

ascending aorta

right auricle

right coronary artery

right coronary vein

right ventricle

pericardium

left common carotid artery

left subclavian artery

aortic arch

left pulmonary artery

left auricle

left coronary artery

left coronary vein

left ventricle

anterior coronary artery

apex

Plate 3 Front View of Heart

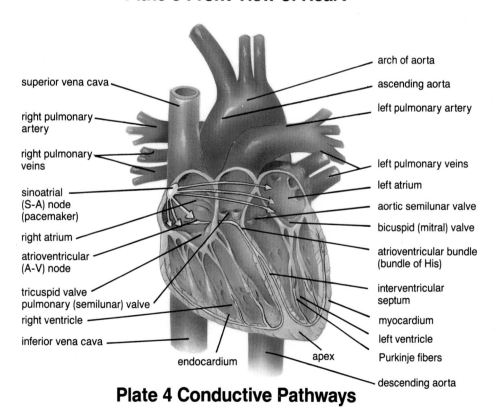

superior vena cava

right pulmonary artery

right pulmonary veins

sinoatrial (S-A) node (pacemaker)

right atrium

atrioventricular (A-V) node

tricuspid valve

pulmonary (semilunar) valve

right ventricle

inferior vena cava

endocardium

arch of aorta

ascending aorta

left pulmonary artery

left pulmonary veins

left atrium

aortic semilunar valve

bicuspid (mitral) valve

atrioventricular bundle (bundle of His)

interventricular septum

myocardium

left ventricle

Purkinje fibers

apex

descending aorta

Plate 4 Conductive Pathways

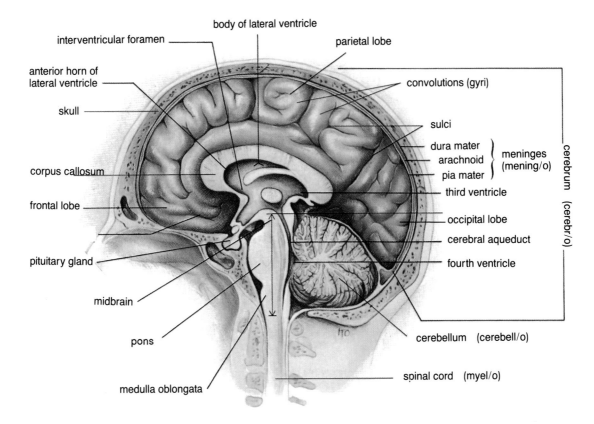

interventricular foramen

body of lateral ventricle

parietal lobe

anterior horn of lateral ventricle

convolutions (gyri)

skull

sulci

dura mater

arachnoid } meninges (mening/o)

pia mater

corpus callosum

third ventricle

frontal lobe

occipital lobe

cerebral aqueduct

pituitary gland

fourth ventricle

midbrain

pons

cerebellum (cerebell/o)

medulla oblongata

spinal cord (myel/o)

cerebrum (cerebr/o)

Plate 5A Section of Brain

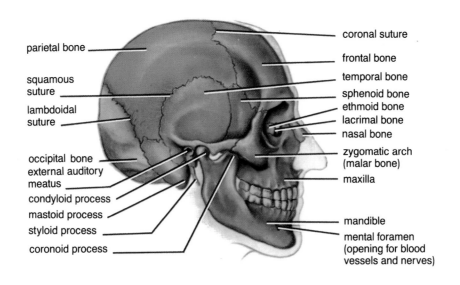

parietal bone

coronal suture

frontal bone

squamous suture

temporal bone

sphenoid bone

lambdoidal suture

ethmoid bone

lacrimal bone

nasal bone

occipital bone

external auditory meatus

zygomatic arch (malar bone)

condyloid process

maxilla

mastoid process

styloid process

mandible

coronoid process

mental foramen (opening for blood vessels and nerves)

Plate 5B Lateral View of Cranium

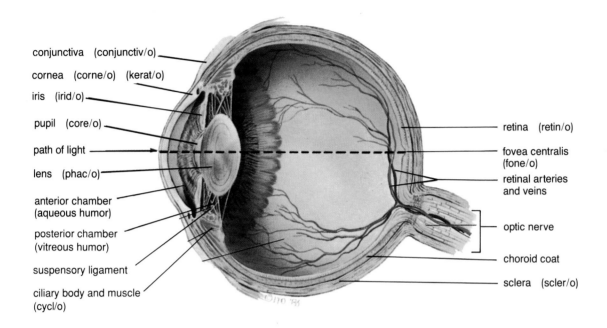

conjunctiva (conjunctiv/o)
cornea (corne/o) (kerat/o)
iris (irid/o)
pupil (core/o)
path of light
lens (phac/o)
anterior chamber (aqueous humor)
posterior chamber (vitreous humor)
suspensory ligament
ciliary body and muscle (cycl/o)

retina (retin/o)
fovea centralis (fone/o)
retinal arteries and veins
optic nerve
choroid coat
sclera (scler/o)

Plate 6A Eye Structure

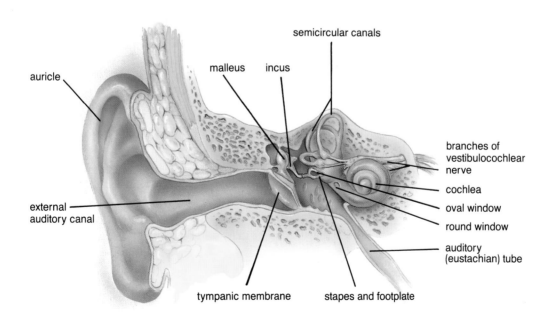

auricle
external auditory canal

malleus   incus
semicircular canals
branches of vestibulocochlear nerve
cochlea
oval window
round window
auditory (eustachian) tube

tympanic membrane   stapes and footplate

Plate 6B Ear Structure

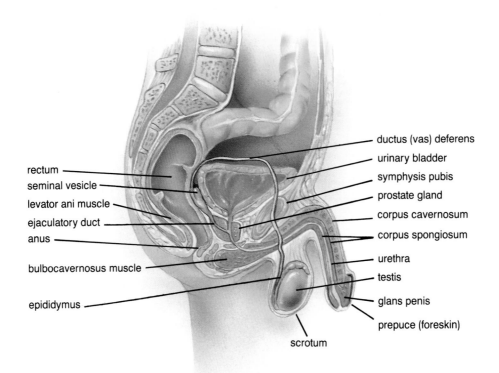

rectum
seminal vesicle
levator ani muscle
ejaculatory duct
anus
bulbocavernosus muscle
epididymus

ductus (vas) deferens
urinary bladder
symphysis pubis
prostate gland
corpus cavernosum
corpus spongiosum
urethra
testis
glans penis
prepuce (foreskin)

scrotum

Plate 7A Male Reproductive

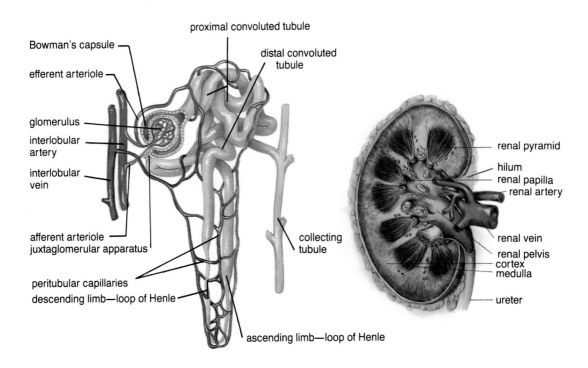

proximal convoluted tubule

Bowman's capsule

distal convoluted
tubule

efferent arteriole

glomerulus
interlobular
artery
interlobular
vein

renal pyramid
hilum
renal papilla
renal artery

afferent arteriole
juxtaglomerular apparatus

collecting
tubule

renal vein
renal pelvis
cortex
medulla

peritubular capillaries
descending limb—loop of Henle

ureter

ascending limb—loop of Henle

Plate 7B Nephron and Cross Section of Kidney

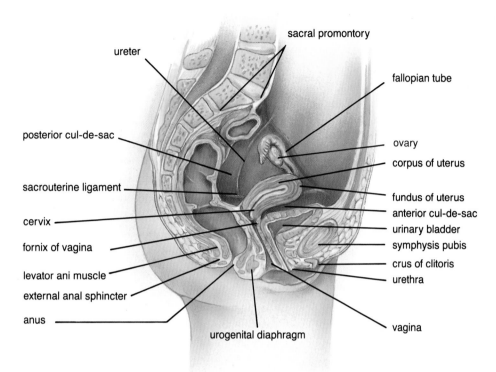

sacral promontory

ureter

fallopian tube

posterior cul-de-sac

ovary

corpus of uterus

sacrouterine ligament

fundus of uterus

anterior cul-de-sac

cervix

urinary bladder

fornix of vagina

symphysis pubis

levator ani muscle

crus of clitoris

external anal sphincter

urethra

anus

vagina

urogenital diaphragm

Plate 8A Female Reproductive

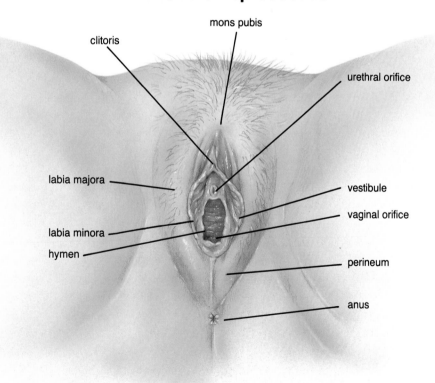

mons pubis

clitoris

urethral orifice

labia majora

vestibule

vaginal orifice

labia minora

hymen

perineum

anus

Plate 8B Female External Genitalia

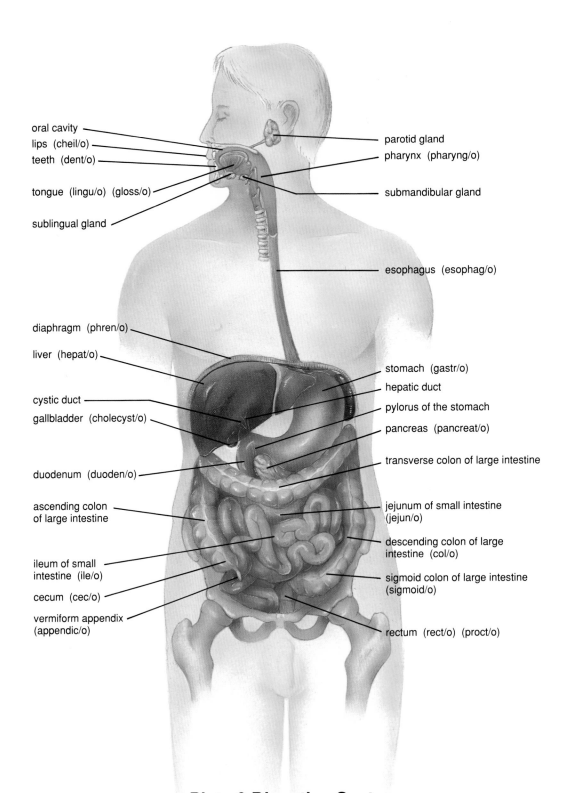

oral cavity

lips (cheil/o)

teeth (dent/o)

tongue (lingu/o) (gloss/o)

sublingual gland

parotid gland

pharynx (pharyng/o)

submandibular gland

esophagus (esophag/o)

diaphragm (phren/o)

liver (hepat/o)

cystic duct

gallbladder (cholecyst/o)

duodenum (duoden/o)

ascending colon
of large intestine

ileum of small
intestine (ile/o)

cecum (cec/o)

vermiform appendix
(appendic/o)

stomach (gastr/o)

hepatic duct

pylorus of the stomach

pancreas (pancreat/o)

transverse colon of large intestine

jejunum of small intestine
(jejun/o)

descending colon of large
intestine (col/o)

sigmoid colon of large intestine
(sigmoid/o)

rectum (rect/o) (proct/o)

Plate 9 Digestive System

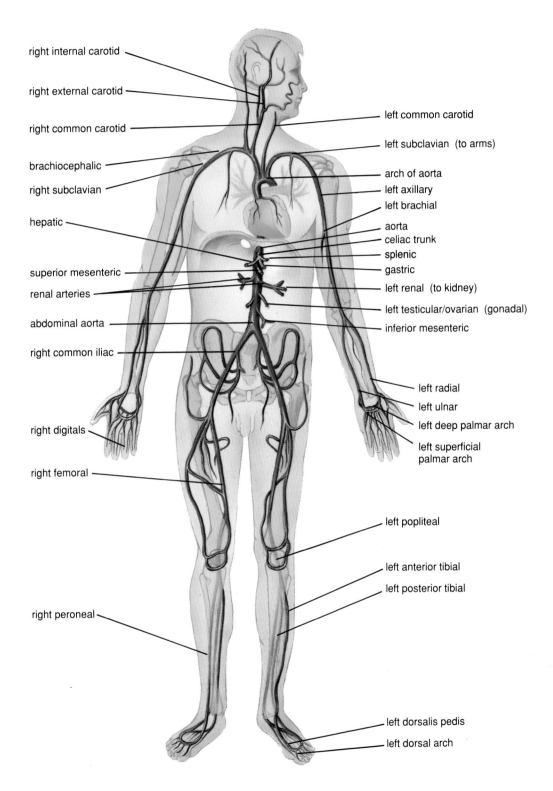

right internal carotid

right external carotid

right common carotid

brachiocephalic

right subclavian

hepatic

superior mesenteric

renal arteries

abdominal aorta

right common iliac

right digitals

right femoral

right peroneal

left common carotid

left subclavian (to arms)

arch of aorta

left axillary

left brachial

aorta

celiac trunk

splenic

gastric

left renal (to kidney)

left testicular/ovarian (gonadal)

inferior mesenteric

left radial

left ulnar

left deep palmar arch

left superficial
palmar arch

left popliteal

left anterior tibial

left posterior tibial

left dorsalis pedis

left dorsal arch

Plate 10A Arterial Distribution

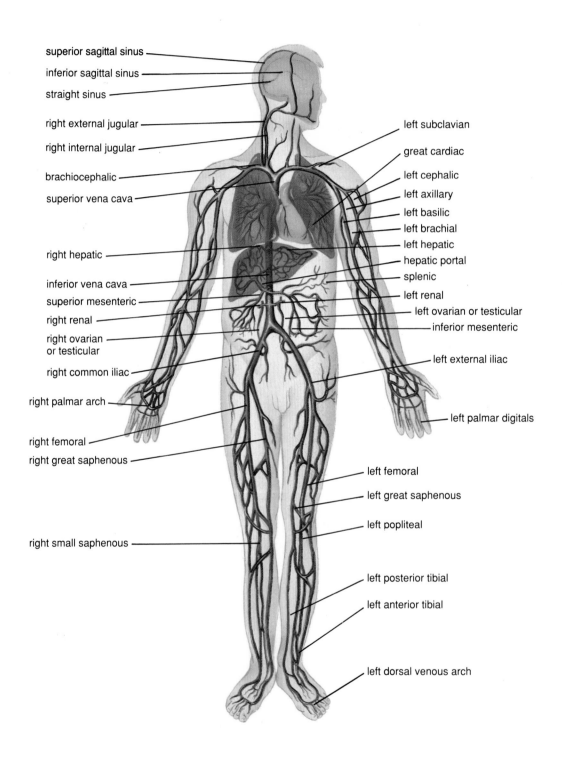

superior sagittal sinus

inferior sagittal sinus

straight sinus

right external jugular

right internal jugular

brachiocephalic

superior vena cava

right hepatic

inferior vena cava

superior mesenteric

right renal

right ovarian
or testicular

right common iliac

right palmar arch

right femoral

right great saphenous

right small saphenous

left subclavian

great cardiac

left cephalic

left axillary

left basilic

left brachial

left hepatic

hepatic portal

splenic

left renal

left ovarian or testicular

inferior mesenteric

left external iliac

left palmar digitals

left femoral

left great saphenous

left popliteal

left posterior tibial

left anterior tibial

left dorsal venous arch

Plate 10B Venous Distribution

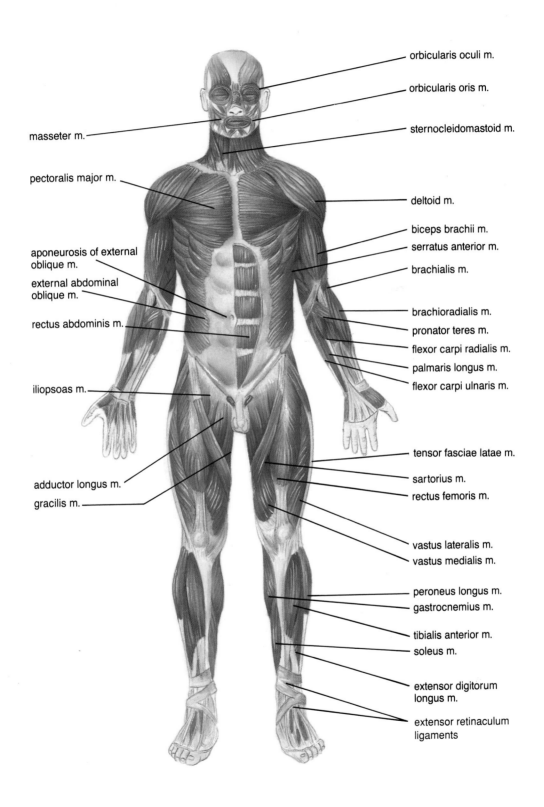

orbicularis oculi m.

orbicularis oris m.

sternocleidomastoid m.

masseter m.

pectoralis major m.

deltoid m.

biceps brachii m.

serratus anterior m.

aponeurosis of external oblique m.

brachialis m.

external abdominal oblique m.

brachioradialis m.

pronator teres m.

rectus abdominis m.

flexor carpi radialis m.

palmaris longus m.

flexor carpi ulnaris m.

iliopsoas m.

tensor fasciae latae m.

sartorius m.

rectus femoris m.

adductor longus m.

gracilis m.

vastus lateralis m.

vastus medialis m.

peroneus longus m.

gastrocnemius m.

tibialis anterior m.

soleus m.

extensor digitorum longus m.

extensor retinaculum ligaments

Plate 11A Muscular System, Anterior

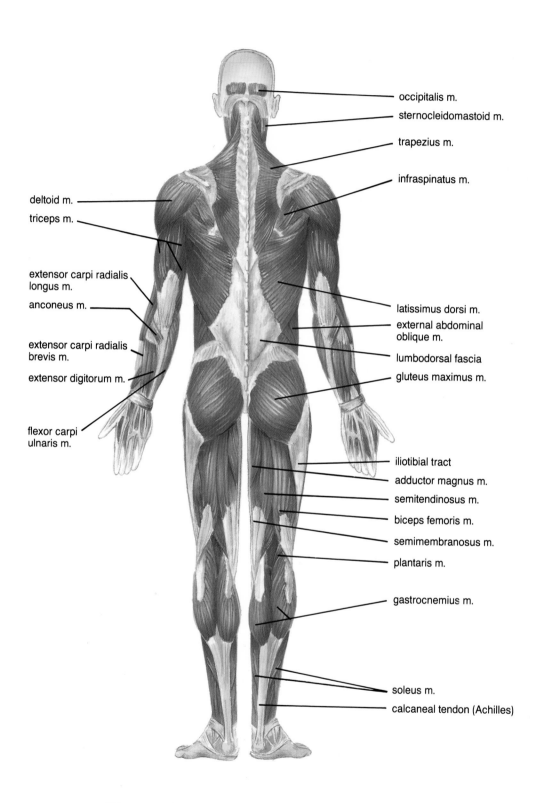

occipitalis m.

sternocleidomastoid m.

trapezius m.

infraspinatus m.

deltoid m.

triceps m.

extensor carpi radialis longus m.

anconeus m.

extensor carpi radialis brevis m.

extensor digitorum m.

flexor carpi ulnaris m.

latissimus dorsi m.

external abdominal oblique m.

lumbodorsal fascia

gluteus maximus m.

iliotibial tract

adductor magnus m.

semitendinosus m.

biceps femoris m.

semimembranosus m.

plantaris m.

gastrocnemius m.

soleus m.

calcaneal tendon (Achilles)

Plate 11B Muscular System, Posterior

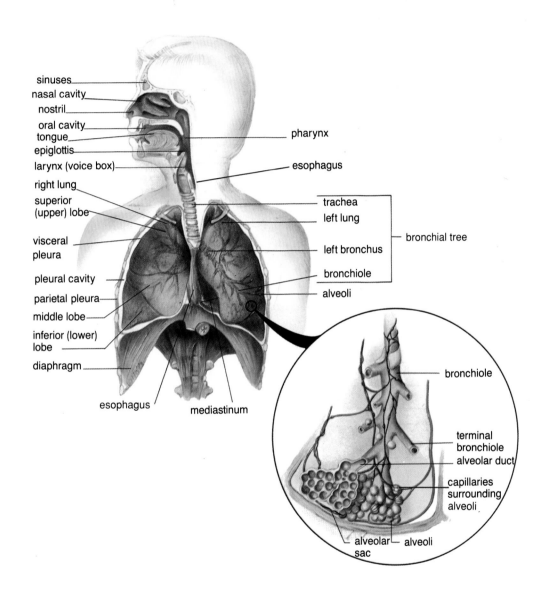

sinuses

nasal cavity

nostril

oral cavity

tongue

epiglottis

larynx (voice box)

right lung

superior
(upper) lobe

visceral
pleura

pleural cavity

parietal pleura

middle lobe

inferior (lower)
lobe

diaphragm

esophagus

mediastinum

pharynx

esophagus

trachea

left lung

left bronchus

bronchiole

alveoli

bronchial tree

bronchiole

terminal
bronchiole

alveolar duct

capillaries
surrounding
alveoli

alveolar
sac

alveoli

Plate 12 Respiratory System

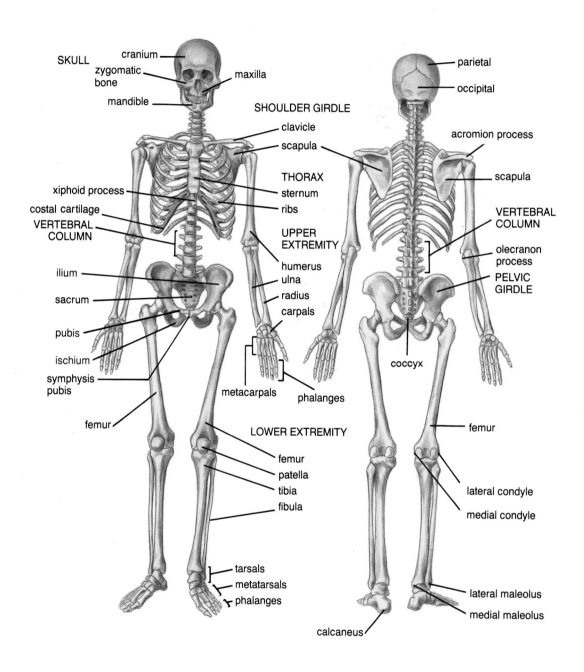

SKULL
cranium
zygomatic bone
maxilla
mandible

SHOULDER GIRDLE
clavicle
scapula

THORAX
sternum
ribs

xiphoid process
costal cartilage
VERTEBRAL COLUMN

UPPER EXTREMITY
humerus
ulna
radius
carpals

ilium
sacrum
pubis
ischium
symphysis pubis

femur

metacarpals
phalanges

LOWER EXTREMITY
femur
patella
tibia
fibula

tarsals
metatarsals
phalanges

parietal
occipital

acromion process
scapula

VERTEBRAL COLUMN
olecranon process
PELVIC GIRDLE

coccyx

femur

lateral condyle
medial condyle

lateral maleolus
medial maleolus

calcaneus

Plate 13 Skeletal System

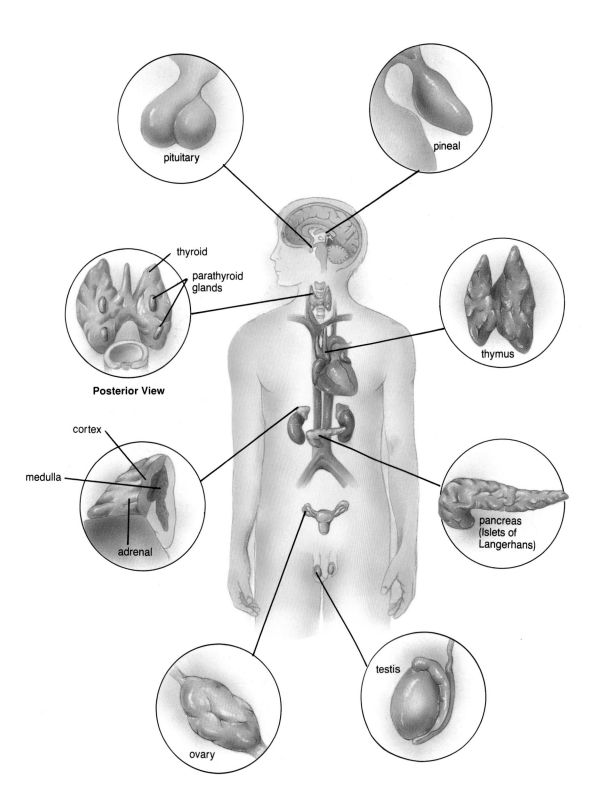

pituitary

pineal

thyroid

parathyroid glands

Posterior View

thymus

cortex

medulla

adrenal

pancreas (Islets of Langerhans)

ovary

testis

Plate 14 Endocrine System

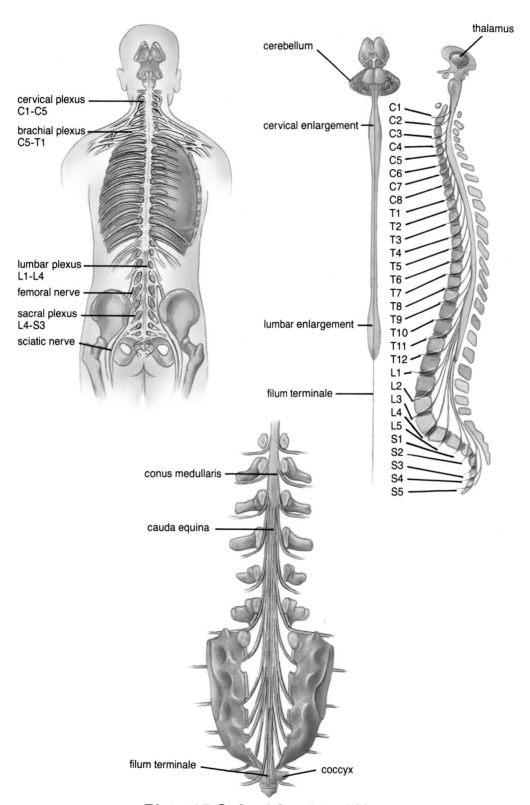

cerebellum

thalamus

cervical plexus
C1-C5

brachial plexus
C5-T1

cervical enlargement

lumbar plexus
L1-L4

femoral nerve

sacral plexus
L4-S3

sciatic nerve

lumbar enlargement

filum terminale

C1
C2
C3
C4
C5
C6
C7
C8
T1
T2
T3
T4
T5
T6
T7
T8
T9
T10
T11
T12
L1
L2
L3
L4
L5
S1
S2
S3
S4
S5

conus medullaris

cauda equina

filum terminale

coccyx

Plate 15 Spinal Cord and Nerves

Procedure #12: Taking a Rectal Temperature

1. Wash your hands and gather the necessary equipment. Your rectal thermometer will either be a glass thermometer or an electronic thermometer.
2. If it is a glass thermometer, remove the thermometer from its container and wipe it with a clean tissue. Check to be sure the thermometer is intact. Place a small amount of lubricant on a tissue.
3. Put on gloves and remove the thermometer from its container.
4. Read the mercury column. It should register below 96 degrees Fahrenheit. If necessary, shake it down by standing away from any objects, grasping the stem of the thermometer tightly, and shaking with a downward motion, Figure 14-5A. If used in your facility, place the thermometer in a disposable plastic cover sheath.
5. If using a glass thermometer, apply a small amount of lubricant to the bulb end. Separate the buttocks with one hand and insert the thermometer about one and one-half inches into the rectum, Figure 14-6.
6. Hold the thermometer in place for five minutes.
7. Remove the thermometer, holding it by the stem. Wipe it from the stem end toward the bulb end and discard the tissue. Wipe lubricant from the patient with a clean tissue.
8. Hold the thermometer at eye level. Locate the column of mercury and read to the closest line. Record your findings on a pad of paper.
9. Wash the thermometer in cold water and soap before returning it to its proper place.
10. Wash your hands.

Procedure #13: Taking an Axillary Temperature

1. Wash your hands and gather the necessary equipment. Your equipment will be the same as for taking an oral temperature.
2. Wipe the axillary area dry and place the thermometer.
   a. The patient's arm is kept close to his body if the axillary site is used, Figure 14-7.
   b. The thermometer r the fold against th groin site is used
3. Leave the thermo ten minutes.
4. Remove, wipe, thermometer. the pad.
5. Clean and re thermomet
6. Wash you

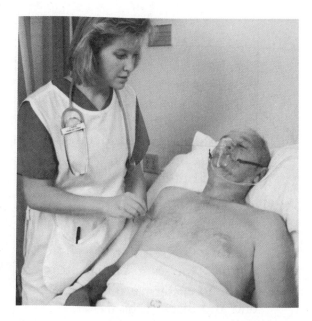

Figure 14-7 When the thermometer is placed in the axilla, it must be held in place for approximately five to seven minutes. (From Hegner and Caldwell, *Nursing Assistant: A Nursing Process Approach*, 6th edition, copyright 1992 by Delmar Publishers Inc.)

Taking an Axillary Temperature

The third and least accurate method of taking a temperature is taken by holding a security or stubby thermometer in place between the inside of the upper arm and the axilla, or armpit. This method is least desirable because of the length of time it takes to register a reading, that is, approximately five to seven minutes, and because its accuracy of can vary and therefore it is usually considered inaccurate.

Abnormal Body Temperatures

As already noted, the average body temperature ranges from 97 degrees Fahrenheit to 99 degrees Fahrenheit, with the average being 98.6 degrees Fahrenheit. While the temperature reading for a rectal temperature usually ranges 99.6 degrees Fahrenheit and 97.6 degrees Fahrenheit for an axillary temperature, any time the body's temperature increases above 99.6 degrees Fahrenheit there is a good indication that the patient may be suffering from some type of infection or other dysfunctional medical condition.

Fever is referred to as *pyrexia* and all fevers denote that the patient's oral temperature has risen above 98.6 degrees Fahrenheit, which is normal. A low fever is one that ranges from 99 degrees to 101 degrees Fahrenheit (37.2 to 38.3 degrees Centigrade). A moderate fever is defined as one ranging between 101 degrees to 103 degrees Fahrenheit (38.3 to 39.5 Centigrade). And a high fever is one ranging between 103 degrees to 105 degrees Fahrenheit (39.5 to 40.6 Centigrade).

A Final Note About Taking the Temperature

Since it is quite rare that the physical therapy aide would be required to measure and record a patient's temperature, it is recommended that you consult the procedure manual in the facility in which you work in order to determine how an oral, rectal, and axillary temperature should be taken.

◆ ◆ ◆

SUMMARY OUTLINE

Understanding the Purpose and Function of Vital Signs
- The physical therapy aide's role

Understanding Vital Signs
- Function of vital signs
- Blood pressure and blood pressure variations

- Measuring the pulse
- Measuring the respirations
- Temperature

CHAPTER REVIEW QUESTIONS

1. Vital signs are important indicators of one's _____ _____.

2. Vital signs include _____, _____, _____, and _____ _____.

3. The amount of force exerted by the heart against the arterial walls, is called _____ _____.

4. _____ pressure occurs when the heart is contracting, while _____ pressure occurs when the heart is relaxing.

5. _____ is defined as the balance between heat lost and heat produced in the body.

6. The process by which oxygen is taken into the body and carbon dioxide is expelled out of it, is called _____.

7. _____ is defined as the pressure of the blood pushing against the walls of an artery as the heart beats and rests.

8. Physical therapy aides should never use their _____ to feel for the patient's pulse.

9. Respiration is characterized according to its _____, and _____.

10. An abnormally low blood pressure is called_____, while an abnormally high blood pressure is called _____.

Observation, Reporting, and Charting

Objectives
After studying this chapter, you will be able to:

1. Describe the purpose of accurate observation, reporting, and charting.

2. Describe the purpose of a medical record.

3. Explain how accurate observation, reporting, and charting affect quality care, future care, reimbursement, staffing, and research.

4. Explain how charting is performed.

5. Differentiate between a medical record and a hospital chart.

6. Discuss how narrative charting is performed.

7. Discuss how problem-oriented record (POR) charting is performed.

8. List and explain the four parts to a "SOAP" format.

9. Discuss the guidelines involved in charting appropriate information.

10. Identify and explain the "ABCs" of charting.

11. Explain how to properly correct charting errors.

12. List the general guidelines for charting.

13. Discuss the role medical terminology plays in charting.

14. Define what a prefix is.

15. Define what a suffix is.

16. Define standard medical abbreviations and terms used by health care professionals.

◆ ◆ ◆

VOCABULARY

Learn the meaning and the correct spelling of the following words and abbreviations:

Observation
Reporting
Charting
Medical record
Quality care
Reimbursement
Hospital chart
Narrative charting
Problem-oriented record
POR
Data base
Problem list
SOAP
Medical terminology
Prefix
Suffix

Accurate, complete documentation in the medical record or patient chart is as important to the welfare of the patient as her care. It is a task completed by nurses and other health team members who provide patient care, and it is based upon the skills involved in careful observation and reporting of the patient's needs and treatment.

Federal and state laws require adequate documentation for an agency to maintain its institutional accreditation and license. Requirements of the medical record include thorough documentation of each patient's condition, what care was provided and why, the total plan of care, and the patient's response to the treatment. In some agencies, such as hospitals and even some physical therapy centers, payment for services can only be received if particular standards for documentation have been met by the agency.

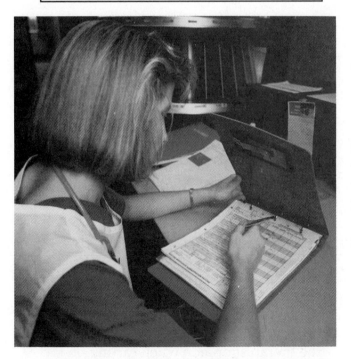

Figure 15-1 Records of patient progress and care are kept in each individual's chart. (From Hegner and Caldwell, *Nursing Assistant: A Nursing Process Approach,* 6th edition, copyright 1992 by Delmar Publishers Inc.)

◆ PURPOSE OF A MEDICAL RECORD

The medical record is a legal document that provides a written record of the patient's problem or condition, treatments, and teaching received, as well as the patient's reaction to that care. It also documents discharge planning, beginning when the patient is first seen in the facility, and terminating upon the patient's discharge from treatment (Figure 15-1).

The medical record also serves as a communication tool among members of the health care team. Nurses, physicians, physical therapists, and others each offer a special expertise. These professions each record their observations and actions in the patient's medical record. The patients benefit most from this because all members of the team communicate through this ongoing written record.

Quality Care, Future Care, Reimbursement, Staffing, and Research

Health care professionals have the responsibility of monitoring their practice for safe, complete, up-to-date care. Physical therapists, nurses, physicians, and others use the medical record to monitor quality.

The medical record is also used to provide a baseline against which other health problems experienced by the same patient may be evaluated. Therefore, what is recorded in the chart during a patient's present care can influence the care the patient receives in the future.

Proper documentation and the medical record is also looked at when payment is to be received by an agency. Insurance companies, Medicare, and Medicaid programs, for example, all require a written record for equipment used and services given before they pay the agency. Incomplete documentation may mean a loss of money for a hospital or other health care agency.

In some cases, patients pay for their care based upon the number of hours of care they require from a health care professional. This type of documentation is generally done on a planning sheet. Using data from patient records, administrators can justify staffing patterns and plan budgets for future care accordingly.

Another reason for keeping accurate documentation and medical records has to do with research. Medical record personnel and other health care professionals review records to determine trends in certain diseases. By doing so, the medical record also helps scientists work toward a cure for specific diseases.

♦ CHARTING

Charting is one of the most important activities performed by the health care provider after giving care to the patient. As we have already stated, it is the method used to document the observations health care providers make about the patient's condition, the care and treatment that was given, and the patient's response to the therapy. It provides a written history of the patient's illness and can be used as evidence of what occurred or what was done. When a therapist or aide makes certain observations about the patient or administers care or treatment but does not chart these, the legal implication is that they were not done or did not exist. Accurate and complete charting gives evidence of the quality of care rendered to the patient and is often the health care professional's best defense when something goes wrong.

When you are working in hospitals and health care facilities, you will be expected to use and understand medical terms or the technical language used in the healing arts. Medical terminology conveys precise information to others regarding the biological structures of the body and medical activities. It is used extensively for diagnosis, in treatment reports, in the physician's progress reports, and in reports of various examinations and procedures. Although medical terminology is generally not used by the therapist or aide when carting on the treatment notes, a number of standard abbreviations may be.

♦ REPORTING AND RECORDING PATIENT CARE

The Medical Record and Hospital Chart

The medical record of the patient's care while in the hospital or while coming to the health care facility, is called the hospital chart or medical record. If the patient is in the hospital, this chart consists of a collection of sheets or forms used to document and record information about the patient. If the patient is being seen in an out-patient physical therapy office or facility, the chart generally consists of only those sheets pertaining to the patient's history and physical therapy treatment (Figure 15-2).

Since a patient's chart contains much information of a private nature, the chart is handled in the same way as other confidential information. Only those people who are involved in the care of the patient are authorized to read the chart or have access to it (Figure 15-3). Although the patient, family members, relatives, friends, lawyers, insurance agents, and others may have an interest in reading or gaining copies of records in the chart, they must go through the legal channels of obtaining administrative approval of the hospital or facility before they can see chart information. The chart is the property of the facility, not of the patient or the physician.

Following the discharge of the patient, the hospital chart or medical record is sent to the Medical Record department for safekeeping. Even charts of patients who die must be kept and not destroyed. In some cases, the old chart from a previous admission is requested by the doctor when treating the patient again. And old charts may also be used by a hospital to provide needed information regarding insurance claims. Charts may also be obtained to

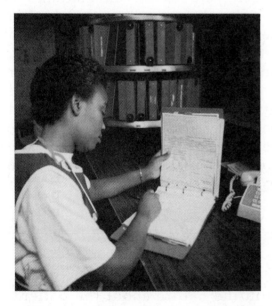

Figure 15-2 Record your observations and actions on the physical therapy progress sheet. (From Hegner and Caldwell, *Nursing Assistant: A Nursing Process Approach*, 6th edition, copyright 1992 by Delmar Publishers Inc.)

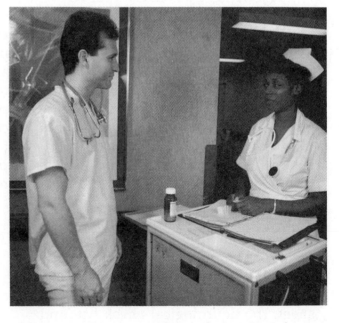

Figure 15-3 Report significant observations that can contribute to the ongoing care and evaluation. (From Hegner and Caldwell, *Nursing Assistant: A Nursing Process Approach*, 6th edition, copyright 1992 by Delmar Publishers Inc.)

be used in court cases as legal evidence of events in the patient's hospitalization or of treatment or care provided.

There are two basic approaches to charting by those giving care to patients. The first, which is the most traditionally used type, is called *narrative* charting, which focuses on the patient's disease. The second type, called *problem-oriented record*, or *POR* charting, is a newer method that focuses on the problems experienced by the patient as a result of being ill. Each health facility uses chart forms designed to meet the needs of that particular institution, and you must use your own institution's chart forms. Although the chart forms may differ in some specific details, most have a similar format and use either the traditional approach or the POR form of charting.

♦ TRADITIONAL NARRATIVE CHARTING

Narrative charting is most often used in hospitals. This is because the hospital care of patients has traditionally been divided into medical care and nursing care with each recorded in separate parts of the patient's chart. Doctors complete the history and physical examination forms, write orders for medical treatment on the order sheet, and record notes concerning the patient's progress on a special form. The nurses record vital signs on the graphic sheet and document their nursing care on the nurse's notes and the medication report. Intake and output forms, the diabetic record sheet, the neurological check list, and other special forms, are all used as required (Figure 15-4).

Although there are some variations in the forms used, the traditional hospital chart contains general forms in addition to whatever special forms may be required in the treatment. These usually include the physician's orders sheet, a graphic sheet, a medical administration record, nurse's notes, a history and physical form, physician's progress sheets, laboratory sheets, and admission forms. Special forms that might be found in the chart include a social history form, respiratory and physical therapy forms, consultation sheets, and surgical or treatment consent forms.

♦ PROBLEM-ORIENTED RECORD (POR) CHARTING

Since the late 1960s, a new system of recording has gained acceptance as a method of focusing on patient care, not medical or nursing care. This new method, called *problem-oriented record* charting, or *POR*, is generally used more frequently by small medical facilities or specialty clinics, such as the physical therapy center, since it provides a method of communicating *what, when,* and *how* things are to be done in order to meet the specific existing needs of the patient. The problem-oriented record contains four basic parts: the data base, the problem list, the plan, and the progress notes. The precise form these records take will vary greatly between agencies.

The Data Base

The data base contains information of a routine nature about the patient, including a general health history, the findings of the physical examination, and the results of physiological and laboratory tests. It also contains information about the patient's lifestyle, family

PATIENT PREFERS TO BE ADDRESSED AS:

Carl

FROM: ☐ E.R. ☐ E.C.F. ☒ HOME ☐ M.D.'S OFFICE

COMMUNICATES IN ENGLISH: ☒ WELL ☐ MINIMAL ☐ NOT AT ALL

☐ INTERPRETER (NAME PERSON) ☐ NONE

MODE OF TRANSPORTATION:

☒ AMBULATORY ☐ OTHER ____ SMOKER: Y ☐ N ☐

☐ WHEELCHAIR ____

☐ STRETCHER ____

☐ OTHER LANGUAGE (SPECIFY) Spanish

HOME TELEPHONE NO. (842) 7806

WORK TELEPHONE NO. (614) 7707

ORIENTATION TO ENVIRONMENT:

☒ ARMBAND CHECKED ☒ CALL LIGHT

☒ BED CONTROL ☒ PHONE

☒ TV CONTROL ☒ SIDE RAIL POLICY

☒ BATH ROOM ☒ VISITATION POLICY

☒ PERSONAL PROPERTY POLICY ☒ SMOKING POLICY

PERSONAL BELONGINGS: (CHECK AND DESCRIBE)

☐ CLOTHING pajamas. Bathrobe, slippers

☐ JEWELRY 1 plain yellow band

☐ MONEY $200

☐ WALKER ____

☐ WHEELCHAIR ____

☐ CANE ____

☐ OTHER ____

DENTURES:

☒ UPPER ☐ PARTIAL

☐ LOWER ☐ NONE

CONTACT LENSES:

☐ HARD ☐ LT ☐ RT

☐ SOFT

GLASSES: ☒ Y ☐ N HEARING AID: ☐ Y ☒ N

PROSTHESIS: ☐ Y ☒ N

(DESCRIBE) ____

DISPOSITION OF VALUABLES:

☐ PATIENT

☒ HOME GIVEN TO: R. Garcia

RELATIONSHIP: Wife

☐ PLACED

IN SAFE ____

(CLAIM NO.)

IN CASE OF EMERGENCY NOTIFY:

NAME: Rosa Garcia

RELATIONSHIP: Wife

HOME TELEPHONE NO. (842) 7806

WORK TELEPHONE NO. ( ) ____

VITAL SIGNS

TEMP: 98.4 ☒ ORAL ☐ RECTAL ☐ AXILLARY

PULSE: 76 ☒ RADIAL ☐ APICAL RESPIRATORY

RATE ____

B/P: 176/114 ☐ RT ☒ LT ☐ STANDING ☐ SITTING ☒ LYING

HEIGHT: 5' 10" WEIGHT: 210 lbs ☐ BEDSIDE

☒ STANDING

ALLERGIES:

MEDICATIONS: ☐ NONE KNOWN

☐ PENICILLIN ☐ TAPE

☐ SULFA ☐ OTHER (LIST)

☐ IODINE

☒ ASPIRIN

☐ MORPHINE

☐ DEMEROL

FOOD: ☐ NONE KNOWN

(SHELLFISH, EGGS, MILK, ETC.)

milk

MEDICATIONS: (PRESCRIPTIVE) (NON PRESCRIPTIVE)

	DOSE/FREQUENCY	LAST DOSE (DATE/TIME)
1.		
2.		
3.		
4.		
5.		
6.		

DISPOSITION OF MEDICATIONS:

☒ NONE BROUGHT TO HOSPITAL

☐ SENT HOME ____

WITH ____

☐ TO PHARMACY: (LIST)

ADMITTING DIAGNOSIS: Hypertension

NURSE'S SIGNATURE B. Rodriguez R.N. RN/LVN DATE 3/8/93 TIME 8³⁰/p

CHARTER SUBURBAN HOSPITAL
16453 SOUTH COLORADO AVENUE
PARAMOUNT, CALIFORNIA 90723
(213) 531-3110

NURSING ADMISSION ASSESSMENT PAGE 1 of 6

Figure 15-4 (A) The patient's history is recorded during the assessment process; (From Hegner and Caldwell, *Nursing Assistant: A Nursing Process Approach,* 6th edition, copyright 1992 by Delmar Publishers Inc.) *(Continued)*

PATIENT ASSESSMENT

PATIENTS STATED
REASON FOR ADMISSION: _uncontrolled hypertension._

PRESENTING SYMPTOMS: _headache, flushed face, elevated B/p._

DETOX ONLY

WHAT IS YOUR DRUG OF CHOICE? HOW MUCH HAVE YOU BEEN USING?
OVER WHAT PERIOD OF TIME, AND THE LAST TIME YOU USED? _____

HAVE YOU EVER HAD CONVULSIONS, HALLUCINATIONS OR MEMORY LAPSES? ☐ Y ☒ N
HAVE YOU EVER BEEN IN ANY HOSPITAL OR FACILITY FOR: CHEMICAL DEPENDENCE OR ANY OTHER REASON? ☐ Y ☒ N

PAST MEDICAL ILLNESSES:

☐ RESPIRATORY DISEASE (COPD)
☐ CARDIAC DISEASE (MI, ANGINA, CHF)
☐ DIABETES
☐ CVA (STROKE)
☐ CANCER

☒ HYPERTENSION
☐ OTHER (I.E. SURGERIES)
appendectomy   1977
hemorrhoidectomy 1981

DATE AND REASON FOR PREVIOUS HOSPITALIZATIONS:
acute appendicitis
External / internal hemorrhoids

NEUROLOGICAL:

LOC:
☒ ALERT
☐ LETHARGIC
☐ UNRESPONSIVE

☒ RESPONDS TO VERBAL STIMULI
☐ RESPONDS TO PAIN ONLY

ORIENTATION:
ORIENTED TO: ☒ SELF ☒ PERSON ☒ PLACE ☒ TIME
DISORIENTED TO: ☐ TIME ☐ PLACE ☐ PERSON ☐ SELF

MOTOR ABILITY: ☒ FULL R.O.M.   ☐ LIMITED R.O.M (DESCRIBE) _____

AMBULATION: ☐ NEEDS ASSISTANCE   ☒ INDEPENDENT   ☐ TOTAL BEDREST

COMMUNICATION ABILITIES:

SPEECH:
☒ ADEQUATE
☐ DEFICIENT
☐ UNABLE TO ASSESS
DESCRIBE DEFICIENCIES: _____

HEARING:
☒ ADEQUATE
☐ DEFICIENT
☐ UNABLE TO ASSESS
DESCRIBE DEFICIENCIES _____

VISION:
☒ ADEQUATE
☐ DEFICIENT
☐ UNABLE TO ASSESS
DESCRIBE DEFICIENCIES _____
Wears glasses

CARDIOVASCULAR/PULMONARY:

CHARACTERISTICS OF PERIPHERAL PULSES:

			LT	RT	
0 - ABSENT	4 - BOUNDING	CAROTID	✓	✓	☐ PERMANENT PACEMAKER
① PRESENT	⑤ STRONG	FEMORAL	✓	✓	NECKVIEN DISTENTION:
2 - WEAK	6 - REGULAR	RADIAL	✓	✓	☒ Y ☐ N
3 - THREADY	7 - IRREGULAR	PEDAL	✓	✓	☐ EDEMA ☐ NONE ☐ PITTING + ___

CHARACTERISTICS OF RESPIRATIONS:

☒ REGULAR   ☐ SHALLOW   ☐ ORTHOPNEA   ☐ DYSPNEA / S.O.B. ON EXERTION   ☐ KUSSMAUL
☐ IRREGULAR   ☐ DEEP   ☐ DYSPNEA / S.O.B.   ☐ CHEYNE-STOKES

BREATH SOUNDS: ☒ AUDIBLE BILATERALLY

☐ CRACKLES (LOCATION)   ☐ RHONCHI (LOCATION)   ☐ WHEEZE (LOCATION)   ☐ DIMINISHED (DESCRIBE)

COUGH: ☐ Y ☒ N   ☐ NON PRODUCTIVE   CONSISTENCY: _____
                   ☐ PRODUCTIVE   COLOR: _____

Figure 15-4 (B) The nurse records the patient's history;   (From Hegner and Caldwell, *Nursing Assistant: A Nursing Process Approach,* 6th edition, copyright 1992 by Delmar Publishers Inc.) *(Continued)*

INTEGUMENTARY:

COLOR: ☐ PALE ☑ FLUSHED ☐ CYANOTIC ☐ NORMAL ☐ OTHER _____

TEMP: ☑ WARM ☐ HOT ☐ COOL ☐ DRY/FLAKY ☐ DIAPHORETIC ☐ OTHER _____

INTEGRITY: ☑ INTACT

☐ **WOUNDS/INCISIONS** (LOCATION/DESCRIBE)
_____
_____

☐ **AMPUTATION** (DESCRIBE)
_____
_____

☑ **SCARS** (LOCATION/DESCRIBE)
Rt. inguinal
_____

☐ **RASH** (LOCATION/DESCRIBE)
_____
_____

☐ **ECCHYMOSIS** (LOCATION/DESCRIBE)
_____
_____

☐ **LACERATIONS** (LOCATION/DESCRIBE)
_____
_____

☐ **CONTRACTURE** (DESCRIBE)
_____
_____

☐ **Other** (GFT, AV Shunt, IV Access) (LOCATION/DESCRIBE)
_____
_____

☐ **PRESSURE AREAS**
_____
_____
_____
_____
_____
_____
_____

LABEL FIGURE

W= WOUNDS   L= LACERATIONS
P= PRESSURE AREA   R= RASH
E= ECCHYMOSIS   S= SCARS

LEGEND: STAGES OF PRESSURE AREA

STAGE I: Reddened Area not Relieved by Local Circulatory Stimulation

STAGE II: Superficial Skin Break

STAGE III: Loss of Deep Skin, Drainage Present

STAGE IV: Full Thickness Loss of Skin, Invasion to Deeper Tissues, Necrosis Present

GASTROINTESTINAL:

ABDOMEN: ☑ SOFT ☐ HARD ☐ DISTENDED ☐ TENDER   BOWEL SOUNDS: ☑ PRESENT ☐ ABSENT ☐ HYPERACTIVE ☐ HYPOACTIVE

NUTRITION: SPECIAL DIET ☑ Y ☐ N IF YES, SPECIFY _Low salt_

PREFERENCES/DISLIKES _Dislikes Lamb_   NEEDS ASSISTANCE WITH FEEDING: ☐ Y ☑ N

SPECIAL PROBLEMS (NO TEETH, LETHARGIC, DYSPHARGIA, NG TUBE, ETC.) _____

GYN REPRODUCTION: ☐ N/A DATE OF LMP _____

PROBLEMS (DESCRIBE) _____

BREAST/SELF-EXAM ☐ Y ☐ N

ELIMINATION: ☐ N/A

STOOL: ☑ VOLUNTARY ☐ INVOLUNTARY ☐ CONSTIPATION ☐ DIARRHEA ☑ REGULAR   DATE OF LAST B/M _3/8_

URINE: ☑ VOIDING ☐ INCONTINENT ☐ DYSURIA ☐ NOCTURIA ☐ FOLEY CATHETER ☐ EXTERNAL CATHETER   INSERTED AT C.S.H: ☐ Y ☐ N

SPECIAL PROBLEMS _____

PSYCHOSOCIAL:

☐ APPROPRIATE   ☐ DEPRESSED   ☐ ANGRY   ☐ SAD   ☐ WITHDRAWN   ☐ DEFENSIVE

☐ HAPPY   ☐ ELATED   ☐ CONVERSANT   ☐ NON-CONVERSANT   ☐ COOPERATIVE   ☐ NON-COOPERATIVE

☐ APATHETIC   ☐ FLAT AFFECT   ☑ ANXIOUS   ☐ CALM   ☐ RESTLESS   ☐ COMBATIVE

PATIENT LIVES: ☐ ALONE ☑ WITH SPOUSE ☑ WITH CHILDREN ☐ NURSING HOME (NAME) _____

☐ OTHER

VOCATION/AVOCATION: OCCUPATION _Fireman_

HOBBIES _Woodworking_   INTERESTS _Supports + is active in Boy scouts_

Figure 15-4 (C) The nurse records the patient's previous medical problems; (From Hegner and Caldwell, *Nursing Assistant: A Nursing Process Approach,* 6th edition, copyright 1992 by Delmar Publishers Inc.) *(Continued)*

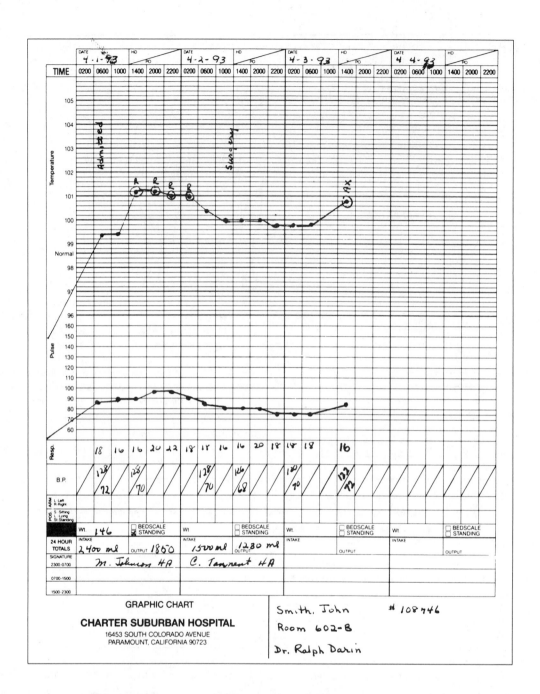

Figure 15-4 (D) The graphic chart is one example of a medical record chart form; (From Hegner and Caldwell, *Nursing Assistant: A Nursing Process Approach*, 6th edition, copyright 1992 by Delmar Publishers Inc.) *(Continued)*

Potterstown General Hospital
Fluid Intake and Output

Name Abrazzi, Cynthia #88-862-457   **Unit** 5-W **Rm** 118-B

Date	Time	Intake			Output			
		Method of Adm.	Solution	Amounts Rec'd.	Time	Urine Amount	Others	
							Kind	Amount
9/12	7 AM	P.O.	Water	6 z	7:15 AM	350 ml		
	8 AM	P.O.	Coffee Orange Juice	240 ml 120 ml				
	10:30 AM	P.O.	Sherbert	120 ml				
					11:30 AM	250 ml		
	12:30 PM	P.O.	Milk	240 ml				
	2	P.O.	Water	150 ml				
Totals	3T			1050 ml		600 ml		

Figure 15-4 (E) The intake/output chart is one example of a medical record chart form. (From Hegner and Caldwell, *Nursing Assistant: A Nursing Process Approach*, 6th edition, copyright 1992 by Delmar Publishers Inc.)

and social relations, and response to illness as determined by an assessment of the patient.

The Problem List

In the POR, a problem is some situation or aspect of the patient's health that interferes with physical or psychological comfort, the ability to function, or threatens survival. From the information provided by the data base, the patient's problems are identified and listed on a form that is usually the first documentation in the patient's chart. The list of problems is dynamic and new problems are added as they develop, while others become inactive as they are resolved. If POR is used in your agency, the problem list provides you with immediate information about the patient's needs for care.

Progress Notes: The SOAP Format

The POR progress notes are a section of the chart that contains the findings, assessment, plans, and orders of the doctors, nurses, and other therapists involved in the care of the patient. All chart on the same form and the progress notes are charted using the SOAP format show below (Figure 15-5):

S = Subjective information obtained from the patient

O = Objective information based on the health team's observations of the patient, the physical examination, or diagnostic and laboratory tests

A = Assessment, which refers to the analysis of the patient's problem

P = Plan of action to be taken to resolve the problem

Progress notes contain the date and the title of the problem with the information recorded in the SOAP format. It is not necessary to chart all problems each day or each time the patient comes into the office nor will it be possible to include each SOAP element in each note. After the initial plan, additional plans may be changed and revisions

made as a result of the evaluation of the previous action.

♦ CHARTING APPROPRIATE INFORMATION

Charting is a skill that takes time to master. As a student, you may feel overwhelmed by instructions to chart your observations of the patient and the care that you provided. You may find it difficult to think of something significant to write down if the patient is doing well, or you may be overwhelmed by so much information that you are afraid of omitting some action that might be important.

Your charting should provide a record of the patient's condition and activities or events that occurred; it is not a diary of the aide's activities. It should focus

---

NURSING NOTES

DATE **Dec. 31** NOTES

3 P.M.

PROBLEM: PAIN IN CHEST

S: "I HAVE A TERRIBLE PAIN IN MY CHEST. I'M GOING TO DIE."

O: GRASPS CHEST

A: IN PAIN, EXPRESSING FEAR OF DEATH

P: CHARGE NURSE NOTIFIED IMMEDIATELY
B. LESLIE, H.A.

3:05 P.M.

S: "HURRY UP, I'M GOING TO DIE"

O: LABORED BREATHING

A: MEDICATION NEEDED TO RELIEVE PAIN

P: NITROGLYCERINE 0.4 MG. SUBLING GIVEN

3:25 P.M.

E: MEDICATION RELIEVED CHEST PAIN AND BREATHING IS LESS LABORED.
P. RYDER, R.N.

Atlantic Hospital	Bruce, James 123456 146-B S. White, M.D. Patient Record

Figure 15-5 A sample charting using the SOAP approach. (From Hegner and Caldwell, *Nursing Assistant: A Nursing Process Approach*, 6th edition, copyright 1992 by Delmar Publishers Inc.)

on the patient and your notes should describe the patient's needs, problems, and activities in terms of the patient's behavior and treatment.

Behavior of the patient consists of two types of information. The first type, called *subjective* information, is in the form of statements made by the patient such as complaints of pain or other verbal reports of emotions or thoughts. *Objective* information, the second type of patient behavior, takes the form of the actual things that can be measured or observed by another person. This might include redness or swelling of a limb or the inability of a patient to feed himself. The POR form of charting emphasizes the behavioral approach in charting by including subjective and objective information in the SOAP format.

♦ THE ABCS OF CHARTING

Your charting should be characterized by the ABCs: be accurate, be brief, and be complete. When these guidelines are followed and are coupled with recording objective behavior observed by you and the subjective information supplied by the patient, the charting gives a meaningful description of the patient's condition.

Be accurate. Accuracy in charting requires that you be specific and definite in using words or phrases that convey the meaning you want to express. This means avoiding the use of such words as *appears* or *seems* in phrases. In charting behavior, the patient either is or is not doing something.

Be brief. Not every behavior of the patient or observation made by the therapist or yourself, is charted. To do so would result in such lengthy notes that no one would have time to read them to find out what was going on. Important information would be difficult to find in the mass of material. Charting must be concise, and that means that you must select the pertinent and more significant behavior and observations to record.

Be complete. The completeness of your charting should never be sacrificed to the principle of keeping it brief. Not only do you record information about the patient's needs and problems, but the care and treatment provided for those needs or problems must be included.

What constitutes complete charting may vary between facilities. Some may require only a monthly summary for patients in stable condition, while others may require continual documentation of the patient's condition.

♦ CORRECTING CHARTING ERRORS

At times, an error is made in charting. Since the chart is a legal document, the error should not be removed by erasing or painting it out with liquid correcting fluid. Instead, a line is drawn through the incorrect word or phrase with the word *error* written above it. The error is then initialed by the person who wrote it. Only errors in charting, such as a misspelled word, use of the wrong word, or an entry made on the wrong chart, are handled in this way by the person doing the charting. It is not to be used to delete a charting entry or phrase made by someone else that may differ from what you observed.

♦ GENERAL GUIDELINES FOR CHARTING

Charting is a relatively simple task and one that can be completed with ease if general guidelines are followed. The following information will assist you if your facility requires that you chart in the patient's medical record:

1. Charting should only be done by the person who made the observations or performed the task and is legally responsible for the accuracy and quality of the care.
2. Never chart or sign for someone else unless you are prepared to be responsible or vouch for the accuracy of the information.
3. Check with the hospital or health care facility to learn the color of ink used there for charting. Usually blue or black ink is specified because it can be microfilmed.
4. Print the proper headings on all new pages added to the chart and make sure the patient's name and other vital information is listed on each page of the chart.
5. All entries on the patient's chart should be printed or handwritten. After completing the account sign the chart with one initial and your last name and your title.
6. Never use ditto marks in your charting.
7. Record *after* completing each task for the patient and sign your name correctly after each entry.
8. Use the present tense. Never use the future tense, as in "patient to be ambulated."
9. It is not necessary to use the term "patient" on the chart, since the chart concerns the patient and all notations are about him.

10. Never leave blank lines in the charting. Draw a line through the center of an empty line or part of a line. This prevents charting by someone else in an area signed by you.
11. Always be exact in noting the *time, effect,* and *results* of all treatments and procedures.
12. Chart the time that the patient leaves the unit or facility for treatment.
13. Use standard abbreviations.
14. Spell correctly. If you are not sure about the spelling of a word, use the dictionary to look it up.
15. Never erase. Erasures provide reason for questioning if the chart is used in a court of law.

♦ MEDICAL TERMINOLOGY

Medical terms form a large part of the technical language used by members of the health care team. The main purpose of medical terms is to communicate ideas in such a way that everyone will understand exactly what is meant. Generally, words in our language have a number of different meanings, and their use can lead to their misunderstanding. The word "hand," for example, is easy to understand, since everyone knows what the speaker is referring to. Or do they? Is the speaker talking about someone's hand or appearance, or the hands on a watch? Medical terms have a specific meaning that is accepted by everyone in the field. Bronchitis, for example, means an inflammation of the bronchi, and the bronchi are the air passages of the lungs. In addition, it is more convenient to write "bronchitis" than "inflammation of the bronchi." The use of medical terminology also allows us to convey confidential information about the patient to other health

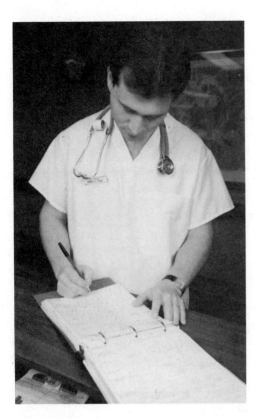

Figure 15-6 A knowledge of medical terminology will help make charting and record keeping easier. (From Hegner and Caldwell, *Nursing Assistant: A Nursing Process Approach,* 6th edition, copyright 1992 by Delmar Publishers Inc.)

care professionals and still protect the patient's privacy (Figure 15-6).

Many of the medical terms we use today are from Latin and Greek sources. Often they are composed by two or more words or word elements. The word elements are the *prefix,* the stem word, and the *suffix,* and when added to the word, they change the meaning.

Not all medical terms contain all three elements, as shown in Table 15-1.

To assist you in your study of medical terminology, a listing of stem words and suffixes is included here so that you can try combining them to form different words (Tables 15-2 and 15-3). Included among the suffixes are those used to name various types of surgical operative procedures.

♦ STANDARD MEDICAL ABBREVIATIONS

Many of the medical terms derived from Greek and Latin have been abbreviated for convenience. The specific meaning of such terms have been accepted universally as part of the *"Language of Medicine,"* and the abbreviations are used throughout the United Staes by those in the health care professions. In addition, many physicians, nurses, therapists, hospitals, and clinics use abbreviations that are specific to their location.

The standard abbreviations listed here are considered to be the most frequently used (Tables 15-4 and 15-5). It is important that you begin to learn and use them as soon as possible. Other groups of abbreviations have been included, but it may not be necessary for you to learn all of these at this time. They include abbreviations related to

---

Composition of Medical Terms

Word	Prefix	Stem	Suffix	Meaning
appendicitis		appendix	-itis	inflammation of appendix
diarrhea	dia-		-rrhea	flow through
arthroscopy	arthro-		-scopy	visualization into a joint

Table 15-1

Common Stem Words

Term	Meaning
append-	appendix; blind pouch
arterio-	artery; carrying blood away from the heart
arthro-	joint
cardio-	heart
cholecysto-	gallbladder
colo-	large intestine
cranio-	skull
encephalo-	brain
gastro-	stomach
laparo-	abdominal wall
leuko-	white
myelo-	spinal cord; bone marrow
thoraco-	chest or rib cage
tracheo-	windpipe

Table 15-2

Common Medical Suffixes

Term	Meaning
-ectomy	to remove a part
-emia	blood
-esthesia	without feeling
-gram	the record made
-graph	the machine
-graphy	process of
-itis	inflammation
-ology	the study of
-oma	tumor
-orrhaphy	surgical repair
-ostomy	to make an opening
-otomy	to cut into
-pexy	to anchor or fixate
-plasty	to repair; revision

Table 15-3

time, to body position or direction, to anatomical regions, to measurements, and to the general administration of medications.

Recording Time

In some medical facilities, time is recorded according to the 24-hour clock, a method commonly used in the military services. The hours are counted from 1 to 24 and the minutes from 1 to 59. Four digits are used; the first two numbers indicate the hour, and the third and fourth numbers indicate the minutes. For example, 8:00 A.M. is written as 0800 and 10:30 P.M. would be written as 2230. With the 24-hour clock, the 12 P.M. hours are added to any time after 12 noon.

Common Medical Abbreviations

Abbreviation	Meaning	Abbreviation	Meaning
abd	abdomen	(O)	orally
ADL	activities of daily living	O_2	oxygen
ad lib	as desired	OB	obstetrics
amb	ambulatory; ambulate; ambulation	OOB	out of bed
		OR	operating room
BM	bowel movement	P	pulse
BP; B/P	blood pressure	po	orally (per os); by mouth
C	celsius	per	through; by
$\bar{c}$	with	postop	after surgery
Ca	cancer; calcium	preop	before surgery
C/O	complains of	PRN	as necessary
DC; dc	discontinue	pt	patient
Dx	diagnosis	PT	physical therapy
ECG; EKG	electrocardiogram	R	respirations
EEG	electroencephalogram	Rx	prescriptions
ER	emergency room	RBC	red blood cells
F	Fahrenheit	RR	recovery room
Fx	fracture	$\bar{s}$	without
GI	gastrointestinal	sol	solution
H_2O	water	spec	specimen
I&O	intake and output	ss	one-half
ICU	intensive care unit	stat	immediately
inv	involuntary	T	temperature
K	potassium	UA	urinalysis
lab	laboratory	URI	upper respiratory infection
Na	sodium	wt	weight
noc	night	WBC	white blood cell
NPO	nothing by mouth		

Table 15-4

Abbreviations Related to Time

Abbreviation	Meaning
A.M.	before noon
BID	twice a day
H; h	hour
HS; hs	hour of sleep
MN	midnight
P.M.	afternoon
QD	every day
QOD	every other day
QH	every hour
Q2H	every two hours
Q3H	every three hours
Q4H	every four hours
Q6H	every six hours
Q8H	every eight hours
QID	four times a day
TID	three times a day

Table 15-5

Twenty-four-hour Clock Charting Compared to Regular Time Charting:

24-Hour Clock	Regular Time
0100	1 A.M.
0200	2 A.M.
0300	3 A.M.
0400	4 A.M.
0500	5 A.M.
0600	6 A.M.
0700	7 A.M.
0800	8 A.M.
0900	9 A.M.
1000	10 A.M.
1100	11 A.M.
1200	12 P.M.
1300	1 P.M.
1400	2 P.M.
1500	3 P.M.
1600	4 P.M.
1700	5 P.M.
1800	6 P.M.
1900	7 P.M.
2000	8 P.M.
2100	9 P.M.
2200	10 P.M.
2300	11 P.M.
2400	12 MIDNIGHT

Table 15-6

Terms Indicating Position or Direction

Term	Meaning
anterior	front of body or structure
posterior	back of body
superior	toward head
inferior	lower part; away from head
proximal	nearest head
distal	away from head
inguinal	lower abdomen, near groin
lumbar	the loin; middle of the back
ventral	front of body
dorsal	back of body or structure
lateral	toward the side
decubitus	lying down; bedsore
medial	toward the midline
peripheral	away from the head
sagital	dividing into right and left halves
transverse	dividing into upper and lower halves

Table 15-7

Quadrants of the Abdomen

Right upper quadrant	RUQ
Right lower quadrant	RLQ
Left upper quadrant	LUQ
Left lower quadrant	LLQ

Table 15-8

Anatomical Regions of the Abdomen

Right hypochondriac area
Epigastric area
Left hypochondriac area
Right lumbar region (in back and side)
Umbilical (naval) area
Left lumbar area (side and back)
Right iliac
Hypogastric area
Left iliac
Genitourinary area

Table 15-9

Abbreviations Related to Measurements

Abbreviation	Meaning
cc	cubic centimeter
cm	centimeter (0.39 inch)
℥	dram (abour 4 ml or 1 teaspoon)
gm; g	gram
gr	grain (15 gr=1 Gm)
gtt	drop
kg	kilogram (about 2.2 pounds)
L	liter (1000 ml; one quart)
meq; mEq	milliequivalents
mg	milligram
m	minim
oz; ℥	ounce (about 30 ml or 30 gr)
tsp	teaspoon (about 4 ml or 4 cc)
tbsp; T	tablespoon (about 15 ml or 1/2 oz)
U	unit (amount as stated or defined)

Table 15-10

Abbreviations Related to Medications

Abbreviation	Meaning
aa	of each
a.c.	before meals
amp	ampule; sealed glass flask
bucc	buccal; between cheek and gums
cap	capsule
comp	compound; two or more substances
dil	dilute
elix	elixir; solution containing alcohol
ext	extract
H (H)	hypodermic, under the skin
ID	intradermal, between layers of skin
IM	intramuscular, between muscle layers
IV	intravenous, within veins
OD	right eye
OS	left eye
OU	both eyes
p.c.	after meals
pp	postprandial, after eating
tab	tablet

Table 15-11

◆ ◆ ◆

SUMMARY OUTLINE

Purpose of Observation, Reporting, and Charting
- Accuracy
- Federal and state compliance

Purpose of a Medical Record
- Legal implications
- Communication

Quality Care, Future Care, Reimbursement, Staffing, and Research
- Safety
- Payment for services
- Staffing
- Research

Charting
- Purpose of charting
- Reporting and recording patient care
- The medical record and hospital chart
- Traditional narrative charting
- Problem-oriented record (POR) charting
- Using the SOAP format
- Charting appropriate information
- The ABCs of charting
- Correcting charting errors
- General guidelines for charting

Medical Terminology
- Purpose of using medical terminology
- Parts of a word
- Common terms and abbreviations used by health care professionals

CHAPTER REVIEW QUESTIONS

1. Briefly explain the purpose of a medical record.
2. The medical record serves as a _____ tool among members of the health care team.
3. List five reasons for keeping an accurate medical record:
   a._____ d._____
   b._____ e._____
   c._____
4. Briefly explain the difference between a medical record and a hospital chart.
5. A patient's medical record or chart is considered a _____ document.
6. Identify the two basic types of charting used by most medical facilities.
   a._____
   b._____
7. What does the abbreviation SOAP refer to?
8. What do the "ABCs" of charting refer to?
   a._____
   b._____
   c._____
9. Briefly explain how to correct a charting error.
10. What is the main purpose for using medical terms?
11. The _____ is located at the beginning of a word, and the _____ is located at the end of the word.
12. Match the following terms with their meaning:
    cardio   gallbladder
    gastro   white
    leuko   stomach
    arthro   heart
    cholecysto   joint
13. Match the following suffixes with their meaning:
    emia   tumor
    itis   to cut into
    oma   blood
    ectomy   to remove a part
    otomy   inflammation
14. Match the following abbreviations with their meaning:
    amb   nothing by mouth
    ADL   whenever necessary
    NPO   four times a day
    PRN   ambulate
    QID   activities of daily living

15. Match the following abbreviations with their meaning:

cc	milligram
gtt	centimeter
kg	drop
mg	cubic centimeter
cm	kilogram

16. Match the following regular times with 24-hour clock time:

11 P.M.	2400
8 A.M.	1900
1 P.M.	2300
12 midnight	0800
7 P.M.	1300

SECTION VI

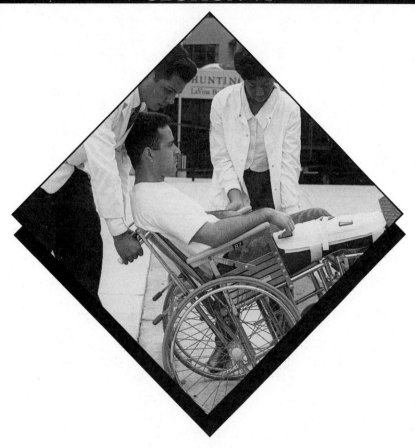

PATIENT CARE SKILLS

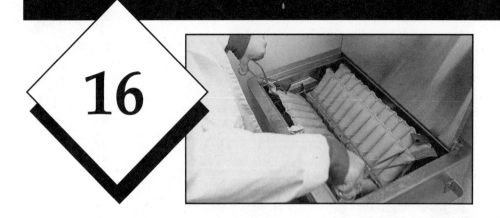

Preparation for Patient Care

Objectives
After studying this chapter, you will be able to:

1. List and explain the three fundamental components to providing care to patients undergoing physical therapy modalities.

2. Describe the role body mechanics play in physical therapy.

3. Explain the purpose of patient preparation and identify the physical therapy aide's role in preparing the patient for physical therapy treatments.

4. Describe patient preparation for transporting patients via a cart and a wheelchair.

VOCABULARY

Learn the meaning and the correct spelling of the following words and abbreviations:

Environment
Gurney
Cart
Body mechanics
Lifting
Squatting
Transferring
Verbal command
Transport
Wheelchair
Draping
Descending
Ascending

The most fundamental component in providing proper care to patients undergoing physical therapy modalities are the skills involved with managing the patient's environment, body mechanics, and communication. Safe and correct implementation of a treatment program can only be achieved when all the components of the procedure are given proper attention. Generally speaking, a few minutes taken at the start of a procedure to plan the steps involved and to prepare for the actual procedure increases the likelihood of a safe, efficient, and effective implementation.

◆ MANAGEMENT OF THE ENVIRONMENT

Managing and maintaining the organization of the work area provides the greatest protection of the patient and staff, and creates an environment for efficiency. Achieving these goals is the responsibility of all staff members. However, you should always remember that the person using the area or the equipment is the individual most responsible for making sure that all equipment is returned to its proper storage place in proper functioning condition and that the area is left clean and ready for the next patient.

All equipment should be periodically checked and inspected for wear and malfunction. It should also be inspected prior to patient use to ensure the patient's safety.

Whenever electrical equipment is used, always make sure to plug and unplug the electrical cord by holding the plug properly. Pulling on the cord generally weakens its attachment to the plug.

When large pieces of equipment, such as the diathermy machine, is used in the treatment of a patient, always remember to position the equipment and patient to allow easy accessibility. Should the patient need assistance quickly, improperly placed equipment may tend to hamper the ability to provide assistance quickly and efficently. The floor should also remain uncluttered in order to avoid any tripping by the patient or the staff.

Preparing the Area

Prior to initiating any patient care, transfer, or treatment, the bed or gurney and surrounding areas must be readied. Enough room should be provided for unimpeded movement. Staff and patients should be able to move around and maneuver within the area without bumping into or tripping over any equipment or other supplies.

Equipment and furniture not needed as part of the transfer or treatment, such as any diathermy machines or mobile foot stools, should be moved far enough out of the area to not present a danger to either the patient or yourself.

After the area has been properly arranged, you should prepare the specific equipment necessary for the treatment. This will avoid the possibility of leaving a patient alone or unguarded or interrupting the treatment once it has begun. Any supplies necessary in a treatment area, such as linens or pillows, should also be prepared before the patient arrives in the treatment area.

♦ BODY MECHANICS

The use of proper posture and body mechanics is necessary in order to limit stress and strain on the musculoskeletal structures. Whenever you are required to lift, push, or pull a patient, the stresses and strains upon the musculoskeletal system tend to increase. Proper posture and the use of body mechanics are based upon the alignment and functioning of the musculoskeletal system. They include the understanding of four very important principles, including (1) using larger and stronger muscles to perform heavy work; (2) maintaining the center of gravity of the body close to the center of the base of support; (3) keeping the combined center of gravity of the aide and patient centered within the base of support; and (4) having a base of support that is of the appropriate size and shape.

Lifting

All lifting should be initiated from a squatting position. The aide's feet are generally placed in a stride position, slightly apart, in order to widen the base of support in the anterior and posterior and lateral directions. The trunk must be erect so that the muscles have only to maintain the erect position and not have to work extra hard in order to extend the trunk during the lifting motion. Beginning from a squatting position allows you to reach the object or person to be lifted. Do not squat so deeply that the leg muscles are put at a disadvantage in regaining the upright position.

You should always be as close as possible to the object or person to be lifted since this allows the center of gravity to be maintained within the base of support. Bending the hips and knees in a squat allows the aide to get close enough to the object or person to permit lifting using the strong leg muscles. Always remember that when you carry patients or objects, keeping them close to the midline of your body, also helps to maintain the combined center of gravity within the base of support.

Transferring

The act of transferring a patient requires special movements that move the center of gravity away from the center of the base of support, possibly causing a loss of balance. By increasing the size of the base of support and setting your feet in stride and slightly apart, you are provided with a larger base of support. Your feet should also be free to move as the situation requires, allowing the base of support to be reestablished under the moving center of gravity. Crossing the legs during movement should be avoided since it tends to decrease the size of the base of support and may also lead to tripping.

Whenever possible, always use quick shuffling movements when required to move your feet.

Moving Large Pieces of Equipment or Furniture

If you are required to move a large piece of equipment or furniture or to guard a patient during ambulation, always remember to position yourself facing the direction of the movement in order to determine if the path is free from obstruction. In addition, being behind an object to be moved allows for more freedom in the lifting or pushing motion and uses larger muscles and body weight more efficiently.

If you are required to guard the patient during gait training, make sure you position yourself at an approximate 45 degree angle, slightly to the side and rear of the patient. If the patient happens to fall forward or backward, your position is close enough to the plane of the fall to support the patient before she falls directly to the floor. If the patient falls from side to side, your position will again allow proper support and break the fall. Again, the base of support must be wide enough to support shifts in the center of gravity if the patient should start to fall. Your feet should not be crossed during ambulation nor should they interfere with the patient's feet or ambulatory devices.

In all cases, movements should be properly planned and the area prepared for use prior to starting. Utilizing proper body mechanics and safety precautions will enhance the safety and effectiveness of the patient's treatment as well as assist you in providing that treatment.

◆ VERBAL COMMANDS

Patients must know what they are expected to do and when they are to do it during transfers and treatment. This understanding is paramount to the patient's effective participation in his treatment. Verbal commands on the part of the aide focus the patient's attention on specifically desired actions. Instructions to the patient should be simple and in language he can understand in order to avoid confusion. If the patient understands medical terminology, medical terms may be used. In most cases, however, lay language will be required. In some cases, the need for foreign language instructions may also be necessary.

Whenever you are asked to provide commands, you must make sure they are specific. Counting to "five" does not tell a patient to do anything specific. If the patient is to look up at the count of five, count to five and then say, "look up." "Look up" is a specific command; it tells the patient what to do without requiring him to translate the word "five" into the specific command "look up."

As a physical therapy aide, you should describe to the patient the general sequence of events that will occur. In addition, the patient should also be instructed in his expected responses. This helps the patient to learn the skill for future independent use and thereby to increase the safety of the immediate task performance. Therefore, always make sure you determine that the patient understands your instructions. Asking the patient "Do you understand the instructions?" does not always ensure understanding. Having the patient repeat the instructions in the proper order, provides an opportunity for mental rehearsal of the task in addition to indicating an appropriate level of understanding.

Always remember to speak clearly and vary your tone of voice as the situation requires. Sharp commands will generally receive quicker responses, while a soft command will elicit a slower response. Make sure that the patient can hear the commands. If she cannot hear or does not understand the spoken word, you may use gestures and demonstrations to convey the necessary meaning.

♦ PATIENT PREPARATION

For the most efficient use of treatment time, it is important that patient preparation be completed prior to transport and treatment. To do so, you should notify the nursing staff or your department's transport person of the preparation requirements well in advance of the scheduled treatment time. You must convey to the appropriate personnel that the patient should be properly dressed for transfer and treatment; this is necessary for the patient's right to modesty, for enhanced and beneficial treatment, and for safety.

All hospital gowns have been designed for ease in dressing and accessibility during nursing care. They may not provide the most effective draping during the movements required for transfers and treatment, but proper securing of the ties may assist in providing some additional coverage. A robe, housecoat, or two hospital gowns, one opening in the front and the other opening in the back, may also be used. If necessary, a sheet or towel may also be used for draping.

Patient preparation also involves dressing the patient in the appropriate attire such as slacks or shorts if the lower extremities must be observed or examined. If a female patient's upper trunk must be observed, a halter top is considered appropriate. Shoes and socks that offer support are also required if the patient is to ambulate or practice standing transfers. When a patient is dependent and working on a mat program only, slippers may be used as they are easier to take off and put on as necessary. In all cases, the decision about proper attire must be dictated according to the patient's needs, his ability to manipulate the clothing, and the requirements of the treatment.

Preparing the patient for her treatment also involves taking into consideration the variety of settings in which he or she may be receiving treatment. In some cases, either intravenous tubes, chest tubes, catheters, or combinations of any one of these could be present. Therefore, whenever you are required to position, transfer, or treat the patient, care must be taken not to disrupt the set-up of vital medical equipment.

During and after patient transport, transfers, or repositioning, attention should always be paid to appropriate draping. In some cases, even shorts or a halter top may limit observation. Draping by sheet may be necessary. The aim is to never expose any part of the body, except for the part that is receiving treatment. The purposes of draping are to protect a patient's modesty, provide warmth, and protect wounds, scars, and stumps. Edges should be tucked under the patient to avoid inadvertent exposure. When repositioning a patient, advance planning is required in order to maintain appropriate draping during the movement.

◆ TRANSPORTING

Transporting, or taking the patient from one area to another, is frequently necessary. A cart, gurney, or wheelchair may be necessary for safety or because of hospital regulations. The patient should be transferred in an appropriate manner with proper draping during the transfer and transport. Always remember to lock the brakes on the cart or wheelchair before beginning the transfer and to adjust the patient's clothing, draping, and medical accessories so that they will not become tangled in the wheels or drag on the floor during the transport. A mattress pad on the cart and a wheelchair cushion may also be used for the patient's comfort and protection. Additional pillows and padding can be used for comfort and protection as necessary.

Safety belts should also be used to secure the patient whenever it becomes necessary to transport or transfer him. There may be circumstances that require the use of restraints that the patient cannot release. If a cart has side rails, they should also be used. Arms and legs should be kept within the cart or wheelchair so that they do not get injured during the transport.

Procedure #14: Descending a Wheelchair From a Curb

1. Position the wheelchair so that the patient is facing away from the curb, Figure 16-1.
2. While facing the wheelchair, carefully step off the curb backwards.
3. Holding onto the handles of the wheelchair, slowly lower the rear wheels to the street by rolling them smoothly off the edge of the curb, Figure 16-2.
4. Continue to slowly roll the wheelchair backward without allowing the front wheels to fall until the front wheels are clear of the curb.
5. Slowly lower the front wheels until all four wheels are securely on the lower level, Figure 16-3.

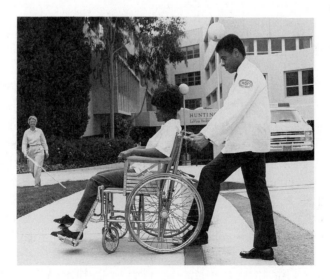

Figure 16-1 Starting position to descend curb backward.

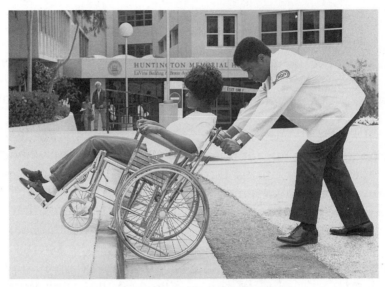

Figure 16-2 Rear wheels lowered to the street.

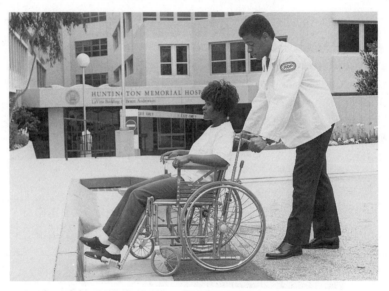

Figure 16-3 Completion of descending wheelchair from the curb in a backward manner.

Transporting Via a Cart

Carts or gurneys may be moved so that the patient is moving feet first, with the aide or therapist pushing from the head of the cart. The pace should be slow and steady; quick, jerky movements should be avoided so as not to upset a patient or make him nauseated. Always remember to maintain control of the cart at all times. This means turning corners cautiously and avoiding bumping into walls or other objects.

Transporting Via a Wheelchair

Using a wheelchair properly requires that the patient be seated well back on the seat and that the lower limbs be placed on the footrests or leg rests. Wheelchairs should also be pushed at a slow and steady pace, avoiding any quick or jerky movements. Control of the wheelchair, especially when turning corners, should always be maintained in the same manner as a cart or gurney.

Procedure #15: Alternate Method for Descending a Wheelchair from a Curb

1. Approach the curb forwards, Figure 16-4, then tilt the wheelchair backward so that the front wheels are about eight inches off the ground.

2. The wheelchair is then rolled slowly and smoothly off the curb onto the lower level, Figure 16-5 and 16-6.
3. The front wheels are then lowered to the ground.

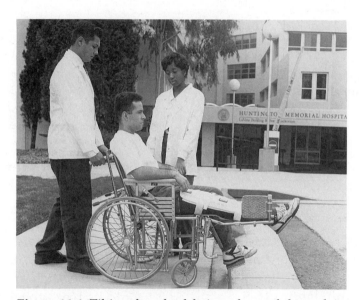

Figure 16-4 Tilting the wheelchair to descend the curb in a forward manner.

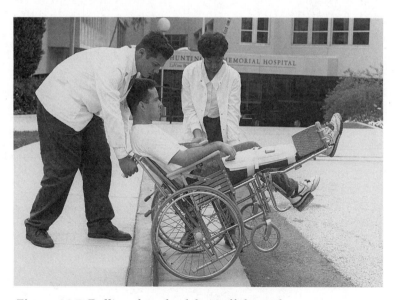

Figure 16-5 Rolling the wheelchair off the curb.

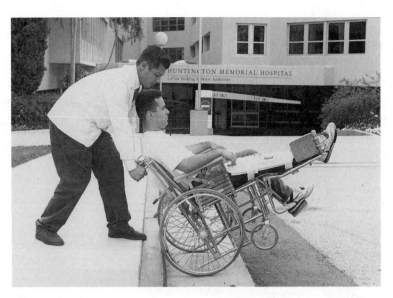

Figure 16-6 Completion of descending the curb in a forward manner.

Procedure #16: Ascending a Wheelchair up a Curb

1. Tilt the wheelchair backward onto the rear wheels, Figure 16-7.
2. Standing on the curb, carefully lift and roll the wheelchair backward up the curb, Figure 16-8.
3. When all four wheels are clearly over the curb, the front wheels can be lowered, Figure 16-9.

Procedure #17: Alternate Method for Ascending a Wheelchair Up a Curb

1. Approach the curb forwards.
2. While facing the curb, carefully tilt the wheelchair backward onto its rear wheels, so that the front wheels can clear the curb.
3. The wheelchair is then wheeled forward, placing the front wheels on the upper level as soon as they are clearly over the upper level.
4. Complete the procedure by continuing to wheel the wheelchair forward until the rear wheels contact the curb, and then lifting and rolling the rear wheels up and over the curb.

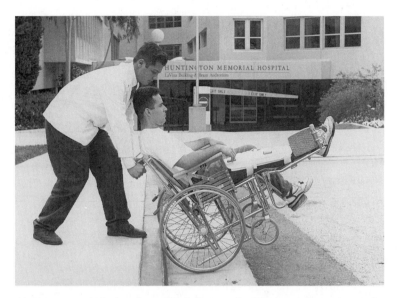

Figure 16-7 Tilting the wheelchair to begin ascending the curb in a backward manner.

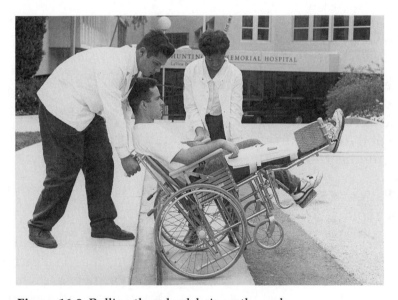

Figure 16-8 Rolling the wheelchair up the curb.

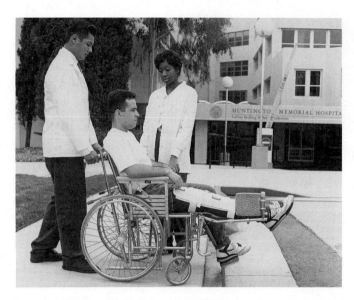

Figure 16-9 Completion of ascending the curb backward.

♦ ♦ ♦
SUMMARY OUTLINE

Purpose for Preparation of Patient Care Management of the Environment
- Managing the environment
- Maintenance of the environment
- Care of the equipment

Preparing the Patient Area
- Preparing the room
- Checking the equipment

Body Mechanics and Patient Preparation
- Lifting
- Transferring

- Moving large pieces of equipment or furniture

Verbal Commands
- Purpose of using verbal commands
- Providing patient instructions

Patient Preparation
- Notification of staff
- Dressing and undressing and appropriate attire

Transporting the Patient
- Transporting via a cart or gurney
- Transporting via a wheelchair
- Descending and ascending a wheelchair from a curb

CHAPTER REVIEW QUESTIONS

1. The three components of preparation for the patient undergoing physical therapy treatments, include _____, _____, and _____.
2. Preparing the patient's area for treatment always involves creating a _____ environment.
3. _____ _____ is necessary in order to limit stress and strain on the body's musculoskeletal structures.
4. The proper practice of _____ _____ involves the implementation of _____ important principles.
5. All lifting should be initiated from a _____ position.
6. The physical therapy aide should always be as _____ as possible to the object or person being lifted.
7. Whenever transferring is required, the center of gravity should be _____ from the center of the base of support.
8. When guarding a patient during gait training or ambulation, the physical therapy aide should always position herself at an approximate _____ degree angle to the side and rear of the patient.
9. _____ _____ are always used to focus the patient's attention on specifically desired actions.
10. The physical therapy aide should always describe the general _____ ____ _____ that the patient is expected to follow.
11. Patient preparation should always be completed _____ to transport or treatment.
12. Three modes of transporting a patient include a _____, _____, and a _____.
13. The physical therapy aide should always remember to _____ the brake whenever transferring a patient is required.

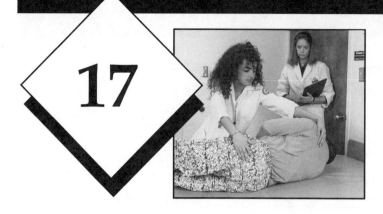

17

Turning and Positioning the Patient

Objectives

After studying this chapter, you will be able to:

1. Describe the purpose of turning and repositioning the debilitated patient and explain the physical therapy aide's role in its function.

2. Describe how to turn a patient in the supine position.

3. Describe how to turn a patient from a supine position to a prone position.

4. Describe how to turn a patient from a prone position to a supine position.

5. Explain how a patient is turned using a floor mat.

6. Explain how to turn a patient from a supine position to a side-lying position.

7. Describe a side-lying position.

8. Explain how to return a patient from a sitting position to a supine position.

VOCABULARY

Learn the meaning and the correct spelling of the following words and abbreviations:

Debilitation
Circulation
Supine
Prone
Floor mat
Gravity
Extremity
Pivoting
Side-lying

Because of the nature and debilitation of some illnesses and injuries, patients frequently are unable to turn in bed or position themselves properly. Frequent turning or repositioning of the dependent patient prevents the development of pressure sores and skin breakdown. A patient who is confined to the bed for any period of time should be turned or repositioned at least every two hours. If a patient has problems such as poor circulation, fragile skin, or decreased sensation, more frequent repositioning may be required. And whenever repositioning or turning is undertaken, time should also be allocated to proper observation and inspection of the skin over the area in which the patient may have been lying. By taking a few extra moments to examine the area for color and integrity, you may prevent the possibility of skin breakdown later on.

When sitting, a patient must be able to relieve pressure on the buttocks and sacrum at least every 10 minutes. Push-ups using the armrests, leaning first to one side and then to the other, and leaning forward are ways in which to relieve

pressure in the sitting position.

Proper positioning involves making the patient as comfortable as possible, thus preventing the development of any deformities and pressure sores as well as providing the patient access to her environment. In order to achieve these goals, the patient and environment must be properly handled. This means that when turning and repositioning is required, the patient must be lifted rather than dragged across the sheets to prevent any skin irritation. Wrinkles in the sheets, blankets, and clothes, should be avoided since they can increase the potential for pressure on a small area causing skin irritation. Pillows and rolled blankets or towels may also be used to support body parts to avoid possible strain on ligaments, nerves, and muscles, Figure 17-1.

When using pillows as a means of support or to provide relief to bony areas or areas of potential skin breakdown, it is important to place them proximally and distally to the involved area.

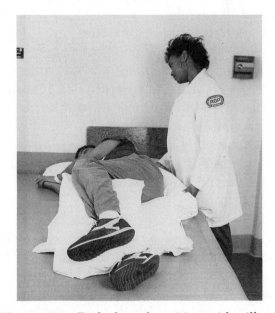

Figure 17-1 Right lateral position with pillow placed under the upper knee.

♦♦♦

Procedure #18: Positioning the Patient in the Supine Position

1. Wash your hands, identify the patient, and provide for privacy.
2. Place the patient's shoulders so that they are parallel to the hips, with the spine straight.
3. Place a pillow under the patient's knees in order to relieve strain on the lower back, Figure 17-2.

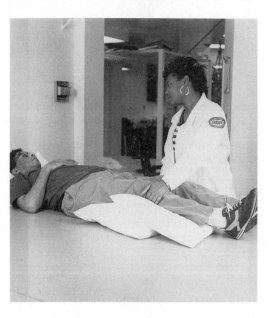

Figure 17-2 Supine position with pillow placed under the lower legs.

♦♦♦

♦ TURNING AND THE SUPINE POSITION

When sheets or blankets are used, they should not be tightly tucked in at the foot of the bed, as this may contribute to a decreased ankle dorsiflexion motion. Footboards are occasionally used to maintain the foot in its neutral or anatomical position. These are usually ineffective since the patient tends to push against the board and the ankle is again in plantarflexion. For some patients, stimulation to the sole of the foot causes a reflex that also will result in ankle plantarflexion.

It is important that you position yourself on the side to which the patient is going to be turned, Figure 17-6. If the bed is narrow or does not have a guardrail, someone should stand next to the patient in order to prevent him from falling while you are moving to the other side of the bed. The second person can assist with the positioning of the pillows and turning the patient. If a pillow is to be placed under the patient for the final positioning, make sure it is positioned so that it will be in the proper position as the patient is rolled.

If the patient has control of his head, chances are that he will be able to assist in turning both his head and neck in the direction of the roll as it is initiated, Figure 17-7. If he does not have this control, you or the therapist must be aware that the face will be subject to some rubbing on the mattress or mat during the roll. When you are ready to initiate the movement, make sure you let the patient know; give a preparatory count and then a specific verbal command. The verbal command should be one which is a direct clue to the task.

If you are working with a therapist, she will be the one to initiate the actual roll by placing her hands on the patient's back. Once the patient reaches the halfway point, he may finish the roll uncontrolled as a result of the pull of gravity. Therefore, the therapist will

Procedure #19: Turning the Patient From a Supine Position to a Prone Position

1. Wash your hands, identify the patient, and provide for privacy.
2. Explain the procedure to the patient.

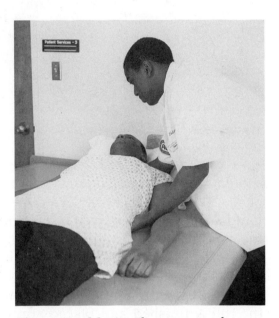

Figure 17-3 Moving the upper trunk.

3. Position yourself on the side to which the patient is going to be turned.
4. If the patient is to roll to the left, position him at the right side of the bed or mat. If he is going to be rolled to the right, position him at the left side of the bed or mat.
5. Move the patient to the edge of the bed in three separate stages; first move the upper trunk (Figure 17-3), then move the lower trunk (Figure 17-4), and finally, move the legs (Figure 17-5).
6. Adduct the left upper arm so that the hand can be placed under the left hip with the palm against the hip.
7. The right lower leg is then crossed over the left lower leg so that the right ankle is resting on top of the left ankle.
8. The right arm is then adducted so that the hand is at the hip with the palm against it.

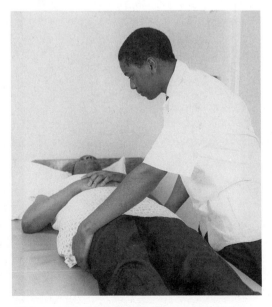

Figure 17-4 Moving the lower trunk.

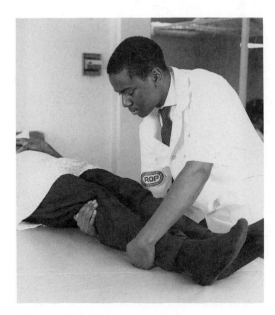

Figure 17-5 Moving the legs.

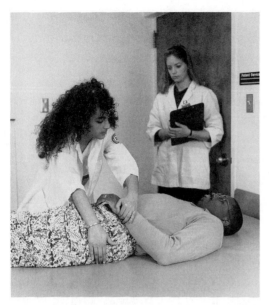

Figure 17-6 Positioning yourself on the side to which the patient is being turned.

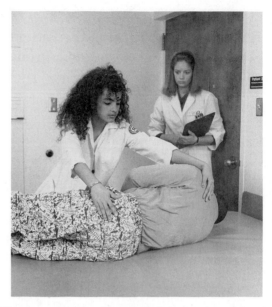

Figure 17-7 Positioning the upper extremity prior to rolling the patient.

begin to rotate her hands as the patient reaches the side-lying position so that they are on the anterior surface of the patient, controlling the second half of the roll (see Figures 17-8 and 17-9).

Once the roll has been completed, the first body segment to be repositioned is the head. It must be placed in a comfortable position, facing to one side. There

should be no pressure on the eyes, nose, or mouth. After this has been done the hands should be removed from under the hips and placed in a position of slight abduction, approximately 20 to 30 degrees. Finally, the feet should be uncrossed if they remain crossed after the roll is finished and placed approximately six to eight inches apart.

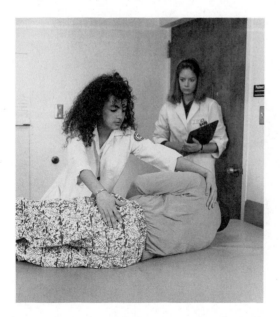

Figure 17-8 Physical therapist's hand position for first part of roll.

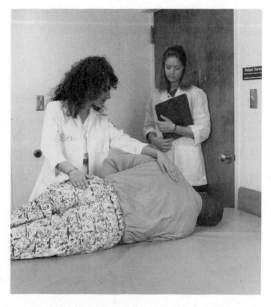

Figure 17-9 Physical therapist's hand position for second part of roll.

◆ TURNING IN THE PRONE POSITION

Patients that are positioned in the prone position lie with their shoulders parallel to their hips and the spine straight. The head may be turned to either the right or left side, or may be maintained in the midline with a small pillow or towel placed under the forehead in order to increase comfort.

Turning from the Prone Position to the Supine Position

In many ways, rolling the patient from the prone position to the supine position is simply the reverse of rolling from the supine to the prone position. The patient's initial position is prone. The beginning steps of moving to one side of the bed and of placement of the patient's hands remain the same. The crossing of the lower extremities is usually unnecessary.

Procedure #20: Positioning the Patient in the Prone Position

1. Wash your hands, identify the patient, and provide for privacy.
2. Place the patient's arms along side his trunk or above his head.
3. Place a pillow under the patient's trunk, either lengthwise or crosswise. Lengthwise may be more comfortable if the patient has limited neck mobility. Crosswise positioning, using a pillow, may be more comfortable for a patient suffering from low back pain.
4. Position the patient's feet over the end of the table, Figure 17-10. A pillow may be placed under the lower legs to avoid the possibility of plantarflexion of the ankle, Figure 17-11.

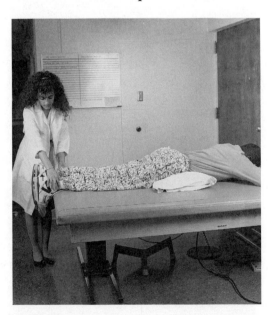

Figure 17-10 Prone position with arms overhead, pillow under hips, and feet off end of table.

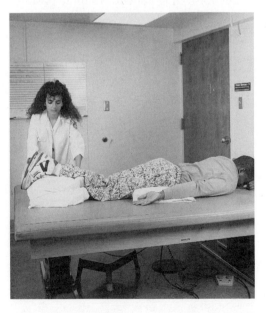

Figure 17-11 Prone position with arm alongside and pillow under legs.

Procedure #21: Turning a Patient from a Prone Position to a Supine Position

1. Wash your hands, identify the patient, and provide for privacy.

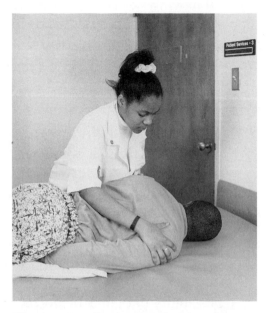

Figure 17-12 Positioning head and upper trunk for rolling patient to supine position.

2. If you are working with a therapist, she should stand on the side to which the patient will roll.
3. Position the patient's head so that he is looking up and over his shoulder as he is being turned toward the therapist (Figure 17-12).
4. Guard the patient on the appropriate side of the bed while the therapist moves to the other side of the bed.
5. The therapist then reaches over the patient and places her hands on the patient's anterior surface. As the patient reaches the side lying position, Figure 17-13, the therapist rotates her hands so that they are on the posterior surface of the patient and she can then control the second half of the roll. From another angle, the complete procedure can be seen in Figures 17-14, 17-15, and 17-16.

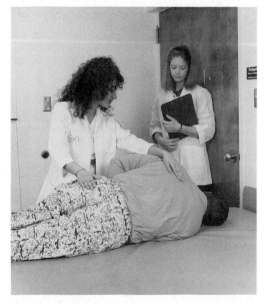

Figure 17-13 Positioning lower trunk for rolling patient to supine position.

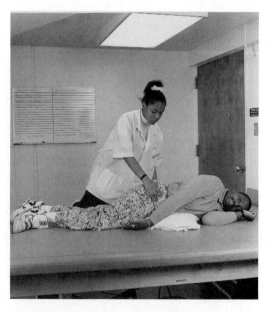

Figure 17-14 Starting position to roll patient from prone to supine position.

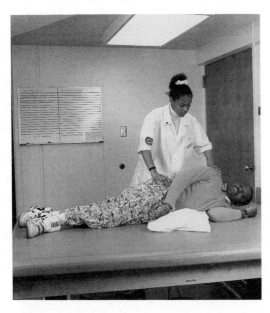

Figure 17-15 Physical therapy aide's hand position to initiate rolling patient to supine position.

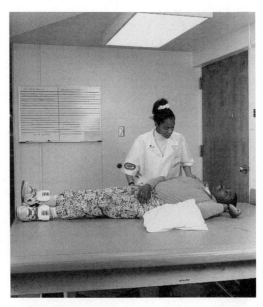

Figure 17-16 Physical therapy aide's hand position to complete rolling patient to supine position.

◆◆◆

◆ **TURNING ON THE FLOOR MAT**

When you are required to turn a patient on the floor mat, the same steps are followed as when turning a patient on a bed.

◆ **TURNING FROM A SUPINE POSITION TO A SIDE-LYING POSITION**

In the side lying position, the patient remains resting on his side for some time. Therefore, adjustments involving rolling may have to be made during the procedure. Side-lying can be accomplished from either the supine or the prone position; however, it may be more comfortable for the patient and easier for yourself if the patient rolls to side-lying from the supine position.

When the patient is to be positioned on his left side, his initial position is supine and to the right side of the mattress. The left arm is abducted to a 45 degree angle. The right lower leg is crossed over the left lower leg at the ankle, and the right hand is placed against the right hip with the palm against it.

Procedure #22: Turning the Patient on the Floor Mat

1. Wash your hands, identify the patient, and provide for privacy.

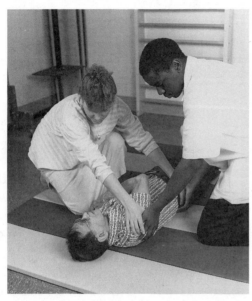

Figure 17-17 Starting position for turning patient on the floor mat.

2. Position yourself on the side to which the patient is going to be turned.
3. Assume a half-kneeling position with the "down" knee at the level of the patient's hips and the "up" knee at the level of the patient's shoulders, Figure 17-17.
4. Place your left hand on the patient's right hip, Figure 17-18, being very careful to hold the patient's right hand on top of the hip.
5. Place your right hand on the patient's right shoulder, Figure 17-19. The hand position must rotate at the midpoint of the roll.
6. Move out of the patient's way as he is turned in order to allow him to complete the roll without rolling onto you.

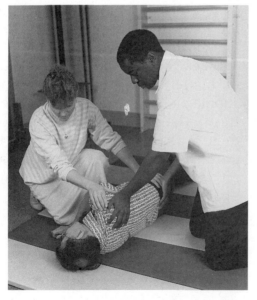

Figure 17-18 Turning patient from a supine position to a prone position on the floor mat.

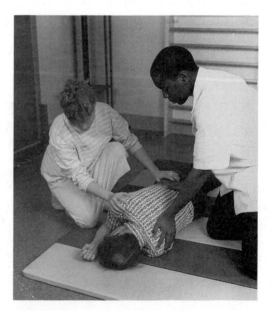

Figure 17-19 Completing the turn from the supine to the prone position on the floor mat.

Procedure #23: Turning the Patient from a Supine Position to a Side-lying Position

1. Wash your hands, identify the patient, and provide for privacy.
2. Assume a position on the side to which the patient is turning.
3. With your left hand, grasp the patient's right hip, being careful to hold his right hand between your hand and his hips.
4. With your right hand, grasp the patient's right shoulder.
5. Roll the patient until he reaches the side-lying position, Figure 17-20.

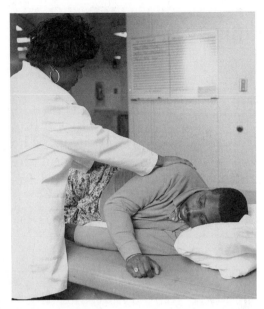

Figure 17-20 Turning the patient to the side-lying position.

Procedure #24: Positioning the Patient in the Side-lying Position

1. Wash your hands, identify the patient, and provide for privacy.
2. Place a pillow under the patient's head. If the patient is being placed in side-lying forward, place the pillow in front of him and bring the uppermost arm forward to rest on the pillow, Figure 17-21. If the patient is being placed in side-lying inclined backward, place the pillow behind him, with the upper most arm extended and supported by the pillow.
3. If necessary, rotate the upper trunk by bringing the lowermost shoulder forward.
4. Flex the uppermost leg and rest it on the pillow.

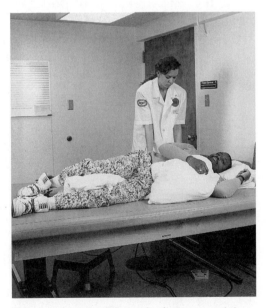

Figure 17-21 The side-lying position, inclined forward.

5. To avoid excessive pressure on the bottom leg, do not allow the uppermost leg to lie directly on top of the bottom leg.

♦ RETURNING FROM A SITTING POSITION TO A SUPINE POSITION

There are several methods that can be used to bring a patient back to a sitting position from a supine position. The method generally depends upon the patient's functional abilities and his medical problem. In all cases, however, a patient should never be left unguarded in the sitting position if he cannot maintain the position safely.

If a patient has enough strength, he can come to the sitting position by doing a sit-up in bed. If slight assistance is necessary, such as for a medical problem involving general weakness, a trapeze bar can be used. In some cases, a patient can do a sit-up or use a trapeze bar

Procedure #25: Returning the Patient from a Sitting Position to a Supine Position

1. Wash your hands, identify the patient, and provide for privacy.
2. Put your arm behind the patient's back and push or pull to assist him up, Figure 17-22.
3. If a trapeze bar is not available, you can stabilize your arm in front of the patient and allow him to pull himself up using your arm.
4. Do not do the patient's work by pulling your arm back as he holds onto your arm; rather, allow the patient to achieve the full sitting position, Figure 17-23.

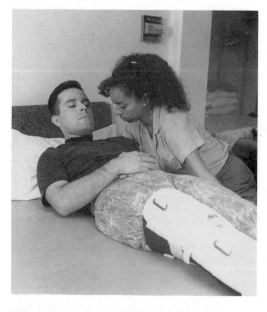

Figure 17-22 Starting position to come to a sitting position.

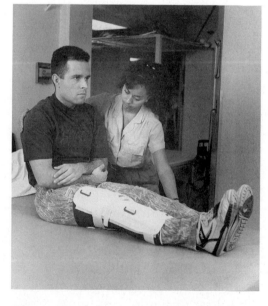

Figure 17-23 Completion of coming to a sitting position.

Procedure #26: Alternate Method for Returning the Patient from a Sitting Position to a Supine Position

1. Wash your hands, identify the patient, and provide for privacy.
2. Have the patient assume a side-lying position, Figure 17-24.

3. Assist the patient to flex the hips and knees to a 90 degree angle. This places the lower legs over the edge of the bed.
4. The patient then pushes or pulls himself to a sitting position, Figures 17-25, 17-26, and 17-27.

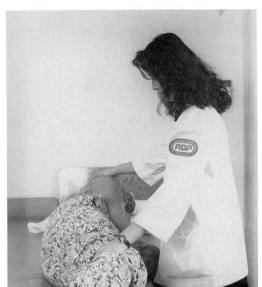

Figure 17-24 Pivoting on bed to lower the legs.

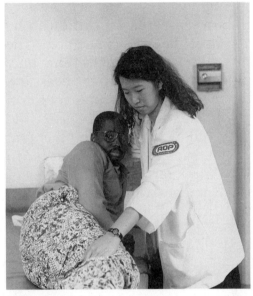

Figure 17-25 Physical therapy aide assisting patient to raise trunk.

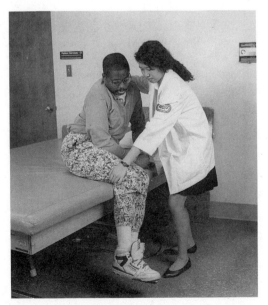

Figure 17-26 Physical therapy aide assisting patient to adjust position.

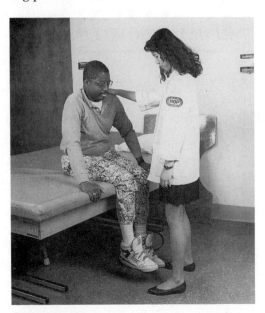

Figure 17-27 Achieving a full upright sitting position.

while you provide assistance at the same time.

Another method of assisting the patient to the sitting position, is teaching him to use his lower extremities as counterweights. If the legs are lowered over the edge of the bed, this will assist the patient to come to a sitting position. There are two ways of performing this maneuver.

If the patient is able to pivot in the bed so that he is lying across it, his legs can then be put into a position to be lowered over the edge of the bed. The trunk should be raised at the same time as the legs are lowered. If necessary, you can assist him by putting your arm under his legs in order to assist the lower leg and by placing your other arm behind his back and head in order to assist the trunk raising, or both. Any of these movements will reduce the strain on the patient's abdominal and hip flexor muscles. For some patients who are too weak to pivot in the bed, assistance may be necessary throughout the entire maneuver.

♦ ♦ ♦
SUMMARY OUTLINE

Turning and Repositioning the Patient
• Purpose of turning the patient
• Purpose of repositioning the patient

Turning and the Supine Position
• Placement of pillows
• Moving the trunk
  • Moving the extremities

Turning in the Prone Position
• Placement of pillows
• Moving the extremities

Turning from the Prone Position to the Supine Position
• Moving the trunk
• Positioning extremities
• Starting the roll

Turning on the Floor Mat

Turning from Supine Position to Side-lying Position
• Side-lying position: inclined forward
• Side-lying position: inclined backward

Returning from a Sitting Position to a Supine Position

CHAPTER REVIEW QUESTIONS

1. Frequently turning and repositioning a dependent patient prevents _____ and _____.
2. When sitting, a patient should be able to relieve pressure on the buttocks and sacrum at least every ____ minutes.
3. Placing a patient in a _____ position means that the shoulders are parallel with the hips.
4. If a patient is to be rolled to the left, she should begin the roll on the _____ side of the bed.
5. Placing a patient in a _____ position means that the shoulders are parallel to the hips with the spine straight.
6. Whenever the physical therapy aide turns the patient from a supine position to a prone position, the lower extremities should be _____ in order to prevent them from dragging.
7. When turning a patient, the physical therapy aide should always remember to position herself to the _____ in which the patient is going to be turned.
8. In turning the patient from a supine position to a side-lying position, the patient's left arm should be _____ to a _____ degree angle.
9. The side-lying position requires the use of _____ for proper placement of the patient's head, trunk, and extremities.
10. If a patient is able, the physical therapy aide should allow him to _____ in turning and repositioning.

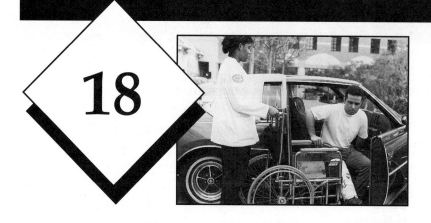

18

Transferring the Patient

Objectives

After studying this chapter, you will be able to:

1. Discuss the importance of properly transferring a patient.

2. Describe the role body mechanics play during the transfer procedure.

3. Identify different types of transfers.

4. Briefly discuss the difference between an unassisted and an assisted bed to wheelchair transfer.

5. Explain an assisted wheelchair to parallel bar transfer.

6. Describe an assisted wheelchair to treatment table transfer.

7. Describe a modified standing transfer.

8. Briefly discuss the following transfers: standing toilet, standing car, and bathtub transfer.

9. Explain the difference between an assisted and an unassisted sitting transfer from the bed to the wheelchair.

10. State the purpose and use of a drawsheet transfer.

11. Define a pneumatic lift transfer and briefly discuss its purpose, operation, and usage.

12. Briefly discuss the physical therapy aide's role in a one-person transfer from the floor to the wheelchair.

Transferring a patient in and out of a wheelchair, bed, car, or any other immobile object requires an understanding of two basic theories: first, you should have a thorough grasp of the importance of safety and efficiency, and, second, you will need to have a complete understanding of the importance of body mechanics and the role it plays in the correct and safe transferring of your physically "challenged" or disabled patients.

The purpose of body mechanics is to provide you with the knowledge and understanding of how to correctly position and move your own body, that is, your trunk, legs, and arms, in order for you to achieve the best possible leverage with the least stress and fatigue. Both you and the patient should be able to move in ways that take advantage of gravity and momentum.

Most transfers that require little, if any, active participation by the patient, are called "dependent" transfers. These would include any transfer that required the use of the aid of one or more individuals, such as yourself, to complete the transfer. Transfers falling into this category include a sliding transfer from a cart or gurney or a bed, a three-man carry, a dependent standing pivot transfer, and the pneumatic lift transfer. Transfers that require some patient participation include the two-man lift, the sliding board transfer, and the assisted standing pivot transfer.

It should be noted that the goal of any assisted transfer is to gradually reduce the assistance necessary until such time as the patient can perform the transfer independently. Assistance may be provided through the use of physical assistance with a maneuver, or verbal reminders of the steps involved. It is also important to always keep the patient informed about the transfer and what he can expect to do. Explanations should be understandable, and commands and counts used to synchronize the actions of all participants should be clear, firm, and concise.

◆ TYPES OF TRANSFERS

There are two basic types of transfers: standing and sitting. In a standing transfer, the patient takes his or her weight on one or both legs and comes to an upright position prior to sitting down again in the new place. In a sitting transfer, the patient does not rise, but moves her hips sideways from one surface to another, generally by taking the weight through the arms. Normally, sitting transfers are used by patients who cannot stand such as those patients suffering from paralysis or having an amputation of the lower extremity(ies).

◆ PREPARATION FOR BEGINNING TRANSFERS

Prior to beginning any transfer, there are certain preparations that will need to be made. First, you should always check the equipment and its position. Make sure it is stable and firm. If you are using a bed during the transfer, you will want to make sure that if it is on casters, they are locked. If not, make sure the bed is pushed against a wall. If you are using a wheelchair, you must make sure that its brakes have been locked.

Always make sure that the transfer surfaces you are using are of the same height. A hospital bed, for example, can be lowered to the height of a wheelchair; also, by placing a raised seat on a toilet seat, you can bring it up to the height of a wheelchair seat. Also remember to keep the transfer surfaces as close together as possible. Removable armrests and swing-away detachable footrests on the wheelchair

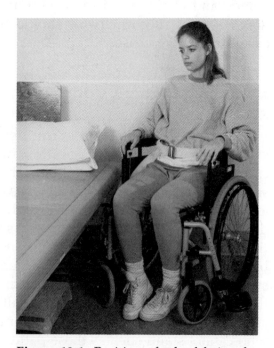

Figure 18-1 Position of wheelchair relative to bed.

allow it to be positioned close to the bed or toilet. A sliding board, or a thin board that is placed across the two surfaces over which a patient may slide, can also be used to close the gap between them completely.

When positioning your equipment, always remember that it must be placed according to the patient's physical limitations or disability. The patient with one side stronger than the other, such as a hemiplegic, will generally prefer to move toward her stronger side during the transfer. If the wheelchair faces the foot of the bed when this patient transfers out of the bed to her wheelchair, then the wheelchair will need to face the head of the bed when the patient wants to return to bed (see Figure 18-1).

Footwear, both for your patient, and yourself, is extremely important during the transfer. Always make sure that both of you are wearing shoes that fit snugly and have a low, wide heel. Also, in case the patient has been prescribed a brace or other prosthesis, make sure that it has been applied prior to the transfer.

Since the patient should know what she is expected to do during the transfer, it is important that you carefully explain and teach the process one step at a time. Instructions should be simple and repeated whenever necessary. They should also be consistent from one time to another. Never try to hurry the patient; allow him time enough to complete each step in a systematic and methodical manner.

Since safety and efficiency is of the utmost importance during the transfer procedure, you should always make sure that you place yourself in the right position for assistance to the patient and for safety for both of you during the procedure. This is accomplished by standing close to the patient. If you

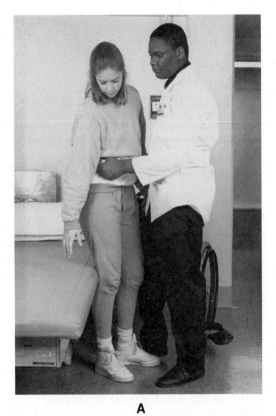

A

allow yourself to stand apart from him, the strain on your back is much greater. Therefore, stand with a broad base of support, keeping your feet slightly apart with one foot ahead of the other. This position allows you to maintain your balance and affords you the ability to quickly and easily shift your weight whenever necessary.

Whenever you are required to transfer the patient from the bed to a wheelchair, you should always remember to assist her at the waist, and never hold onto her at the shoulder. If a transfer belt is available, you may use it to assist in the transfer. Make sure it is securely fastened around the patient's waist since this will give you a better grip on the patient without restricting the use of her arms (see Figure 18-2).

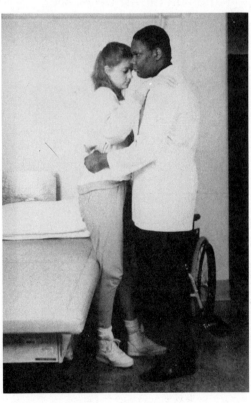

B

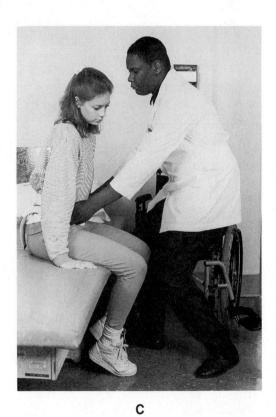

C

Figure 18-2 (A) Lifting with a transfer belt; (B) Pivoting; (C) Transferring from the wheelchair to the bed using a transfer belt.

Procedure #27: Unassisted Bed to Wheelchair Transfer

1. Have the patient slide forward to sit on the edge of the bed and put his feet on the floor with the stronger leg slightly behind and apart from the weaker one. Then have him lean forward, see Figure 18-3A.
2. The patient then stands by pushing down with his arms and, at the same time, straightening his legs.
3. After the patient stands, have him reach for support to the far side armrest of the wheelchair. Then have him step or pivot his back to the wheelchair, see Figure 18-3B.
4. To complete the transfer, the patient bends forward to improve his leverage and balance and, at the same time, slowly lowers himself to sit by bending his hips and knees and easing himself down. At the same time, he supports himself with his hands on the armrests, see Figure 18-3C.

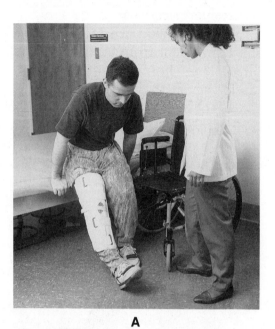

A

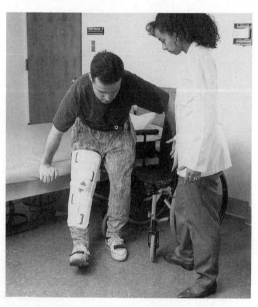

B

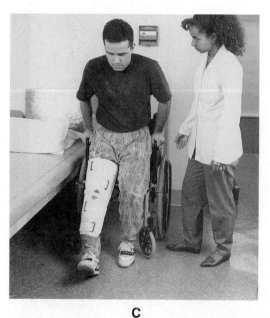

C

Figure 18-3 Unassisted standing transfer from bed to wheelchair.

As we have previously discussed, the use of proper body mechanics is of the utmost importance when transfer techniques are employed. Therefore, when you are required to implement these techniques, always make sure that you keep your back straight, with your hips and knees slightly bent. Straightening your legs as you help the patient into the standing position will prevent you from injuring or straining your back as you complete the transfer. Lifting with your legs is also much less strenuous than lifting with your back muscles. Let the patient see the surface to which he is being transferred, and never obscure his vision since not being able to see the place in which he is going can sometimes frighten him.

Finally, you should always remember that the exact manner in which the patient is to be transferred will always depend upon his abilities, the environment, and any other circumstances unique to that particular patient. Following simple and proper transferring techniques will assist both you and the patient to complete the procedure in a safe and efficient manner.

◆   STANDING TRANSFERS

Bed to Wheelchair: Unassisted

Some patients will have the ability to transfer themselves unassisted from the bed to the wheelchair. If this is the case, the rule of thumb is if the transfer is being completed for the first time, you

---

Procedure #28: Assisted Bed to Wheelchair Transfer

1. Keeping your back straight and your feet slightly apart, bend your hips and knees in order to become more level with the patient.
2. Using your transfer belt or gripping the patient around the waist with one hand and under the thighs with the other, assist the patient to come into a sitting position at the edge of the bed.
3. While bending your hips and knees, place your feet so that you have a good broad base of support and your knees are blocking the patient's knees. Lift the patient by the waist or by the belt as you straighten your hips and knees and carefully rise with the patient into the standing

position. Remember to keep slightly to the side in order to give the patient room enough to move and thus enable him to see the area to which he is being transferred.
4. Position yourself so that you are standing close to the patient, making sure that you still have a broad base of support and, if necessary, are still using your knees to support the patient's knees. Together, allow both yourself and the patient to pivot or turn, slightly shifting the weight from one side to the other and taking tiny steps.
5. As the patient bends forward to sit, slowly bend your hips and knees, gently easing the patient to the seat and helping him in sliding back into the wheelchair.

will want to stay close and supervise the patient during the procedure. Once you have properly instructed him on the technique and have seen him complete the task, you should allow him to finish the transfer on his own.

Bed to Wheelchair: Assisted

If your patient does not have the sufficient strength necessary to bring himself from a lying position to a sitting position, you will need to assist him during the bed to wheelchair transfer.

Wheelchair to Treatment Table: Assisted

Whenever your patient is required to use a treatment table, you should always make sure that there is a stool with four rubber-tipped legs available for his use. Before beginning the procedure, make sure that the wheelchair is placed sideways next to the treatment table, with the patient's stronger side nearest the table.

To dismount from the table, assist the patient to move to the edge, slide down onto her feet, and proceed with the basic transfer.

Standing Toilet Transfer

The same minimum locomotion potentials that are necessary for a patient's standing transfer from a bed to a wheelchair are required for a standing transfer from the wheelchair to a toilet. The patient should have the use of one good leg, and one good arm with a hand able to grip firmly and a good sitting balance.

Procedure #29: Assisting the Patient from a Wheelchair to the Parallel Bars

1. Wash your hands, identify the patient, and provide for privacy.
2. Make sure the wheelchair brakes are applied and that the footrests are swung out to the side.
3. Assist the patient to the front edge of the wheelchair.
4. With his feet flat on the ground and under his hips, ask the patient to place his hands on the bars.
5. Assist the patient to complete the maneuver by bending your hips and knees in order to bring your self to the patient's level, Figure 18-4.
6. Block the patient's knees in order to prevent him from falling.

7. Using the patient's belt or his waist, assist him to rise with you from his wheelchair to the bars.

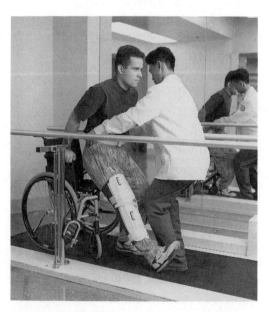

Figure 18-4 Standing from a wheelchair to the parallel bars.

Bathrooms may vary in size and the arrangement of fixtures. While the patient may have to practice the transfer technique in the hospital bathroom, the method which he ultimately learns should be suitable for his bathroom at home.

Preferably, the toilet seat should be approximately 50 centimeters above the floor. If it is lower, a raised toilet seat may be used without any difficulty (see Figures 18-5A, 18-5B, and 18-5C).

A 45 degree angle wall handrail or a right-angle handrail should be placed on the wall that is closest to the side of the toilet bowl. The rail is mounted on the

---

Procedure #30: Assisting Patient from the Wheelchair to the Treatment Table

1. Wash your hands, identify the patient, and provide for privacy.
2. Place a step stool alongside the treatment table.
3. If the patient has one weak leg, use your knees to block hers, while she steps onto the stool with her strong leg.
4. If a transfer or gait belt is available, use it to assist in the transfer.
5. Complete the transfer by assisting the patient to turn her back toward the treatment table and helping her into a sitting position.

Procedure #31: Modified Standing Transfer

Depending upon the patient's specific disability or injury, some variations of the standing transfer technique may be necessary. A patient suffering from hemiplegia, for example, may have total or partial paralysis in one arm and one leg. If indeed, this is the case, the following procedure may be followed (assume the nonfunctional side is the right side):

1. To sit up in bed, the patient moves toward his left side.
2. The patient then grips his weak right arm with his strong left hand and places it across his abdomen.
3. The patient then moves his left foot under the knee of the weak right leg. He then slides his good foot down under the calf to the ankle. Crossing the ankles so that the involved leg can be supported by the non involved one, he lifts or slides both legs over the edge of the bed.
4. Holding onto the edge of the mattress with his left hand and bending his head forward, the patient should lean with his weight against the left forearm and left elbow as he brings the left leg to the floor.
5. The patient completes the transfer by pushing on his left forearm and coming into a sitting position while straightening his left elbow.

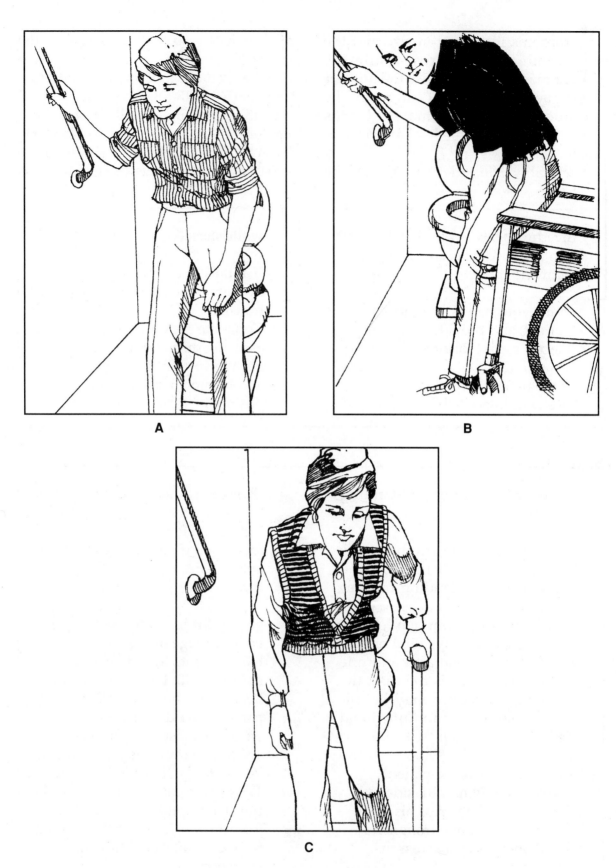

Figure 18-5 Unassisted standing transfer from the toilet to the wheelchair.

♦♦♦

Procedure #32: Assisting the Patient with a Standing Toilet Transfer

1. Wash your hands, identify the patient, and provide for privacy.
2. Bring the patient's wheelchair as close to the front edge of the toilet as possible. Make sure that the patient's stronger side is brought nearest to the toilet.
3. Lock the wheelchair brakes and swing the footrests to the out-side.
4. Have the patient grasp the handrail firmly and assist him to pull himself up to a standing position.
5. Assist the patient so that his body weight is borne entirely or as much as possible on his stronger leg, and his trunk is bent slightly downward. This will establish the patient's center of gravity closer to the grip on the wall bar.

♦♦♦

wall with the lower part of the bar placed about five centimeters behind the front edge of the toilet. The length of the bar can vary from 50 to 90 centimeters.

Standing Car Transfer

Patients who have disabilities involving paralysis of the lower extremities may still be able to drive a car with an automatic transmission. With the aid of special hand controls, the patient can apply the brakes and accelerate the car with his hands.

The car transfer is an advanced and more difficult mode of transfer and is generally only accomplished unassisted by patients with strong upper extremities and good body control.

♦ BATHTUB TRANSFERS

For patients who may be spending either a prolonged period of time in the hospital or whose disability may be chronic, or long lasting, certain daily tasks, such as bathing, must be addressed. For the patient who is confined to a wheelchair, the standing transfer from a wheelchair to a bathtub may be a bit more difficult than some of the other standing transfers already discussed. This patient will need good balance and sure footing; therefore, the person who may be able to perform a standing transfer from a wheelchair to a bed may not be able to use this type of transfer. If the patient is unable to perform this transfer, the use of a sliding board may help to diminish the risk of falling.

The major difference with this type of transfer is that, unlike other transfers, it is generally made toward the weaker side. The reason for this is that it seems to be much easier for the patient to get into the bathtub than to get out of it. Therefore, when the patient returns from the bathtub to the wheelchair, he can move with his better side first.

Procedure #33: Standing Car Transfer

1. Whether or not the patient is the driver or the passenger, he should always enter the car through the right front door, since the steering wheel on the left side frequently hampers or inhibits the transfer. In addition, if the patient is a passenger, the rear doors may not open wide enough to allow proper positioning of the wheelchair for the transfer.

2. The door should be opened as wide as possible, Figure 18-6A. If he wishes the patient may use the edge of the door after the window has been rolled down, the back of the car seat, the door frames of the car, or the seat of the wheelchair for support, Figure 18-6B.

3. The patient turns his back to the car seat and sits down, Figure 18-6C. He then swivels on the seat in order to bring both feet inside, lifting up his involved leg with his hands, if necessary.

4. To leave the car, the patient reverses the process.

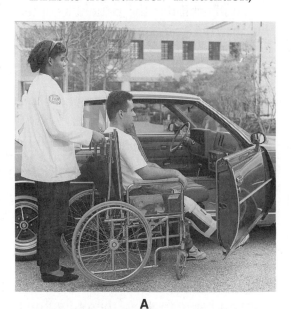

A

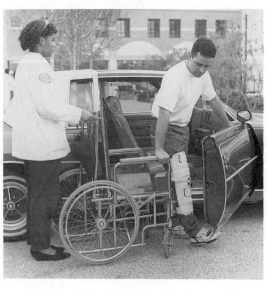

B

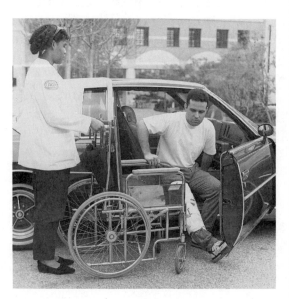

C

Figure 18-6 Standing transfer, from the wheelchair to a car.

Procedure #34: Assisting the Patient with a Bathtub Transfer

1. Wash your hands, identify the patient, and provide for privacy.
2. Place a sturdy chair of the same height as the bathtub edge inside the tub, on a bath mat, see Figure 18-7, and another one beside the tub. Make sure both chairs have rubber tips on the legs, in order to avoid any possibility of slipping.
3. Place a tread tape under the bath mat in the tub to avoid any slipping of the mat.
4. If necessary, have the patient hold onto the bars on the walls for greater security.
5. Assist the patient to assume a sitting position on the chair in the tub.

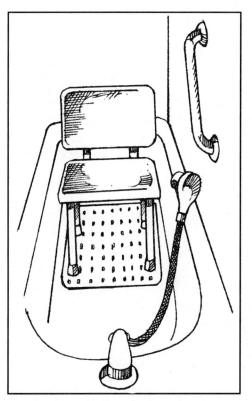

Figure 18-7 Bathtub with chair and bath mat in it.

Procedure #35: Assisting the Patient with a Bathtub Transfer Using a Sliding Board

1. Wash your hands, identify the patient, and provide for privacy.
2. Obtain a sliding board. It is usually made out of lightweight pine, approximately two centimeters in thickness in the middle and beveled lengthwise approximately one centimeter at both ends.
3. If the patient is sitting in a wheel chair, bring it as close to the edge of the tub as possible.
4. Apply the wheelchair brakes and remove or swing the footrests out to the side.
5. Place one end of the board securely under the patient's buttocks on the wheelchair seat and the other end on the chair in the bathtub.
6. Pushing down on the board with one hand, place the other hand on the wheelchair seat, and assist the patient to slide over to the edge of the bathtub, and to place the leg closest to the bathtub in it.
7. The patient then grips the handrail on the edge of the tub and slides his buttocks onto the chair in the tub.
8. The transfer is completed by the patient bringing his second leg over the edge of the bathtub.

Oftentimes, it may be difficult to place the proper chair beside the bathtub in the bathroom. The patient may also experience difficulty in sliding across the chair and the edge of the bathtub onto the chair in the tub. If this is the case, it may be easier to teach the patient a sliding-board transfer.

♦ SITTING TRANSFERS

Patients experiencing weakness or paralysis in both lower extremities are generally unable to support their body weight with their legs, even for only a few moments. Therefore, it may be necessary to complete a transfer from a sitting position.

Bed to Wheelchair: Unassisted

Whenever the patient is to be moved unassisted from the bed to the wheelchair, the wheelchair should be placed against the bed sideways. The armrest and the footrest of the wheelchair that are located nearest the bed should be removed and the brakes locked.

Bed to Wheelchair: Assisted

If the patient's arms are not strong enough to lift his body, he may have to be assisted in moving from the bed to the wheelchair.

Finally, you should always remember that the same principles of good body mechanics that are applied for a sitting transfer from the bed to the wheelchair, whether assisted or unassisted, also apply to sitting transfers from the wheelchair to the toilet or from the wheelchair to a car.

♦ DRAWSHEET TRANSFERS

In some cases, when a patient is totally paralyzed or experiences such weak-

**Procedure #36: Unassisted
Transfer from Bed to Wheelchair:**

1. The patient learns forward and pushes down with his fists into the mattress, carefully shifting his hips until they are angled toward the wheelchair. With the arm closest to the wheelchair, he supports himself on the wheelchair seat.
2. Still leaning forward, the patient pushes down forcefully with one arm on the bed and the other on the wheelchair seat and slides his

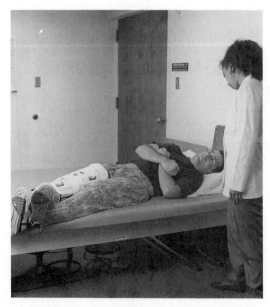

A

buttocks from one surface to the other. As the patient shifts his position, he adjusts his legs. He should avoid pushing on the backrest of the wheelchair for support during the transfer.

3. To complete the transfer, the patient then replaces the armrest, and, pushing down on it with his hands, slides back into the chair and adjusts his legs with his arms, if necessary, Figure 18-8.

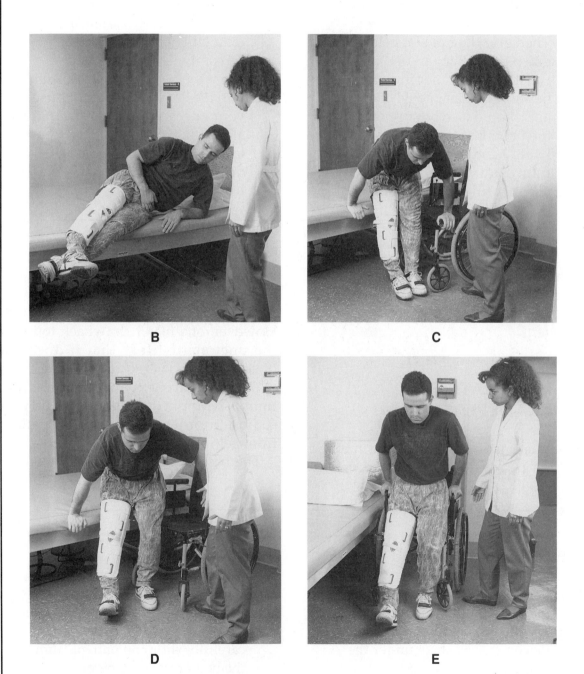

B

C

D

E

Figure 18-8 Unassisted sitting transfer from the bed to the wheelchair.

♦♦♦

Procedure #37: Assisted Transfer from Bed to Wheelchair

1. To assist the patient in this transfer, you will first have to bring yourself to the level of the patient. To perform this task, you should bend at your hips and knees to lower yourself. Then grip the transfer belt or grasp the patient around her waist and assist her in angling her hips toward the wheelchair. You should also be supporting the patient's knees with your knees in order to prevent her from sliding forward.

2. Again, using the transfer belt or griping the patient at her waist, assist her in sliding her buttocks to the wheelchair. At the same time, allowing her to see the surface toward which she is being transferred. Throughout this procedure, always make sure that you are assisting the patient to lean forward, so that she can maintain her trunk balance.

3. To complete the transfer and assist the patient to move back into the chair, you should push your knees against hers, continually making sure that she keeps leaning forward and pushes down on the armrests with her hands.

♦♦♦

ness that she cannot participate in the transfer at all, other means of transferring may have to be employed. One such method, is called the drawsheet transfer.

♦ PNEUMATIC LIFT TRANSFER

A pneumatic lift provides a method for one person to transfer a dependent patient or a patient who is larger than herself. This mechanical system has caster wheels, which make it easier for positioning and moving the patient. However, one major drawback to using the pneumatic lift is that it does not have brakes. Therefore, the aide must make sure that safety measures are continuously applied throughout this procedure in order to prevent the patient from getting hurt.

The base of the pneumatic lift can be

♦♦♦

Procedure #38: Assisting the Patient with a Drawsheet Transfer

1. Wash your hands, identify the patient, and provide for privacy.
2. Roll the patient to one side.
3. Place a folded sheet under the patient's back.
4. Gently roll the patient to the other side of the bed and unfold the drawsheet.
5. Two persons must perform the transfer, one on each side of the patient's bed. They hold either side of the drawsheet and carefully slide the patient from the bed to the gurney or treatment table.

♦♦♦

widened to fit around the patient's wheelchair or any other piece of equipment. It is generally in the narrow position when the patient is being moved, in order to make the maneuvering easier.

The long lever attached to the base is turned and moved from one side to the other to increase or decrease the width of the base (see Figure 18-9).

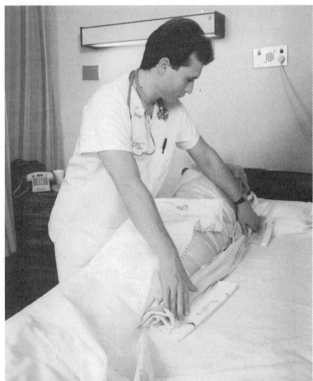

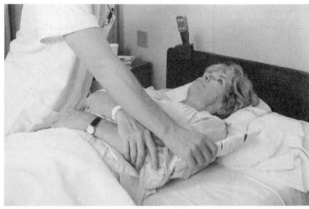

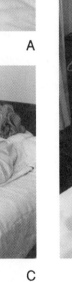

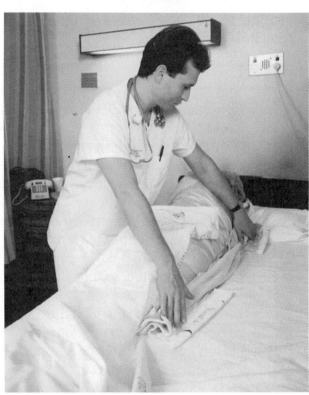

A

B

C

D

Figure 18-9 Lifting a patient using a mechanical lift. (From Hegner and Caldwell, *Nursing Assistant: A Nursing Process Approach*, 6th edition, copyright 1992 by Delmar Publishers Inc.) *(Continued)*

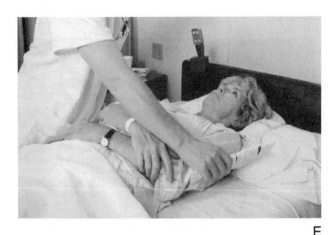
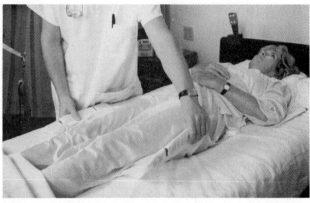

E   F

Figure 18-9 Lifting a patient using a mechanical life. (From Hegner and Caldwell, *Nursing Assistant: A Nursing Process Approach,* 6th edition, copyright 1992 by Delmar Publishers Inc.)

Procedure #39: Transferring the Patient Using the Pneumatic Lift

1. The valve on the front of the upright is closed in order to allow the lift to be raised and then opened slowly in order to lower the patient. After checking that the valve is closed, the aide "pumps" the handle to raise the lift.
2. The sling on which the patient rests is then attached to the spreader bar on the lift by chains, with the length of the chain adjusted to the patient's height. A short segment of the chain is then attached to the upper part of the sling, and a longer segment of the chain, is attached to the lower part of the sling in order to suspend the patient in a sitting position.
3. The hooks are then attached to the sling from the inside to the outside. By doing this, the patient is less likely to be injured by the hook.

4. The sling is then positioned so that the seams are away from the patient. This is done in order to avoid pressure areas. Slings are made of a variety of fabrics and may either be one piece or two piece. When the patient is in bed, the sling is placed under her by rolling her to one side, positioning the sling, and then rolling her to the other side. The sling may be left under the patient when she is in the wheel-chair; therefore, it is extremely important to avoid pressure from the seams.
5. Once the patient has been positioned on the sling, the lift is moved into position so that the spreader bar is across the patient. Both ends of each chain are then attached to their respective sides of the sling. The valve should be closed and the patient raised slowly. Remember that care should be taken in order to ensure that a safe sitting position is achieved as the patient is raised.

6. The patient is then moved into position over the seat of a locked wheelchair.
7. The valve is opened slowly in order to lower the patient into the wheelchair.
8. In order to properly seat the patient in the wheelchair, you will have to apply slight pressure in the horizontal plane at the patient's knees and thighs. This pushes the patient into the seat completely, with her back resting firmly against the back of the wheelchair.
9. Once the patient has been seated in the wheelchair, the valve is closed in order to avoid striking the patient should the lift arm continue to lower. The chains are then removed from the sling. The transfer is completed by moving the lift away from the wheelchair and placing the patient's feet properly onto the footrests.

♦♦♦

♦ ONE MAN TRANSFER FROM FLOOR TO WHEELCHAIR

Occasionally a patient may fall out of or tip over the wheelchair. If the patient is unable to transfer from the floor to the wheelchair, you may have to perform a one man transfer.

♦♦♦

Procedure #40: One Man Transfer from Floor to Wheelchair

1. When using this transfer, the wheelchair should be positioned on its back, at the patient's buttocks. The patient's ankles are then placed over the front edge of the wheelchair seat. You will then have to perform a series of short lift and scooting maneuvers in order to move the patient into the wheelchair. This is accomplished by placing one arm under the patient's knees and the other under her upper trunk and neck.
2. After you have placed yourself into a half-kneeling position to help provide a stronger lifting posture, lift the handles of the wheelchair, bringing it to an upright position. As you are bringing the wheelchair up, begin to move out of the half-kneeling position to a standing position.
3. As the wheelchair begins to approach the upright position, shift one arm to guard the patient's upper trunk. This will prevent you from falling forward.

♦♦♦

CHAPTER REVIEW QUESTIONS

1. Transferring patients requires an understanding of _____, _____, and _____ _____.
2. _____ _____ require little, if any, active participation by the patient.
3. The goal of any assisted transfer is to _____ the assistance and _____ independence.
4. The two basic types of transfers are _____ and _____.
5. It is important to always check the _____ of the wheelchair before starting any transfer to or from it.
6. A _____ _____ may be used to assist the patient transferring from the bed to the wheelchair.
7. When transferring from the bed to the wheelchair un assisted, the patient should slide _____ to the edge of the bed.
8. When assisting the patient to transfer from the bed to the wheelchair, the physical therapy aide should always keep his back _____ and hips and knees _____.

9. When using the parallel bars, the patient always starts from a
    _____ position.
10. A standing toilet transfer requires the use of a _____ degree
    angle wall handrail.
11. When making a standing car transfer, the patient always enters
    the car through the _____ front door.
12. A bathtub transfer is generally made toward the patient's
    _____ side.

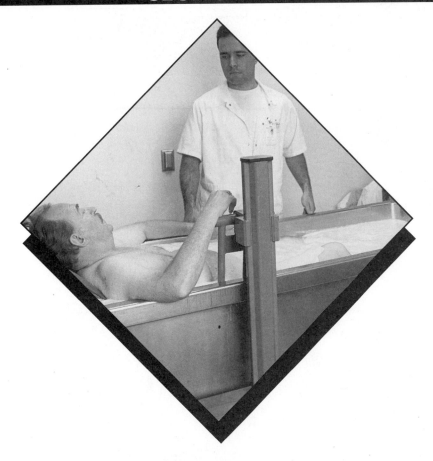

PHYSICAL THERAPY MODALITIES

19

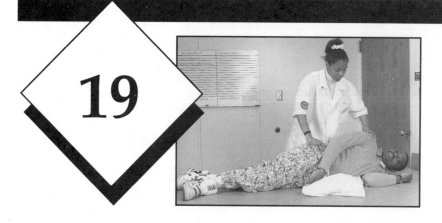

Therapeutic Exercises

Objectives

After studying this chapter, you will be able to:

1. State the ultimate goal and purpose of any therapeutic exercise program.

2. Discuss the physical therapy aide's role in assisting the patient with therapeutic exercises.

3. Describe the purpose of range of motion exercises and explain the difference between passive and active range of motion.

4. Briefly discuss how muscle strength is graded.

5. Compare the difference between skill and coordination exercises.

VOCABULARY

Learn the meaning and the correct spelling of the following words and abbreviations:

Therapeutic
Strength
Endurance
Mobility
Flexibility
Relaxation
Coordination
Range of motion
Active range of motion
Passive range of motion
Progressive resistive
Isometric exercise
Sensory input
Skill

As a physical therapy aide, one of the more difficult tasks you might be expected to perform is the actual teaching of an exercise program to your patients. Most of the time, it does not suffice to show the patient just once how to do the exercises. You may have to reemphasize certain very specific details, correct the patient's performance frequently, and adjust to his physical condition at a particular time. Much effort and dedication on the part of the physical therapist and the aide are often necessary in order to improve the patient's performance. In order to assist the patient with his exercise program, you must first have a basic understanding of the importance placed on it.

The ultimate goal of any therapeutic exercise program is its ability to assist the patient in achieving symptom-free movement and function. Such a goal can only be met by establishing the positive effects the program has on the patient. These effects include the benefits derived for the patient's development, improvement, and restoration, or maintenance of normal strength, endurance, mobility and flexibility, relaxation, coordination, and skill.

In order to effectively administer therapeutic exercise to the patient, both the therapist and the aide must know the basic principles and effects of the treatment. While the therapist is the individual responsible for conducting the functional evaluation of a patient prior to beginning the exercise program, it is generally the aide who assists the patient in carrying the exercise program out. While each patient reacts differently to an exercise program and needs individual consideration in the program outline, there are some well-established physiological principles that should always be followed. Let's take a look at some of the most important principles.

First, let's note that the purpose and goal of the exercise program must be very clearly defined for the patient. For example, it has to be decided whether the patient's general physical condition should be improved or whether the range of motion of a specific joint should be increased or a specific muscle be strengthened. The program has to be designed accordingly.

Secondly, the amount of stress that the exercise program places on the patient in general or on a specific joint or muscle must be determined according to the patient's tolerance and the strength of the specific muscle or the condition of the joint.

A third point is that when an exercise program is designed, the type of stress imposed by the exercises should be relevant to the function that is to be enhanced. For example, extending the knee against resistance and gravity will strengthen the quadriceps muscle. There should always be a steady attempt, day by day or week by week, to perform better. In other words, the tolerance of the patient or the strength of the muscle or the range of joint motion should constantly be challenged, but always at a steady pace. If a person only performs the activity he is accustomed to, that person will never increase his strength, tolerance or skill.

A fourth point to note is that the program should always adhere to well-established physiological principles; that is, the intensity and duration of the stress imposed should increase gradually. In order to achieve an increase in strength, tolerance, or endurance, the exercise program has to be performed, if not daily, at least frequently and at regular intervals.

The final physiological principle deals with never allowing your patient to become exhausted. If the patient still feels fatigued the day following the exercise program, it probably means that the program was too strenuous for her or she has to be given additional rest. The same applies to the specific muscle or joint that was exposed to the exercise stress.

Should the muscle become painful or weaker or the joint more swollen and painful the day following the exercises, the program must be eased or decreased temporarily.

Improvement is not entirely a physiological function; psychological factors also play a key role in the patient's exercise program. Many of the problems your patients may be facing are long-lasting and are therefore more apt to be the cause of discouragement. Patients entrusted to your care will need much encouragement. Also remember that a substantial number of patients you will encounter may have ailments that cannot be entirely cured; however, the patient's functioning nearly always can be improved. The patient has to be made aware of this by his or her physician. This potential for improvement only, and not a complete cure, may sometimes hinder the patient's motivation to perform the prescribed program.

◆ FORMS OF EXERCISE

There are various forms of exercises that may be used according to the effect they are designed to achieve. These generally include exercises for range of motion of a joint, exercises to increase strength, and exercises to improve skill or coordination.

Range of Motion Exercises

When a joint is not being regularly moved, it may become stiff and the range of motion is, therefore, decreased. You may have noticed the desire to stretch after you have been lying in one position for a long period of time. With advancing age, tightness and stiffness of the joints sets in more readily, and it becomes more difficult to restore normal range of motion. If a patient is unable to move one arm or leg after a stroke because no impulses are able to travel from the brain to the peripheral motor nerves, the joint's range of motion decreases and the tissue around the joint contracts and shortens. In the case of a temporary or permanent paralysis, the treating person has to move the patient's limb through various ranges of motion. In this instance, one speaks of *passive range of motion* exercises. If the

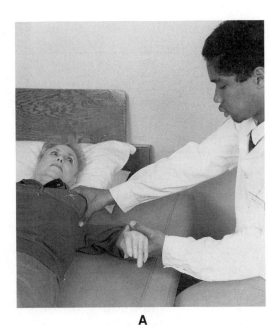
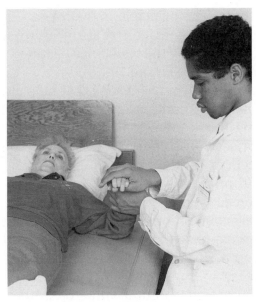

A

B

Figure 19-1 Example of range of motion exercise for shoulder flexion.

patient is able to move the limb by active muscle contraction, we say the exercises are *active range of motion.*

Range of motion exercises can be performed by a physical therapy aide after she has been instructed how to perform them by a physical therapist. Whenever these exercises are to be performed, great care must always be taken not to damage or further contract the involved joints. It is easier to prevent contractures than to restore normal range of motion after the contracture has occurred (see Figure 19-1).

Exercises to Increase Strength

Whenever a muscle or a group of muscles are forced into inactivity, the strength of those muscles will gradually fade away. If total inactivity is forced upon a patient, the rate of decrease in muscle strength is approximately 7.5 percent per day.

Muscles that are forced into inactivity become flabby and eventually decrease in size. In case the peripheral nerve or the lower motor neuron is damaged and the muscle cannot contract at all for a long period of time, the muscle fibers which cannot contract are replaced by nonfunctional fibrous tissue. In such instances, the muscle cannot be made stronger.

Progressive resistive exercises are designed to increase the strength of the

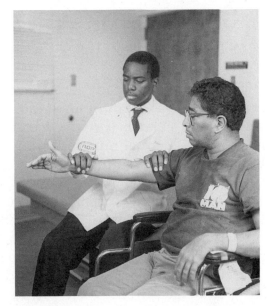

Figure 19-2 Example of resisted exercise for shoulder flexion.

muscles. The principle is that of repetition of maximal contraction against resistance, with the resistance gradually increasing (see Figure 19-2).

Another form of exercise that helps to maintain or, perhaps, even improve the strength of a muscle is called *isometric* exercises. In this type of exercise, the muscle is contracted without bringing about any joint motion. Many claims have been made about this form of isometric contraction. It is said that when these exercises are performed several times a day, muscle strength does increase.

The most important value of isometric exercise is that it can be used when active motion in the joint is not possible or desirable. In addition, isometric exercises may also be used to help facilitate active exercises. Out of fear of causing pain in an inflamed joint, the patient often thinks he is unable to contract a muscle. The use of isometric exercises allows you to show the patient that it is still possible to do the exercises without feeling the pain.

♦ MEASURING MUSCLE STRENGTH

There are a great many methods for measuring the strength of a muscle. It can be done manually or with measuring devices. Manual muscle testing is the more widely used method since all it requires is the examiner's knowledge of the tested muscle's origin and insertion and the direction of its maximal force upon the joint. Usually manual muscle testing is performed by an experienced physical therapist, but this skill can also be acquired by the physical therapy aide.

The most widely used grading of muscle strength in manual muscle testing is as follows:

Normal:	complete range of motion against gravity with full resistance
Good:	complete range of motion against gravity with some resistance
Fair:	complete range of motion against gravity
Poor:	complete range of motion with gravity eliminated
Trace:	evidence of slight contractility; no joint motion
Zero:	no evidence of contractility

Grading becomes very difficult if the patient has an upper motor contracture or suffers from any spasticity or rigidity. No adequate testing can be performed when contraction against resistance or even active motion causes pain.

♦ SKILL OR COORDINATION EXERCISES

Each and every skilled motion or movement we use depends upon the intact functioning of various components or parts of our nervous system. The structures that conduct the sensory input, the structures in the brain that integrate the many stimuli to the appropriate organ, and the skeletal muscle fibers all have to be intact. When we speak of improvement of skill, coordination, and balance, what we are really saying is that we are increasing the control that the individual has over various muscle contractions. In order to achieve a high degree of control over the various

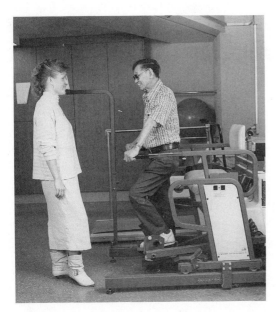

Figure 19-3 Example of using therapeutic exercise equipment.

muscle groups, it takes many years of experience and practice. A young child, for example, has the necessary reflexes, nerve structures, and muscles to perform all the skills adults can perform easily and well; yet the child's movements appear clumsy. The child's gait, or walk, is still broad-based, and therefore, the child tends to fall more frequently than does the adult. When a high degree of precision in muscle control is attained, even strenuous motions appear very easy.

When disease causes movement disorders, there is generally some loss of skill and coordination. Even when a patient loses a limb, such as a leg, there is usually some problem with balance. An artificial limb, regardless of how sophisticated and well-fitting it may be, always lacks one component— the sensory input.

Various exercise programs and equipment are available in print for specific diseases (see Figure 19-3). As with progressive resistive exercise programs, exercises to increase control of muscle action must also be performed. The challenge to improve muscle control has to be steadily increased; otherwise, no improvement can be achieved and the patient stays at the same level of function.

The learning of skills, or, in other words, the acquisition of a better and more precise control of muscle action and muscle coordination, needs constant reinforcement by the person treating the physically limited patient. Control of muscle action can be lost by long-standing disease or after a serious illness. In such instances, skill nearly to the same level as previously achieved can be regained with training. It is always easier to retrain for previously acquired skills than to learn new ones.

♦ ♦ ♦
SUMMARY OUTLINE

Understanding Therapeutic Exercise
- Goal and purpose of therapeutic exercise
- Physical therapy aide's role in providing therapeutic exercise
- Psychological factors involved in therapeutic exercise

Forms of Exercise
- Range of motion exercises
- Exercises to increase strength
- Skill or coordination exercises

CHAPTER REVIEW QUESTIONS

1. If a joint is not regularly moved, the range of its motion may become _____.

2. The use of _____ range of motion is accomplished with the assistance of a treating person.

3. _____ range of motion is used when the patient is able to move the affected body part independently.

4. If total inactivity is forced upon a patient, the rate of _____ in muscle strength is approximately ____ per day.

5. _____ _____ exercises are designed to increase the strength of the muscles.

6. An _____ exercise is generally used to improve the strength of a muscle.

7. Normal muscle strength indicates that there is _____ range of motion against gravity with _____ resistance.

8. Improvement of skill, coordination, and balance indicates an _____ in the patient's control over muscle contractions.

9. Diseases causing movement disorders generally cause some _____ in skill and coordination.

10. An artificial limb, no matter how sophisticated and well-fitted, always lacks _____ _____.

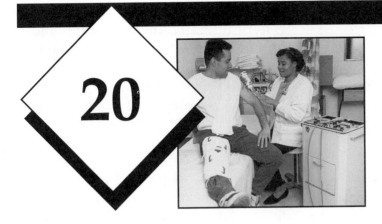

20

Physical Therapy Agents and Modalities

1. Discuss the purpose of employing different agents and modalities in performing physical therapy.

2. Define hydrotherapy and describe its use in physical therapy.

3. Identify and discuss the three different superficial heating agents used in physical therapy.

4. Explain the function of diathermy.

5. Differentiate between microwave and shortwave therapy.

6. Define ultrasound and briefly discuss its application in physical therapy.

7. Contrast the difference between cold therapy and heat therapy and briefly discuss when each should be applied.

VOCABULARY

Learn the meaning and the correct spelling of the following words and abbreviations:

Agent
Modality
Hydrotherapy
Superficial
Hydrocollator pack
Infrared
Electromagnetic
Paraffin
Contraindication
Diathermy
Microwave
Ultrasound
Whirlpool

In order to properly prepare the muscles and joints of a body region for exercise or physical therapy, various modalities, or agents, of heating or cooling these structures may be employed.

Heat helps in the reduction of pain and tightness within the muscles and stiffness in the joints. In the body region in which the temperature is elevated, the blood vessels dilate, making it possible for the flow of blood to that area to increase. All these changes aid in the performance of exercise therapy. Such heat application has basically the same purpose as the warming-up and loosening-up exercises that are used by athletes just before they enter a strenuous event.

Heat can be applied to parts of the body by a number of methods. One such method is by the complete immersion of the body part into heated water. This form of heating is called **hydrotherapy.** In hydrotherapy, the heat delivered to the immersed body part is only one of the therapeutic factors from which the patient can receive benefit.

The goal in the use of heating modalities is to effect a specific temperature elevation and an increased blood flow in the part selected for therapy. Optimal benefit from this type of local application of heat is generally achieved within 20 minutes. After that amount of time, no further local temperature elevation can be achieved. In fact, any more time can cause the increased blood flow to carry the heat away into the entire body.

The various heating agents used in physical therapy can be divided into two types: the one brings heat to the superficial structures and the other brings heat to the deeper structures of a body region.

Both temperature elevation and cooling may be used to create a therapeutic environment for the affected body region or structure. The lowering of tissue temperature is generally achieved through the application of various forms. In essence, the lowering of the temperature of the affected body part helps to decrease the amount of swelling, inflammation, and spasticity to the area involved.

◆ SUPERFICIAL HEATING AGENTS

Modalities found within this group are those which can affect temperature elevation approximately 10 millimeters beneath the skin's surface. They include hydrocollator packs, infrared lamps, and paraffin baths.

Hydrocollator Packs

A hydrocollator pack is composed of a silica gel that has been encased in a canvas bag and can be contoured to the various body regions (see Figure 20-1A). Silica gel is able to maintain a temperature of 104 degrees Fahrenheit (40 degrees Centigrade) for a period of approximately 30 to 40 minutes. The hydrocollator pack should be placed in a water bath at a temperature of about 170 degrees Farenheit. It must then be removed from the water and placed onto the area that afterward will be treated with range-of-motion, active, or resistive exercises. Both the area in which the moist pack will be applied the packs themselves are generally covered with a thick Turkish towel in order to protect the patient's skin from any possible burns and to reduce any emis-

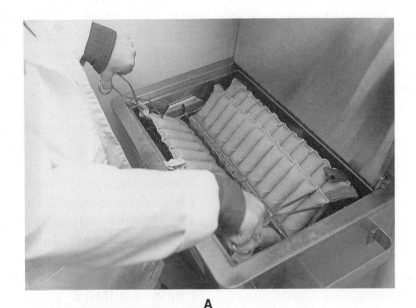

A

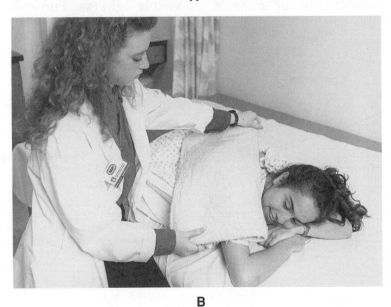

B

Figure 20-1 (A) Hydrocollator packs; (B) in use.

sion of heat from the packs toward the outside. The upper side of the pack can also be covered with a plastic or rubber sheet in order to forestall any heat emission away from the packs, Figure 20-1B.

Generally speaking, it is more advantageous to place the pack on the patient-than to make the patient lie on the pack. The latter invites greater chances for burns. Sometimes the patient's condition may require the placing of the hydrocollator pack under a part of his or her body. If this is the case, special precautions have to be taken, and you should speak with the physical therapist prior to applying the pack.

Heat delivered from the moist hydrocollator pack to the body is a form of conductive heat. The moisture of the pack serves as the conductor to the skin surface. Water is also a good heat conductor. The counterpart of conductors are the insulators. They are responsible for the hampering of the transfer of heat, and some of the more common types include wood, asbestos, plastics, and rubber.

If a patient suffers from a skin disease, hydrocollator packs should never be used. The same is true for areas of impaired blood supply.

When the hydrocollator pack is used as a therapeutic application, it should be removed after a period of 20 minutes and placed in a reheating bath of 170 degrees Farenheit. Thirty minutes later, the packs may again be ready for application.

Infrared Heating

This form of heat is found widely in both nature and in daily life. The most abundant of all infrared sources is the sun. More than half of the sun's total radiation is infrared, and most heated substances emit infrared rays. Infrared is a type of radiant heat and can be transmitted to an object or the body from a distance source through a vacuum.

The physical properties of any radiant energy are that of electromagnetic waves. The spectrum of the electromagnetic waves ranges from electric power supply and radiowaves, with a very long wave length, through the visible light spectrum, to x-rays, which have a very short wave length. The wave length of infrared is longer than that of visible light (see Figure 20-2).

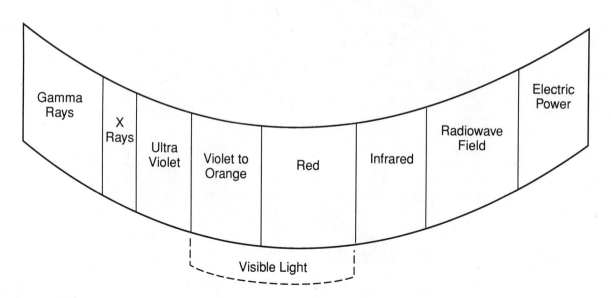

Figure 20-2 The electromagnetic spectrum.

For therapeutic purposes, an artificial source is used for infrared radiation. The infrared lamp (see Figure 20-3), consists of a non-luminous wire core to which electric energy is applied. Infrared can affect temperature elevation down to approximately 10 millimeters beneath the skin's surface.

There are several advantages to using infrared heat as a therapeutic modality. There is no pressure on the body, and the aide attending the patient can easily observe the area without interrupting the treatment.

As with other local heating methods, the optimal local temperature is generally achieved within 20 minutes. Any extension of this time frame may lead to sweating and general heating. The effects of infrared are very similar to those of the heat emitted by the hydrocollator packs. It also should not be applied over areas of impaired vascular supply or impaired temperature sensation.

♦ THE PARAFFIN BATH

The paraffin bath (see Figure 20-4), contains a mixture of one part liquid petrolatum to seven parts paraffin. After these components are placed in the container of the paraffin bath, the mixture has to be heated until the paraffin melts. Before it is ready for use, the temperature of the mixture must drop to approximately 125 to 130 degrees Fahrenheit (51 to 54 degrees Centigrade). A period of two to three hours may be required for this drop to occur.

Procedure #41: Applying an Infrared Lamp

1. Wash your hands, identify the patient, and provide for privacy.
2. Inspect the lamp for good working condition prior to beginning the procedure.
3. Explain the procedure to the patient.
4. Place the lamp 30 inches (about 45 centimeters) from the body area receiving the rays, Figure 20-3.
5. Drape the surrounding body parts not receiving treatment.
6. Make sure that the infrared lamp has been turned on 20 to 30 minutes prior to its use.
7. Instruct the patient to report any feelings of "hot spots" immediately since they may be warning signals of an imminent burn from the infrared lamp.
8. Remove the infrared lamp after 15 to 20 minutes.

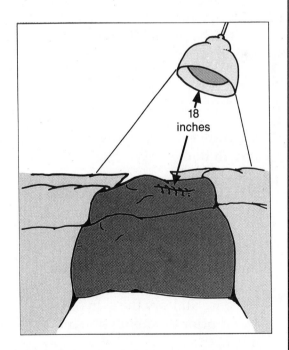

Figure 20-3 Application of the infrared lamp. (From Hegner and Caldwell, *Nursing Assistant: A Nursing Process Approach*, 6th edition, copyright 1992 by Delmar Publishers Inc.)

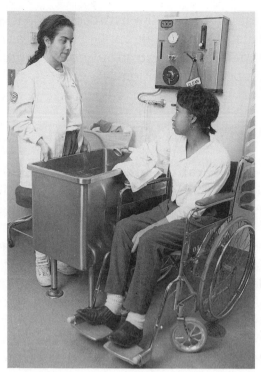

Figure 20-4 Hand immersion into a paraffin bath.

The paraffin bath is most often used to treat small areas, such as the hands and feet. Arthritic joint pain and stiffness in the hands, are frequently indications for paraffin use.

Contraindications for the application of the paraffin bath are similar to those of the hydrocollator packs. Paraffin should never be applied when there is evidence of skin infection, an impairment of sensation, or an impairment of the blood supply in the part to be treated.

♦ DEEP HEATING AGENTS

These types of heating modalities emit energy in the form of electromagnetic or mechanical waves. These waves have the physical properties necessary to elevate the temperature of the tissue as far down as 30 to 50 millimeters beneath the skin's surface. Electromagnetic waves generate heat by the tissue's resistance to electric current, and mechanical waves cause a form of tissue vibration that is able to generate heat.

Deep heating by electromagnetic or mechanical waves, is called **diathermy**. It is a process of heating the tissue with

---

Procedure #42: Applying a Paraffin Bath

1. Wash your hands, identify the patient, and provide for privacy.
2. Explain the procedure to the patient.
3. Instruct the patient to remove all jewelry from his hands.
4. Cleanse and dry the skin of the hand prior to submission into the bath.
5. Instruct the patient to "dip" the hand (or other affected area) quickly in and out of the paraffin

10 to 12 times and to keep the fingers spread in order to allow the paraffin to form a glove.
6. Inform the patient that she may feel a warmth and/or tingling in the fingers and explain that such a sensation is brought on by the dilation of blood vessels from the increased heat.
7. After 20 minutes, the hand is withdrawn from the paraffin, and the glove removed.
8. Remove used paraffin and place it into the paraffin container for future use.

electromagnetic waves by warming up a wire that conducts electric current. The amount of generated heat depends on several factors and is also governed by a simple law of physics found in the study of electrical current. *Joule's Law* states that "a rise in temperature in a conductor is caused by the passage of an electric current; the degree of temperature rise is therefore dependent on the amount of heat being produced." The law further indicates that the amount of heat produced is dependent upon three proportions: it must be directly proportional to the resistance of the conductor in *ohms;* it must be directly proportional to the square of the strength of the current in *amperes;* and it must be directly proportional to the length of time the current flows.

Deep heating, or diathermy by electromagnetic waves, is accomplished through the means of a microwave or a shortwave generator.

♦ MICROWAVES

One of the most frequently used deep heating or diathermy machines currently in use is the microwave diathermy machine (see Figure 20-5).

Microwaves are located on the right of infrared in the electromagnetic spectrum since the wave length is longer than that of infrared rays but shorter than the wave length of electromagnetic waves, which can supply mechanical power. Microwaves are found within the radiowave field frequency.

A microwave machine consists of a generator, which is operated by electrical power; the director, which emits the microwaves; and a spacing gauge. The generator is a magnetron responsible for generating high-frequency electric energy, or microwaves. No part of the machine comes in contact with the patient.

The distance of the director from the body part being treated is of importance. It must be calculated accurately by the spacing gauge. The director should be perpendicular to the treated part. The intensity of the microwaves reaching the part to be treated decreases with the square of the distance between the microwave director and the body part.

Prior to microwave application, the skin of the area to be treated should be clean and dry since moisture and grease would increase the skin's resistance, thereby causing a burn. As with other heating agents, the optimal temperature elevation is obtained within 20 minutes.

Microwaves should never be applied to a patient with a cardiac pacemaker. Since the pacemaker rests beneath the patient's skin continuously sending out electrical impulses to the heat in order to maintain a regular heartbeat, microwaves could seriously interfere with the function of the pacemaker and lead to serious complications or even death.

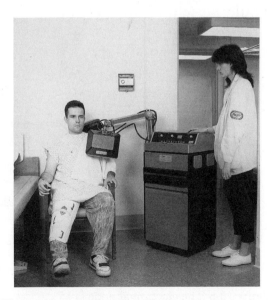

Figure 20-5 Application of microwaves.

♦ SHORTWAVES

Another form of diathermy or deep heat application, is the use of short-waves. The so-called shortwaves have a longer wave length than microwaves, and in the electromagnetic spectrum, they are located to the right of the microwave.

The shortwave diathermy machine consists of an electric power supply unit, an oscillator unit, a shortwave frequency circuit, and a patient output circuit. The widely used household alternating current is transformed by the oscillator unit into electromagnetic waves with the length and frequency of shortwaves. The shortwaves are within the radiowave frequency range.

The application of shortwave diathermy is a bit more difficult than microwave application. The shortwaves are delivered to the patient by contour applicators, inductance cable, or air-spaced electrodes. Therefore, the patient's skin must be protected with a thick Turkish towel since this type of material also absorbs for body's sweat from the surface of the skin.

The body part that is to be treated should be within the electromagnetic field that is generated between the applicator devices (see Figure 20-6). A milliampere meter is located on the panel and indicates the amount of energy being "drained" by the body. A specific meter reading will indicate that the patient output circuit has been tuned to the oscillator unit. This means that maximal flow in the area to be treated can be achieved.

Most recently, the use of shortwave diathermy has decreased, since it is being replaced more and more with microwave therapy. Contraindications for the use of shortwave therapy are generally the same as for microwaves. It must never be used in hemorrhage, acute inflammation or marked circulatory disorders, and never near metallic implants such as cardiac pacemakers.

♦ ULTRASOUND

Another deep heating treatment is the application of ultrasonic waves. Ultrasonic waves are not faster than sound but are of a higher frequency than the sound waves that can be heard by the human ear. The principles of the ultrasound wave involve electricity

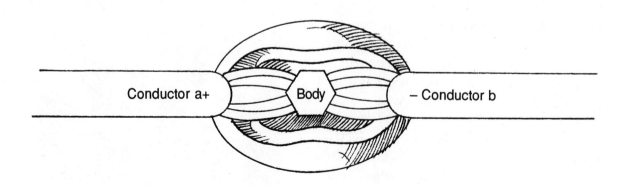

Figure 20-6 The electromagnetic field.

being supplied to a crystal of a certain physical constitution. This crystal, in turn, starts to emit ultrasonic waves that penetrate the superficial tissue and are reflected on the deep tissue. This sets up a very fine vibrating motion within the tissue, which in turn generates heat. A similar effect is the heating up of a wire that is bent back and forth rapidly.

The major difference between electromagnetic waves and ultrasound waves is that the latter are mechanical. The mechanical force of sound and ultrasound waves can be demonstrated by a membrane placed in the course of these waves. A vibrating motion takes place in the membrane. Ultrasound must also be transmitted by a media that is not compressible such as water or mineral oil.

The ultrasound machine contains a power supply and an oscillator circuit (see Figure 20-7). The latter transmits the ultrasound waves generated in the crystal to the ultrasound head. The head is moved in a stroking or circular motion over the part to be treated. These motions help to distribute the energy. A commercially available coupling agent or mineral oil must be applied with the ultrasound. Water

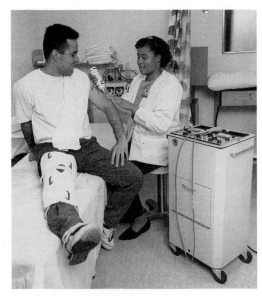

Figure 20-7 Application of ultrasound.

may also be used. While the therapeutic application of ultrasound is still quite limited, in recent years, it has had great diagnostic use in diseases of the heart and eyes.

♦ HYDROTHERAPY

Whirlpool Therapy

The whirlpool (see Figure 20-8) consists of a container filled with water and

---

Procedure #43: Application of Ultrasound

1. Wash your hands, identify the patient, and provide for privacy.
2. Explain the procedure to the patient.
3. Expose only that area which is to receive the ultrasound and drape the surrounding areas with a towel.
4. Apply a small amount of coupling agent, gel, or mineral oil to the ultrasound head.
5. Turn the machine on and set the timer for 15 to 20 minutes.
6. Apply ultrasound by using a vibrating circular motion of the head against the affected area.
7. Upon completion of the treatment, wipe off any excess oil or gel from the affected area of the body and from the ultrasound head.
8. Turn the machine off.

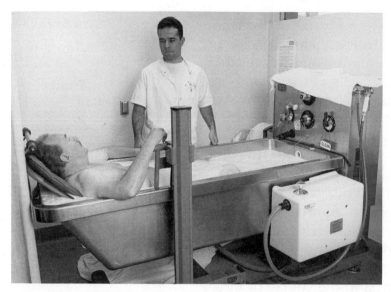

Figure 20-8 Whirlpool application.

an agitator. The agitator causes the water to move in a whirling motion that has a massaging effect on the skin and tends to dilate the blood vessels. This massaging effect also soothes pain and is therefore most widely used for disorders related to joints in the wrists, ankles, and knees, as well as in the treatment of bones after a fracture has occurred.

The whirlpool temperature generally ranges from 98 to 104 degrees Fahrenheit (37 to 40 degrees Centigrade). Much care should be exercised in adjusting the temperature of the water since allowing it to become too high may cause the patient to become disoriented or delirious. Also, submission into the whirlpool bath should never be longer than 20 minutes, and is generally a therapy used most frequently in conjunction with exercise therapy during and after its application.

Therapeutic Pool

The therapeutic pool is generally kept at a temperature of 98 degrees Fahrenheit (37 degrees Centigrade). It is usually structured in such a way as to

---

Procedure #44: Assisting the Patient with a Whirlpool Bath

1. Wash your hands, identify the patient, and provide for privacy.
2. Explain the procedure to the patient.
3. Fill the whirlpool tub with water at a temperature ranging from 98 to 104 degrees Fahrenheit (37 to 40 degrees Centigrade).
4. Assist the patient into the bath.
5. Set the timer for 20 minutes and check on the patient at frequent intervals.
6. Assist the patient out of the whirlpool.

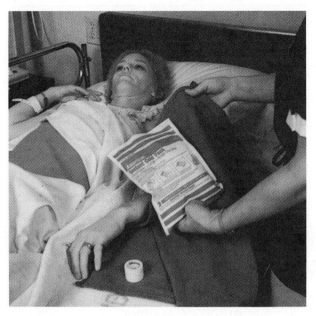
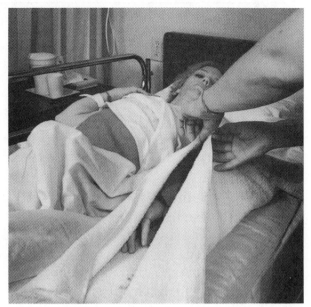

A   B

Figure 20-9 Application of cold pack. (From Hegner and Caldwell, *Nursing Assistant: A Nursing Process Approach*, 6th edition, copyright 1992 by Delmar Publishers Inc.)

have an inclining bottom so that the patient can be placed either in the deep end or in the shallow water.

This type of pool is most widely used for patients who have disorders or afflictions of the lower extremities. It is also used for gradually increasing ambulation after hip, knee, and back surgery.

The patient receiving treatment usually begins therapy by floating in the pool and then standing in deep water. This allows the patient to become buoyant, reducing the weight of the submerged body parts on the legs. Gradually the patient progresses to the shallow side, and as he goes to the shallow water, the weight on the lower extremities increases.

Walking in the therapeutic pool also helps to strengthen the muscles of the lower extremities. To overcome the resistance of the water, increased muscle activity is also required.

The therapeutic pool is a very expedient mode of treating patients, but the same results can be obtained in rehabilitation departments without the use of the pool. If a department does not have one, it does not necessarily mean that the care or treatment is inferior.

◆ COLD THERAPY

Application of cold therapy (see Figure 20-9), is generally done with a large ice cube or a plastic pack of ice cubes which have been frozen at 28 to 32 degrees Farenheit (0 to 2 degrees Centigrade). The ice is placed or rubbed over the affected area until the patient feels some numbness. This usually takes between 10 to 15 minutes. Shortly afterward, a redness of the skin will appear. This is called *erythema*. Exercise therapy is also generally initiated immediately after the application of the ice packs.

♦♦♦

Procedure #45: Applying a Cold Pack

1. Wash your hands, identify the patient, and provide for privacy.
2. Assemble all necessary equipment.
3. Explain the procedure to the patient.
4. Expose the area to be treated and note its condition.
5. Place the cold pack in a cloth covering.
6. Strike or squeeze the cold pack to activate the chemicals inside it.
7. Place the covered cold pack on the proper area and enclose it with a towel. Note the time of the application.
8. Secure the pack with tape or gauze.
9. Leave the patient in a comfortable position with a call light within reach.
10. Check on the patient at least every 10 minutes, and note any changes in the condition of the affected area.
11. If no adverse symptoms occur, remove the pack in 30 minutes.
12. Remove the pack from the cover and dispose of it in the appropriate manner.

♦♦♦

Cold therapy is frequently applied in order to reduce swelling, inflammation and spasticity.

It should always be kept in mind that the use of heating or cooling modalities or agents is considered an axillary measure to therapeutic treatment. Application of heat or cold alone usually does not offer the patient any significant benefit. Heat or cold applications are used as precursors of therapeutic programs such as exercises, gait training, or stretching.

♦ ♦ ♦
SUMMARY OUTLINE

Purpose of Physical Therapy Agents and Modalities

Application of Superficial Heating Agents
- Hydrocollator packs
- Infrared lamps
- Paraffin baths

Application of Deep Heating Agents
- Diathermy
- Microwaves
- Shortwaves
- Ultrasound

Application of Hydrotheraphy
- Whirlpool
- Therapeutic pool

Application of Cold Therapy

CHAPTER REVIEW QUESTIONS

1. _____ helps to reduce pain and tightness within muscles and stiffness in joints.

2. Complete immersion of a body part into heated water, is called _____.

3. A _____ _____ is an example of a superficial heating agent.

4. A _____ _____ is often used to treat small areas, such as the hands and feet, which are afflicted with arthritic joints.

5. _____ _____ _____ emit energy in the form of electromagnetic or mechanical waves, which eventually generate heat beneath the skin's surface.

6. _____ is a process created by the heating of tissues with electromagnetic waves by warming up a wire that conducts electric current.

7. _____ therapy should never be applied to a patient with a cardiac pacemaker.

8. The major difference between electromagnetic and ultrasonic waves is that the latter are _____.

9. A _____ is used to create a massaging effect on the skin and thus tends to dilate the blood vessels, thereby soothing pain in the affected part.

10. A _____ _____ is most widely used for patients suffering from disorders or afflictions of the lower extremities.

11. Cold therapy is frequently applied in order to reduce _____, _____, and _____.

SECTION VIII

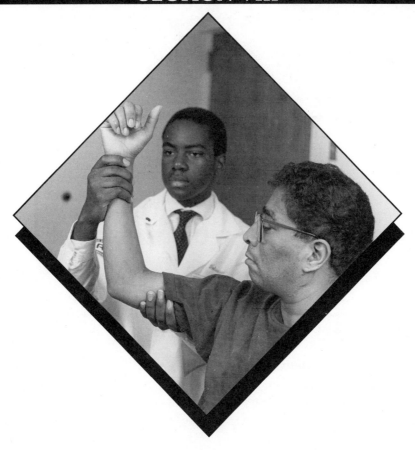

PHYSICAL THERAPY PROCEDURES

◆ ◆ ◆

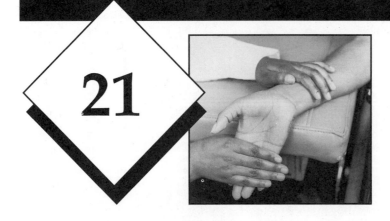

21

Performing Range of Motion Exercises

Objectives

After studying this chapter, you will be able to:

1. Describe the purpose of range of motion exercises.

2. Explain anatomical planes of motion.

3. Briefly discuss diagonal patterns of motion.

4. Identify the seven range of motion exercises used on the lower extremities.

5. Identify the 13 range of motion exercises used on the upper extremities.

VOCABULARY

Learn the meaning and the correct spelling of the following words and abbreviations:

Range of motion
Passive range of motion
Active range of motion
Anatomical position
Diagonal pattern
Flexion
Extension
Abduction
Adduction
Internal rotation
External rotation
Plantarflexion
Dorsiflexion
Inversion
Eversion
Protraction
Retraction

Range of motion exercises involve performing movements of each joint and muscle through the use of available range of motion. The execution of these exercises prevent the patient from developing contractures, muscle shortening and tightness or adhesions in capsules, ligaments, and tendons that could eventually limit mobility. Range of motion exercises involve two principles. First, the joint is ranged with respect only to its actual movement, and second, it must be ranged so that the length of the muscles actually cross the joint. It should also be noted that range of motion exercises provide the patient with sensory stimulation.

There are two types of range of motion exercises. The first, called *passive* range of motion, is generally used when the patient is unable to move a body part or when movement by the patient produces increased spasticity or other undesirable muscle tone, pain, or excessive cardiopulmonary stress. The second type of range of motion exercises are referred to as *active* range of motion. These exercises may be performed when the patient needs some help due to weakness, pain, cardiopulmonary problems, or decreased muscle tone. Unlike the passive exercises, active range of motion is usually performed independently by the patient, generally with the aide or therapist supervising in order to ensure proper performance of the exercises.

Whenever you are required to perform range of motion, you should always make sure that the body part you are working with is gently but firmly supported. The placement of your hand should allow movement of the body part through the full range with minimal hand repositioning. You should also support all segments distal to the joint at which the motion is to occur. Movements should be slow to moderate through all planes of motion available in the joint.

When performing range of motion exercises, remember that each joint should be moved through its full range for both the joint motion and the muscle length. When moving a joint through its full range of motion, multi-joint muscles, or muscles that stretch over more than one joint, must not be lengthened across all the joints over which they act.

You should always remember that maximum range is generally achieved when the body part cannot be moved further due to the restriction of tissues or bone or the patient complaints of pain. When pain is limiting the range of motion, it is time to stop the exercises.

In some cases, involuntary muscle contractions may occur and interfere with range of motion exercises. This generally happens when a patient involuntarily contracts muscles in order to avoid pain. Spasticity may also be felt as gradually increasing resistance to movement occurs. This is followed by a sudden reduction of tone. Movement

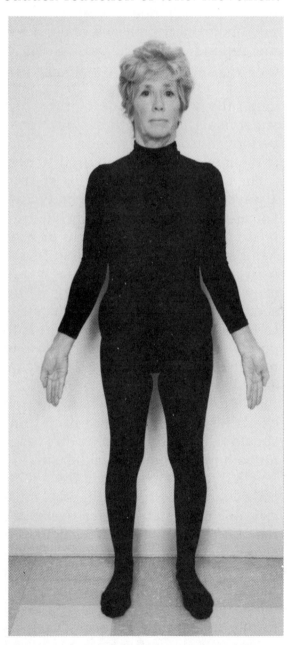

Figure 21-1 The anatomical position. (From Hegner and Caldwell *Nursing Assistant: A Nursing Process Approach,* 6th edition, copyright 1992 by Delmar Publishers Inc.)

through the remaining range of motion is then possible. If spasticity does occur, slow maintained movement will usually allow movement through the full range of motion.

◆ ANATOMICAL PLANES OF MOTION

All motions of the body are described in terms of starting from the anatomical position, that is, the position in which a person is standing upright, eyes looking straight ahead, arms at the sides with the palms facing forward, and the feet approximately four inches apart at the heels, with the toes pointing forward (see Figure 21-1). In this position, three planes are seen. The first, called the *sagital* plane, divides the body into two portions through a longitudinal axis of the trunk. The *mid-sagital plane* is an imaginary line that divides the body through an anterior-posterior mid-axis, thereby dividing it into equal right and left halves. Hence, all motions involving flexion and extension, occur in the sagital plane.

The second plane is called the *frontal plane.* It divides the body into front and back portions. All motions involving abduction and adduction occur in the frontal plane.

The third and final plane defined in the anatomical position is called the *transverse plane.* It divides the body into upper and lower portions and all movements involving rotation occur here.

◆ DIAGONAL PATTERNS OF MOTION

There are two basic diagonal patterns for movements of the extremities, and each of these patterns may be modified by

varying the position or movement of the elbow or knee, thereby providing the patient with the ability to perform both joint range of motion and muscular range of motion exercises. When combining components of motion are performed, the part may not be taken through as full of a range as when anatomical planes of motion are used. However, the mobility necessary for function is maintained.

◆ RANGE OF MOTION EXERCISES: LOWER EXTREMITIES

The following range of motion exercises are generally performed on patients who experience diseases or injuries affecting the lower extremities:

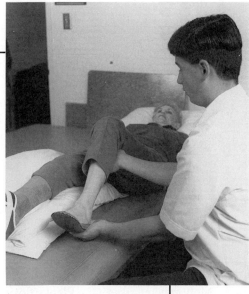

Figure 21-2 Hip and knee flexion and extension.

1. **Body segment:**   **Hip and knee**
                           (see Figure 21-2)

   Joints being ranged: Hip and knee
   Motion being used: Extension and flexion
   Placement of hands: Heel and behind knee

2. **Body segment:**   **Hip** (see Figure 21-3)
   Joints being ranged: Hip
   Motion being used: Extension
   Placement of hands: One on the pelvis for
                           stabilization; the other
                           with the forearm, used
                           to support the patient's
                           lower extremity in
                           anatomical position

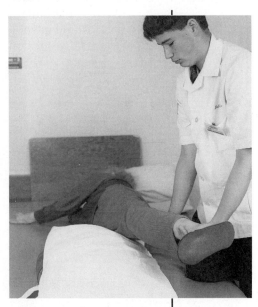

Figure 21-3 Hip extension.

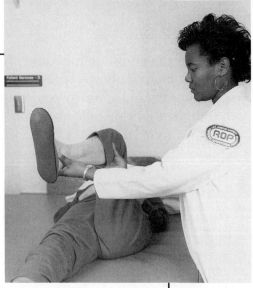

Figure 21-4 Hip abduction and adduction.

3. **Body segment:**   **Hip** (see Figure 21-4)
   Joints being ranged: Hip
   Motion being used: Abduction and
                          adduction
   Placement of hands: Heel and behind knee

4. **Body segment:**   **Hip** (see Figure 21-5)
   Joints being ranged: Hip
   Motion being used: Internal and external
                          rotation; hip and knee
                          flexed at 90 degree
                          angle
   Placement of hands: Heel and behind knee

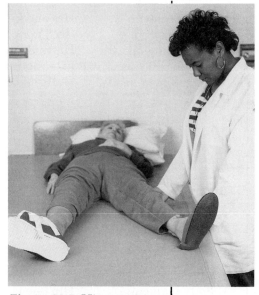

Figure 21-5 Hip rotation.

5. **Body segment:**   **Ankle** (see Figure 21-6)
   Joint being ranged: Ankle
   Motion being used: Plantarflexion and
                          dorsiflexion
   Placement of hands: Heel and dorsum of foot
                          for plantarflexion; heel
                          and lower leg for
                          dorsiflexion

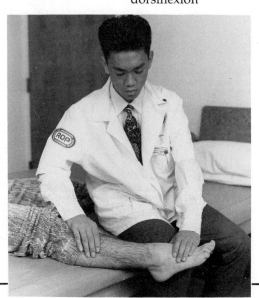

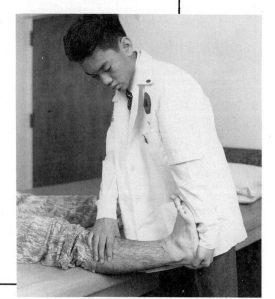

Figure 21-6 (A) Ankle plantarflexion; and (B) dorsiflexion.

6. **Body segment:**   **Foot** (see Figure 21-7)
   Joint being ranged: Foot
   Motion being used: Inversion and eversion
   Placement of hands: One hand stabilizes the lower leg and
                            the other grasps the forefoot

7. **Body segment:**   **Toes** (see Figure 21-7A, B, C, and D)
   Joint being ranged: Toes
   Motion being used: Extension and flexion
   Placement of hands: One hand stabilizes the lower leg and
                            the other grasps the toes

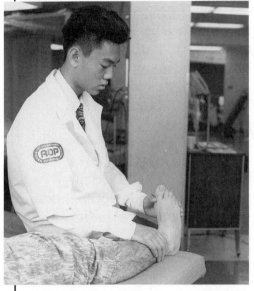

A

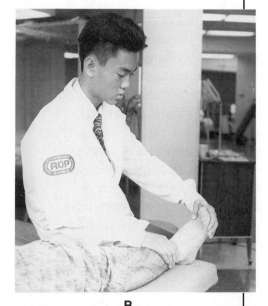

B

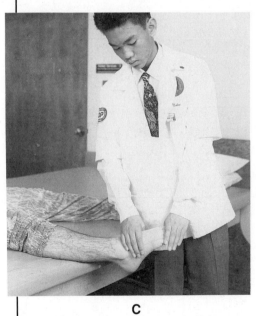

C

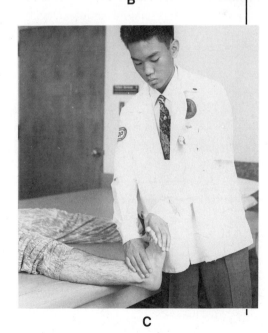

C

Figure 21-7 (A) Foot inversion; and (B) eversion; (C) Toe extension; and (D) flexion .

Procedure #46: Performing Passive Range of Motion on the Lower Extremities

1. Wash your hands, identify the patient, and provide for privacy.
2. Explain the procedure to the patient.
3. Adjust the patient's clothing or top covers and only allow for exposure of the affected area.
4. Supporting the knee and ankle, move the entire leg away from the body center (abduction) and toward the body (adduction).
5. Turn to face the bed. Supporting the knee in a bent position (flexion), raise the knee toward the pelvis (hip flexion). Straighten the knee (extension) as you lower the leg to the bed.
6. Supporting the leg at the knee and ankle, roll the leg in a circular fashion away from body (lateral hip rotation). Continuing to support the leg, roll the leg in the same fashion toward the body (medial hip rotation).
7. Grasp the patient's toes and support the ankle. Bring the toes toward the knee (dorsiflexion). Then point the toes toward the foot of the table (plantar flexion).
8. Gently turn the patient's foot inward (inversion) and outward (eversion).
9. Place your fingers over the patient's toes. Bend the toes away from the second toe (abduction) and then toward the second toe (adduction).
10. Cover the leg with clothing or a top cover and move to the opposite side.
11. Move the patient close to you and repeat steps 4 through 9.

♦ RANGE OF MOTION EXERCISES: UPPER EXTREMITIES

1. **Body segment:** **Scapulo-thoracic** (see Figure 21-8)

   Joints being ranged: Scapulo-thoracic

   Motion being used: Protraction and retraction

   Placement of hands: One hand placed over the acromion and the other placed behind the scapula

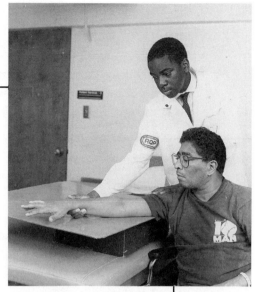

Figure 21-8 Scapulo–thoracic protraction and retraction.

2. **Body segment:** **Shoulder** (see Figure 21-9)

   Joints being ranged: Shoulder

   Motion being used: Extension and flexion

   Placement of hands: One hand supports the wrist and hand while the other supports the upper arm

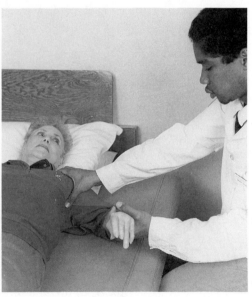
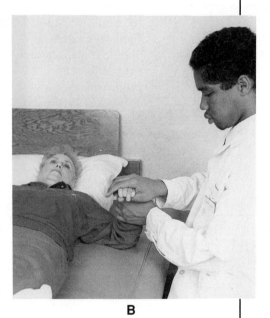

A   B

Figure 21-9 (A) Shoulder extension; and (B) flexion .

3. **Body segment:**   **Shoulder and elbow** (see Figure 21-10)
   Joints being ranged: Shoulder and elbow
   Motion being used: Flexion
   Placement of hands: One hand supports the wrist and hand while the other supports the upper arm

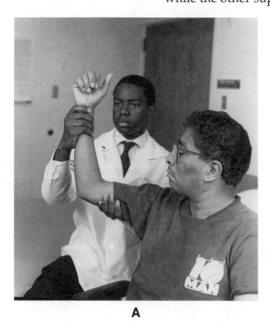 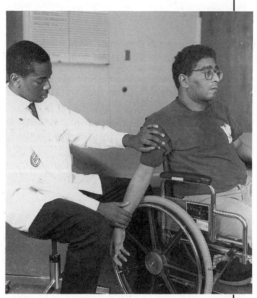

A   B

Figure 21-10 Shoulder and elbow flexion.

4. **Body segment:**   **Shoulder, elbow and forearm** (see Figure 21-11) shoulder and elbow
   Joints being ranged:
   Motion being used: Shoulder and elbow extension with pronation; shoulder and elbow flexion with supination

   Placement of hands: One hand supports the wrist and hand while the other supports the upper arm; the aide's left hand should support the patient's right wrist and hand

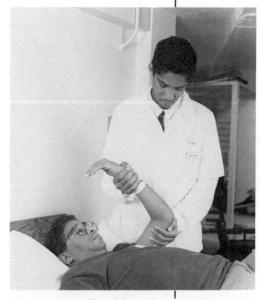

Figure 21-11 Shoulder, elbow, and forearm flexion and extension and pronation and supination.

5. **Body segment:** **Shoulder** (see Figure 21-12)
   Joints being ranged: Shoulder
   Motion being used: Abduction
   Placement of hands: One hand stabilizes the shoulder girdle while the other hand and forearm supports the patient's upper extremity

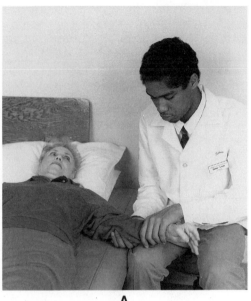
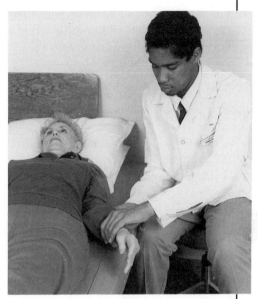

A   B

Figure 21-12 Shoulder abduction.

6. **Body segment:** **Shoulder** (see Figure 21-13)
   Joints being ranged: Shoulder
   Motion being used: Adduction and flexion; the shoulder is abducted 90 degrees while the elbow is flexed to 90 degrees
   Placement of hands: One hand stabilizes the shoulder girdle while the other grasps the forearm

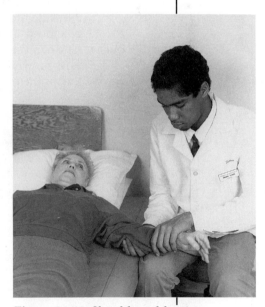

Figure 21-13 Shoulder adduction.

7. **Body segment:**   **Shoulder** (see Figure 21-14)
    Joints being ranged: Shoulder
    Motion being used: Internal rotation; the
                            shoulder is abducted
                            90 degrees while the
                            elbow is flexed to 90
                            degrees
    Placement of hands: One hand stabilizes the
                            shoulder girdle while
                            the other grasps the
                            patient's forearm

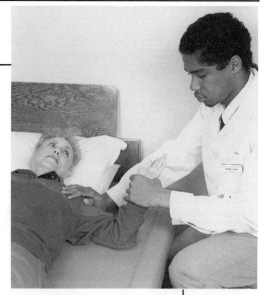

Figure 21-14 Shoulder internal rotation.

8. **Body segment:**   **Shoulder** (see Figure 21-15)
    Joints being ranged: Shoulder
    Motion being used: External rotation; the
                            shoulder is abducted 90
                            degrees while the elbow
                            is flexed 90 degrees
    Placement of hands: One hand stabilizes the
                            shoulder girdle while
                            the other grasps the
                            patient's forearm

9. **Body segment:**   **Wrist** (see Figure 21-16)
    Joints being ranged: Wrist
    Motion being used: Flexion and extension;
                            the elbow is flexed,
                            allowing the fingers to
                            be moved
    Placement of hands: One hand stabilizes the
                            forearm while the other
                            grasps the patient's hand

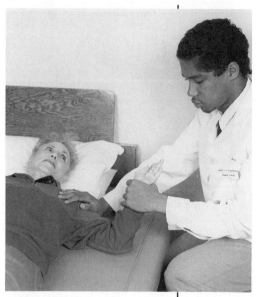

Figure 21-15 Shoulder external rotation.

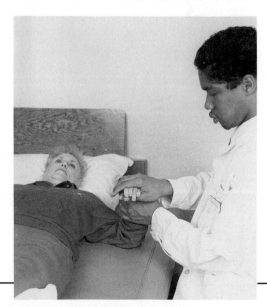

A

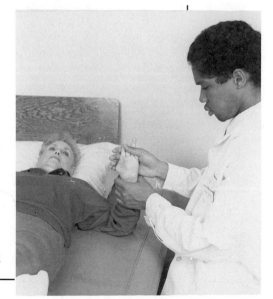

B

Figure 21-16 Wrist flexion and extension.

10. **Body segment:**   **Fingers** (see Figure 21-17)
    Joints being ranged: Fingers
    Motion being used: Flexion and extension; the wrist is in the anatomical position allowing the elbow to be flexed 90 degrees
    Placement of hands: One hand stabilizes the forearm while the other grasps the fingers

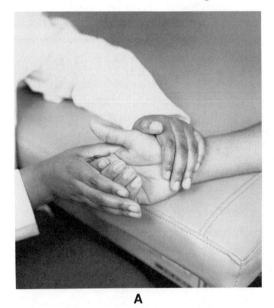

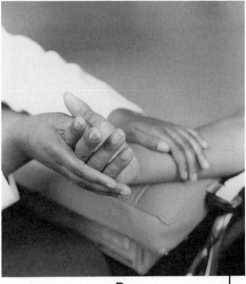

A   **B**

Figure 21-17 Fingers flexion and extension.

11. **Body segment:**   **Wrist and fingers** (see Figure 21-18)
    Joints being ranged: Wrist and fingers
    Motion being used: Wrist extension with finger extension; wrist flexion with finger flexion; the elbow is extended
    Placement of hands: One hand grasps the wrist while the other grasps the fingers

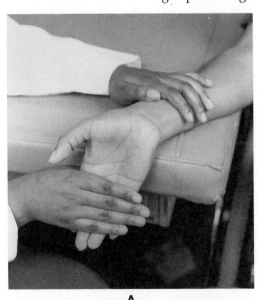

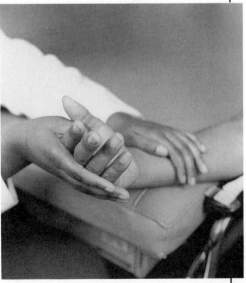

A   **B**

Figure 21-18 Wrist and fingers flexion and extension.

Procedure #47: Performing Passive Range of Motion on the Upper Extremities

1. Wash your hands, identify the patient, and provide for privacy.
2. Explain the procedure to the patient.
3. Position the patient on his back close to you.
4. Adjust the patient's clothing or top cover to keep the patient covered as much as possible.
5. Turn the patient's head gently from side to side (rotation).
6. Bend the patient's head toward the right shoulder and then toward the left shoulder (lateral flexion).
7. Bring the chin toward the chest (flexion).
8. Place a pillow under the shoulders and gently support the head in a backward tilt (hyperextension). Return to the straight position (extension). Adjust the pillow under the head and shoulders.
9. Supporting the elbow and wrist, exercise the shoulder joint by bringing the entire arm out at a right angle to the body (horizontal abduction) and returning the arm to a position parallel to the body (horizontal adduction).
10. With the arm parallel to the body, roll the entire arm toward the body (internal rotation of the shoulder). Maintaining the parallel position, roll the entire arm away from the body (external rotation of the shoulder).
11. With the shoulder in abduction, flex the elbow and raise the entire arm over the head (shoulder flexion).
12. With the arm parallel to the body (palm up— supination), flex and extend the elbow.
13. Flex and extend the wrist. Flex and extend each finger joint.
14. Move each finger, in turn, away from the middle finger (abduction), and toward the middle finger (adduction).
15. Abduct the thumb by moving it toward the extended fingers.
16. Touch the thumb to the base of the little finger, then to each fingertip (opposition).
17. Turn the hand palm down (pronation), then turn it palm up (supination).
18. Grasp the patient's wrist with one hand and the patient's hand with the other. Bring the wrist toward the body (inversion) and then away from the body (eversion).
19. Move the patient close to you and repeat steps 5 through 18.

◆ ◆ ◆
SUMMARY OUTLINE

Performing Range of Motion Exercises
- Muscle movement
- Joint movement
- Passive range of motion
- Active range of motion

Anatomical Planes of Motion
- Anatomical position

Diagonal Patterns of Motion

Range of Motion Exercises
- Lower extremities
- Upper extremities

CHAPTER REVIEW QUESTIONS

1. Range of motion exercises involve performing movements of
   _____ and _____.
2. _____ range of motion is generally used when the patient
   is unable to move the affected body part.
3. _____ range of motion is generally used when the patient
   is able to assist in moving the affected body part.
4. The physical therapy aide should always remember to
   _____ all segments farthest away from the origin of the
   range of motion.
5. In some cases, _____ _____ _____ may interfere
   with range of motion exercises.
6. The _____ position describes the position in which the
   patient stands upright, eyes looking straight ahead, arms at
   sides with the palms forward, and feet approximately four
   inches apart.
7. A _____ plane divides the body into right and left sides.
8. A _____-_____ plane divides the body into exact right
   and left halves.
9. The _____ plane divides the body into front and back
   sections.
10. The _____ plane divides the body into upper and lower
    portions.

11. Match the correct answers in Column A with its
    appropriate response in Column B:

Column A	Column B
thumb	protraction and retraction
foot	extension and flexion
hand	opposition
ankle	abduction
scapulo-thoracic	abduction and adduction
shoulder	inversion and eversion
hip and knee	internal and external rotation
hip	plantarflexion and dorsalflexion

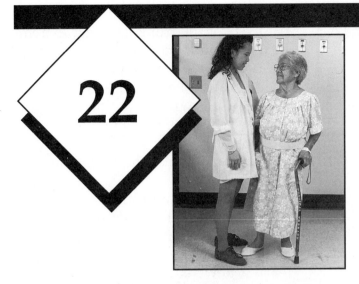

Assisting with Ambulation

Objectives

After studying this chapter, you will be able to:

1. Define the term ambulation and discuss the physical therapy aide's role in assisting the patient with it.

2. Briefly explain how to choose the appropriate ambulatory device for a patient's use.

3. Identify four basic ambulatory devices and briefly discuss the physical therapy aide's role in assisting the patient to use them.

4. Delineate the difference between a two-point gait, a three-point gait, and a four-point gait as each relates to crutch walking.

5. Describe the difference between a swing-to and a swing-through gait, and briefly explain how each relates to crutch walking.

6. Briefly explain the physical therapy aide's role in assisting the patient to walk up and down stairs, using crutches.

Ambulation is a term that means *to walk*. It is a functional activity that some patients may be able to accomplish, but for others, because of physical limitations or disabilities affecting the lower extremities, may be completely impossible or only possible with the aid of an assistive device. The ambulatory aid or device a patient needs depends on the type of disability she may have. Ambulation aids can be prescribed by a physician only after a careful evaluation of the patient's general condition and the specific gait disability.

Generally speaking, assistive devices are used to make safe ambulation possible. The three main indications for such devices include a decreased ability to bear weight on the lower extremities, resulting from structural damage of the skeletal system; muscle weakness or paralysis of the trunk or lower extremities; and poor balance in the upright posture. These devices may also be used to increase the patient's base of support, allowing a redistribution of weight within the base of support and a larger area within which the center of gravity can shift without the patient's losing balance.

Whenever an ambulatory device is used, the amount of energy the patient puts out is generally very high. This, coupled with the necessity of having to learn a new sequence of walking, can cause the patient to tire quite rapidly. Therefore, in early training sessions, the patient usually requires greater concentration in order to learn the proper gait.

Under the supervision and guidance of a physical therapist, you may be allowed to introduce the patient to the proper use of ambulatory aids. You should remember, however, that some of these patients may be so weakened by disease or prolonged bedrest that a preambulatory therapy program may be necessary before ambulation training begins. Such a program may consist of range of motion and strengthening exercises for the upper extremities, especially for the muscles extending to the elbow and the muscles depressing the shoulder.

◆ TIPS ON PREAMBULATION TEACHING

Part of the preambulation program may consist of teaching the patient newly acquired gait patterns. To provide maximum stability, this often begins with bringing the patient to the parallel bars since they require the least amount of coordination by the patient.

By practicing on the parallel bars, the patient can become accustomed to the upright posture and learn the sequence for gait or walking in relative safety. Also, assistive devices or aids may be fitted while the patient stands between the parallel bars.

Whatever device may be prescribed for the patient's use, it is the task of the physical therapy team member to describe and demonstrate its proper use to him, as well as the appropriate gait sequence, before ambulation begins. Usually, a demonstration is the primary method of instruction, but a verbal description reinforces the demonstration. Verbal descriptions should always be kept to a minimum. Observing other patients who may be using the same or similar devices can also be a useful method of instruction.

Once a patient has become proficient on level surfaces, instruction or teaching in the use of stairs, curbs, ramps, and doors can be given. The patient should be taught to climb and descend stairs on the right-hand side since this is the usual method used throughout the United States. Teaching the patient to sit down and stand up when using arm-less chairs, low or soft sofas and chairs, toilets, and car seats may also be necessary. In addition, the patient should also be instructed on how to protect herself during a fall and how to get up after the fall has occurred.

Finally, it is important to teach the patient how to check his ambulatory aid for its safe operation and use. Wing nuts used on crutches, for example, often loosen with prolonged use. The rubber tips of assistive devices will not grip the floor properly if they become too worn or dirt fills their grooves. The patient should also be warned to avoid small throw rugs that may slip or

become entangled when the ambulatory aid is placed on them.

◆ CHOOSING THE APPROPRIATE DEVICE

As we have previously discussed, the type of ambulatory device or aid the patient uses, is generally dependent upon the type or disability she has. Some devices provide more stability and support than others; some require more coordination. As the patient's limitations decrease, she may also progress from a device that provides more stability and support to one that provides less. Other patients may continue to use the same aid throughout the entire time an assistive device is required. Some of the more frequently used devices include parallel bars, walkers, crutches, and canes.

Parallel Bars

Parallel bars, as we have already stated, are generally used as the first step in teaching the patient to ambulate (see Figure 22-1). Because of their stability, they tend to give the patient a sense of security, as well as assisting the patient in initial standing and walking.

The use of parallel bars actually helps the patient to propel himself forward more with his hands than with his legs. To induce him gradually to place more body weight on his lower extremities, encourage him to put the palm of his hands on the bars without gripping them.

The height and width of the bars are extremely important. They should be adjusted to fit the individual patient, with the height being such that the elbows are bent 25 to 30 degrees when

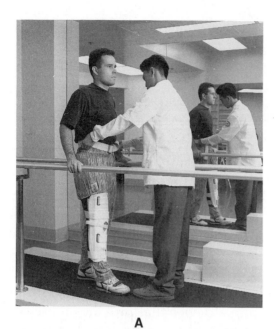

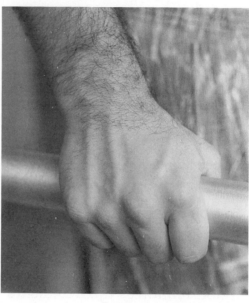

A

B

Figure 22-1 Patient using the parallel bars.

the patient is standing and holding on to the bars with his hands.

Walker

After the patient has been able to master the parallel bars, the next step is to instruct her in the use of a walker. Generally made of aluminum, this device consists of a frame with four adjustable legs (see Figure 22-2). Each of the legs has a rubber tip in order to prevent sliding.

The walker serves the same function as the parallel bars but is not as stable. It can be used at home and in the hospital and can be easily transported. The height of the walker should be adjusted to the individual patient, so that the elbow can be flexed 25 to 30 degrees when the patient is standing with her hands on it.

When ambulating with a walker, the walker is first lifted with both hands and then placed forward 25 to 30 centimeters. Then it is stepped into, first with the stronger leg and then with the weaker leg.

If the patient can only bear weight on one lower extremity or has one leg amputated, she must place the walker

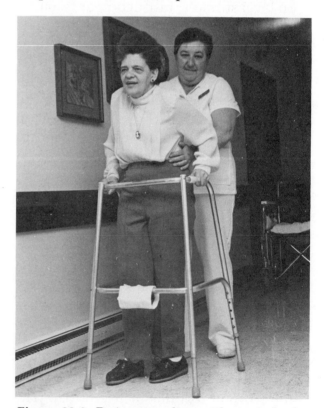

Figure 22-2 Patient standing with a standard walker. (From Simmers, *Diversified Health Occupations*, 2nd edition, copyright 1988 by Delmar Publishers Inc..)

forward and then lift her body weight. This is accomplished by pressing down on the walker while stepping into it with the weight-bearing extremity. The lifting of the body weight is done by the shoulders.

A walker may be used only on level ground and, as we previously mentioned, can be easily transported, however, it is useless on stairs. A hinged walker may be occasionally used for stair walking, but it does not provide as much stability as the standard walker.

Walkers are most helpful in the early stages of training for patients who will eventually be able to use lesser ambulatory aids such as crutches or a cane. However, it is used frequently as a permanent walking aid for elderly people who are confined to a specific area of the home or hospital or who have difficulty with balance and coordination.

♦ CRUTCHES

Once the patient is secure with the walker, he is ready to begin ambulating with crutches.

Procedure #48: Assisting the Patient to Ambulate with a Walker

1. Wash your hands, identify the patient, and provide for privacy. Obtain the necessary equipment.
2. Explain the procedure to the patient.
3. Check the walker. Make sure the rubber suction tips are secure on all the legs. Check for rough or damaged edges on the hand rests.
4. If possible, position the patient in a standing position, a wall or chair may be used for support. Make sure the patient is wearing walking shoes with a one to one-and-one-half inch heel.
5. Check the height of the walker to see if the hand rests are level with the top of the femur and the elbows can be flexed at a 25 to 30 degree angle.
6. Start with the walker in position; the patient should be standing inside the walker.
7. Tell the patient to lift the walker and place it forward so the back legs are even with the patient's toes.
8. Instruct the patient to transfer her weight forward slightly to the walker.
9. Instruct the patient to use the walker for support and to walk into the walker.
10. Repeat steps 7 through 9. While the patient is using the walker, you should walk to the side of and slightly behind her. Be alert at all times and be ready to catch the patient if she starts to fall.
11. Check the patient constantly to see that she is lifting the walker to move it forward. Also make sure the patient is placing the walker just up to the toes and is not attempting too large a step.
12. Note the patient's progress and report any problems to the therapist.
13. Replace the equipment.

There are two basic types of crutches. The first, called *axillary crutches*, can be made of wood or aluminum, and are generally used for patients who will need crutches for a relatively short period of time. They are easier to use than forearm crutches, but are also more restrictive. The second type of crutch, called a *Lofstrand crutch*, are recommended for patients who will need crutches permanently or for long periods of time, and who have the stability, strength, and coordination to use them. These crutches, commonly referred to as "forearm" crutches, allow the patient greater maneuverability and are less wearing on the patient's clothing.

Crutch Walking

The standard axillary crutch is composed of two uprights and an adjustable bottom, which are secured to the uprights with two screws, an axillary crossbar joining the uprights at the upper end, and a handgrip that can be adjusted (see Figure 22-3). They must be rubber-tipped at the bottom in order to not slip on the floor. In crutch walking, the patient shifts about 50 percent of the weight-bearing load from his legs to his arms and crutches. Therefore, the crutches must be fitted to the individual patient.

In the standard position, the tips of the crutches should be approximately 15 to 20 centimeters in front and 15 to 20 centimenters to the side of the toes. A "tripod" base is formed with the patient's feet and the crutches. To place the body center of gravity more toward the base of the tripod, you must ask the patient to bring his hips forward. You should also instruct him to look straight ahead in the direction he will walk, not down at the tip of the crutches and his feet as he may have a tendency to do.

You must instruct the patient not to bear weight on the axillary crossbar

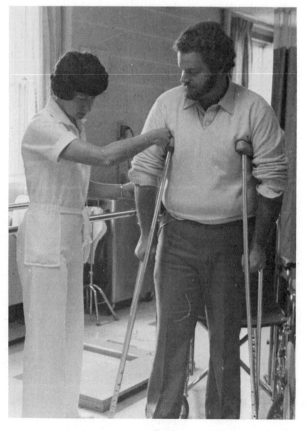

A

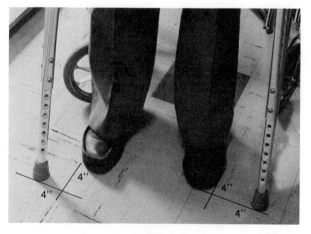

B

Figure 22-3 (A) Standard crutch; (B) Patient standing with axillary crutches. (From Simmers, *Diversified Health Occupations*, 2nd edition, copyright 1988 by Delmar Publishers Inc.)

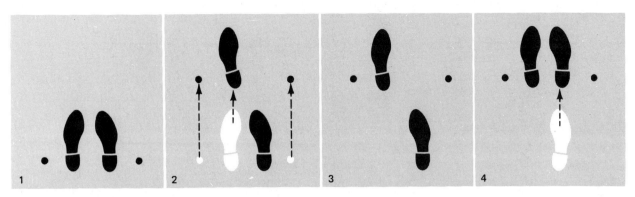

Figure 22-4 The three–point gait. (From Simmers, *Diversified Health Occupations*, 2nd edition, copyright 1988 by Delmar Publishers Inc.)

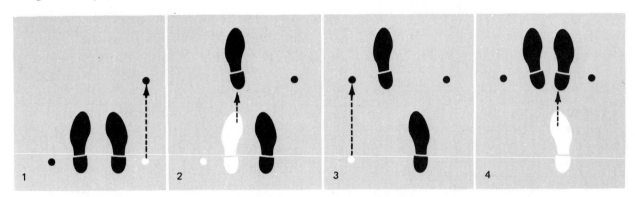

Figure 22-5 The four–point gait. (From Simmers, *Diversified Health Occupations*, 2nd edition, copyright 1988 by Delmar Publishers Inc.)

since this can cause undue impairment of the nerves or arteries that supply the arm and hand, causing the patient to complain of numbness in his arms or hands.

Different types of gaits may be used with crutches, depending upon the patient's disability or limitations. If one leg is not affected and the patient can tolerate full weight bearing, the crutches are moved forward with the affected limb. This is called a three-point gait (see Figure 22-4). This type of gait is generally used for patients who have had hip or knee surgery.

Another gait, called the four-point gait, is usually indicated for a patient who is able to move her legs alternately, but may not be able to bear the full weight on either leg without the support of crutches (see Figure 22-5). With this gait, the legs and crutches move in the sequence of left crutch-right foot, right crutch-left foot. Hence, when the patient is using the crutches in this manner, you can assume that she is actually ambulating with four legs. In the four-point gait, only one leg or crutch is off the floor at one time, leaving three points for support, and thereby creating a very stable and safe gait.

The two-point gait is a modification of the four-point gait and is closest to the natural rhythm of walking. In this gait, the right crutch and left leg move together and the left crutch and the right leg move together (see Figure 22-6).

For patients who may suffer from paralysis of both lower extremities or who are unable to move the legs alternately, the swing-to or swing-through gaits may be used.

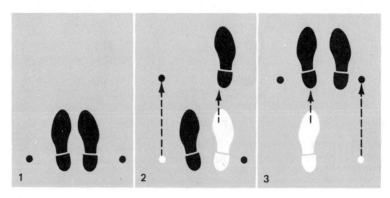

Figure 22-6 The two–point gait. (From Simmers, *Diversified Health Occupations*, 2nd edition, copyright 1988 by Delmar Publishers Inc.)

In the swing-to gait, the patient assumes a standing position and places her full body weight down on the hand-grips of the crutches by extending her elbows, Figure 22-7A. While standing, she thrusts the pelvis forward in order to place the center of gravity behind her hip joints. With the feet placed firmly in line with the crutches, the patient lifts her body and swings forward, Figure 22-7B. At that point, both crutches are moved forward again to end directly under the arm.

The swing-through gait, is similar to the swing-to gait except the feet are placed ahead of the crutches and then the crutches are brought in front of the feet again. This form of gait generally

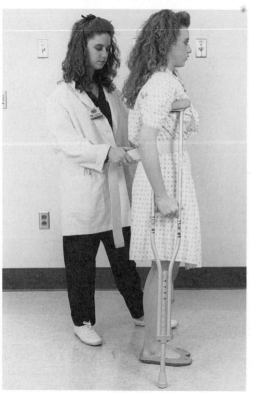

A

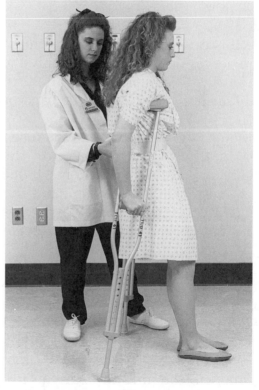

B

Figure 22-7 The swing–to gait.

◆◆◆

Procedure #49: Assisting Patient to Ambulate with Crutches

1. Wash your hands, identify the patient, and provide for privacy. Obtain the necessary equipment.
2. Explain the procedure to the patient.
3. Check the patient's order or obtain authorization from your supervior to ascertain which gait the therapist taught the patient.
4. Check the crutches. Make sure there are rubber suction tips on the bottoms. Check to be sure the axillary bar and hand rest are covered with padding.
5. If possible, position the patient in a standing position leaning against a wall for support. Advise the patient to bear weight on the unaffected leg. A chair can be used for additional support.
6. Make sure that the patient is wearing walking shoes with a one to one-and-one-half inch heel.
7. Check the measurement of the crutches: position crutches four inches to the side of the feet; make sure there is a two-inch gap between the axilla and the axillary bar or rest. If the length must be adjusted, check with your supervisor; the elbow must be flexed at a 30 degree angle. If the hand rest must be adjusted to get to this angle, check with your supervisor.
8. Assist the patient with the required gait. The gait used depends on the patient's injury and condition and is determined by the therapist or physician.
9. To assist the patient with a four-point gait, start in a standing position with the crutches at the patient's sides. The patient must be able to bear weight on both legs.
   a. Move right crutch forward.
   b. Move left foot forward.
   c. Move left crutch forward.
   d. Move right foot forward.
10. To assist the patient with a three-point gait, start in a standing position with the crutches at the patient's side. The patient must be able to bear weight on one leg only.
    a. Advance both crutches and the weak or affected foot.
    b. Transfer body weight forward to the crutches.
    c. Advance unaffected or good foot forward.
11. To assist the patient with a two point gait, start in a standing position with the crutches at the patient's side. The patient must be able to bear weight on both legs.
    a. Move the right foot and left crutch forward at the same time.
    b. Move the left foot and right crutch forward at the same time.
12. To assist the patient with a swing-to gait, start in a standing position with the crutches at the patient's side.
    a. Balance weight on one foot or both feet. Move both

crutches forward.

b. Transfer the weight forward.

c. Use shoulder and arm strength to swing the feet up to crutches.

13. To assist the patient with a swing-through gait, start in a standing position with the crutches at the patient's side.

a. Balance the weight on one foot or both feet.

b. Advance both crutches forward at the same time.

c. Transfer the weight forward.

d. Use shoulder and arm strength to swing up to and through the crutches, stopping slightly in front of the crutches.

14. While using the crutches, do not allow the patient to rest her body weight on the axillary rest. The shoulder and arm strength should provide the movement on the crutches.

15. Check to be sure that the patient is not moving too far at one time. Distances should be limited. If the patient attempts to move the crutches too far forward, it is very easy for her to lose balance and fall forward.

16. Check the patient's progress and report it to therapist.

17. When the patient is finished using crutches, replace all equipment.

requires very strong shoulder and arm muscles. It is a very fast gait, but it can usually be mastered by a young, strong patient.

Crutch Walking and Chairs

Another problem a patient experiences with crutch walking is the use of a chair. In addition to learning how to walk with the crutches, the patient must also be instructed in how to sit down and stand up from chairs of varying heights. Such techniques are taught at the beginning of the crutch ambulation program so the patient can practice them when she stops to rest during an ambulatory session.

It is important to remember that the mode of getting in and out of a chair with crutches will depend greatly on the type of chair and the patient's limitations. Generally speaking, the method safest for the patient is usually the pre-ferred one. The chair should be well supported and should not be allowed to slide. The crutches should be removed from under the arms and held in one hand, freeing the other hand for support when the patient sits down. With her free hand, the patient should push down on the chair seat or armrest in order to support her weight. Finally, she lowers herself into the chair by gradually flexing the elbow. To stand up from the chair, the patient follows the reverse order of sitting down.

If the patient is required to use the Lofstrand type of crutch, she will find greater support than that of the standard axillary type. Instead of one point of support, like the handgrip of a cane, these "forearm" crutches have two points, the handgrip and the forearm cuff (see Figure 22-8). As with the standard axillary crutches, rubber tips prevent slipping on the floor, and the forms of gait are the same as with the axillary crutches.

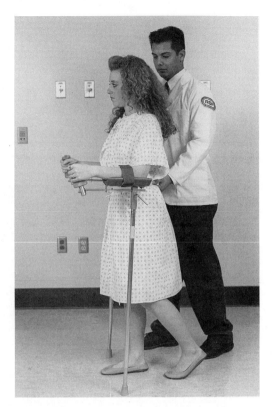

Figure 22-8 Forearm or Lofstrand crutches.

Stair Walking and Crutches

If the patient finds herself in a position where stair walking is required, you will have to remind her that the stress is always on the leg that does the lifting of the body weight by extension in the hip and knee. When walking upstairs, the good leg must be placed on the next higher step first (Figure 22-9A) while the ambulatory aid supports the impaired leg on the step below. The walking aid and the impaired leg must be brought up together (Figure 22-9B). When walking downstairs, the impaired leg comes first with the ambulatory aid while the good leg has to bear the body weight when flexed with the hip and knee (see Figure 22-10).

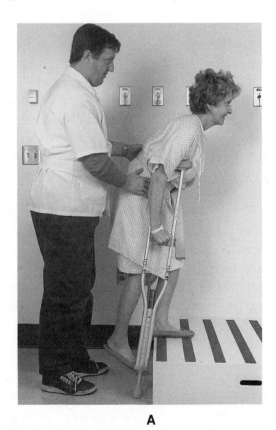

A

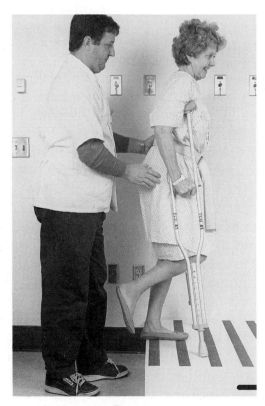

B

Figure 22-9 Going upstairs with crutches.

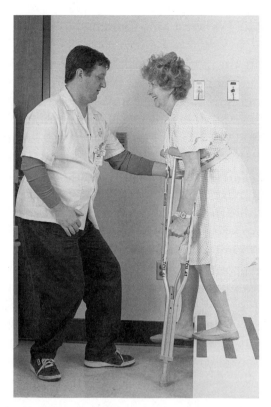

Figure 22-10 Going downstairs with crutches.

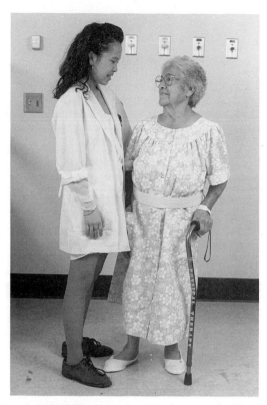

Figure 22-11 The standard cane.

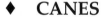 **CANES**

The use of a cane as an ambulatory aid is a convenient device for relieving one extremity of some weight-bearing load. Constructed of either wood or aluminum, this device is also able to provide the patient with continuous stability.

The length of a cane should always be adjusted so that the elbow is bent approximately 25 to 30 degrees when standing with the cane (see Figure 22-11). In most physical therapy departments, adjustable aluminum canes are also available for patient training and measurement.

The cane should always be used in the hand opposite the impaired leg. There are several reasons for this. First, the leg and opposite arm move together in normal walking. Second, a wider base is provided in order to increase stability. Finally, the shift of the center of gravity from one side to the other is eliminated.

When we speak of a cane, we are generally referring to a unilateral walking aid. Therefore, an axillary or forearm crutch can be used like a cane. When these are used properly, approximately 20 to 30 pounds of stress is placed on the cane and about 40 pounds of stress is placed onto the forearm crutch.

In order to assure more stability in elderly people, a three- or four-legged cane may be used. This type of ambulatory aid is most useful on level ground, but its greatest limitation is that it only allows for a slow gait. Hence, if the patient were to try to walk faster, a rocking action from the two rear legs to the front legs or leg might develop. This rocking action defeats the goal of the increased stability, or the very purpose of the use of the cane.

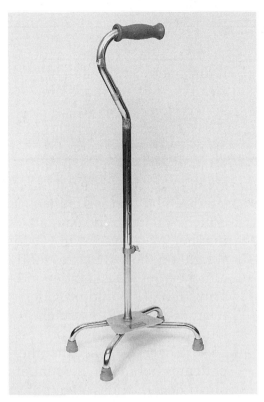

Figure 22-12 The four–legged cane.

The three- or four-legged cane is extremely useful for most elderly people since their gait tends to be slower anyway. Also, people who suffer from hemiparesis after a stroke may derive greater benefit from this type of cane since it can also be used on stairs with a very wide or low step (see Figure 22-12).

Another type of ambulatory walking aid that may be used as a cane, is the hemiwalker (see Figure 22-13A). With this device, the patient holds the walker like a cane (Figure 22-13B), on the opposite side with one hand. Increased stability is gained, but the patient can only ambulate slowly. The walker has four points of contact with the floor, but, again, a faster gait could result in a rocking motion that would eliminate the stabilizing effect.

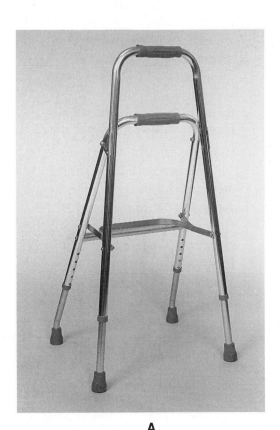

A

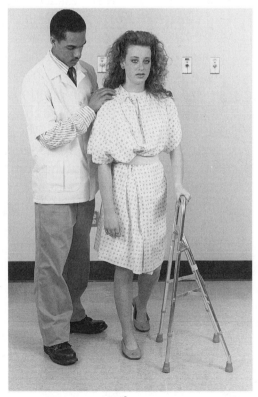

B

Figure 22-13 (A) The Hemiwalker; (B) in use.

Procedure #50: Ambulating a Patient Using Crutches

1. Check the doctor's orders in order to ensure proper authorization for the use of crutches and to determine what type of gait should be taught.
2. Obtain the proper crutches. You will need to make sure that they are the proper size and both bottom ends have rubber suction tips. Also make sure that the axillary bar and handrests are covered with padding.
3. Wash your hands.
4. If at all possible, have the patient stand leaning against a wall for ample support. Advise him to bear weight on the unaffected leg. If necessary, you may use a chair for additional support.
5. Make sure that the patient is wearing sturdy walking shoes, with a heel that is no more than one-and-one-half inches high.
6. Check the measurement of the crutches. This is accomplished by positioning the crutches four inches in front of the patient's feet and moving them four inches to the side of the foot. There should be no more than a two-inch gap between the axilla (armpit) and the axillary bar. The elbow is then flexed to a 30 degree angle. Any adjustment to the handrest should be cleared by your immediate supervisor.
7. Assist the patient with the appropriate gait, that is, four-point, three-point, two-point, swing-to, or swing-through.
8. While ambulating with the crutches, remind the patient that he must never rest his body weight on the axillary rest of the crutches, and his shoulder and arm strength should provide the movement of the crutches.
9. During the ambulation process, be sure to check to see that the patient is not moving too far at one time. If he does attempt to move too far too quickly, slow him down so that he does not lose his balance or fall forward.
10. At the completion of the ambulation, report the patient's progress and tolerance to the activity to the therapist or your immediate supervisor. At that time, a determination will be made as to whether or not the patient is ready for a more advanced gait.
11. After the patient has finished the crutch walking, replace the crutches to their proper location.
12. Wash your hands.

Procedure #51: Ambulating a Patient Using a Cane

1. Check the doctor's orders to make sure the patient should be ambulated with a cane and determine what type of gait should be taught.
2. Obtain the appropriate cane. Check its size and make sure that it has a rubber suction tip. If the patient needs additional stability, use a tripod or quad cane.
3. Wash your hands.
4. If at all possible, try to position the patient in a standing position, using the wall or a chair for additional support. Make sure the patient is wearing shoes with a heel no more than one to one-and-one-half inches high.
5. Check the height of the cane to make sure that the top of it reaches the femur and that the patient's elbow is flexed at a 25 to 30 degree angle.
6. Instruct the patient to use the cane on the unaffected side.
7. Assist the patient with her gait, as necessary.
8. While ambulating with the cane, try to make sure that the patient does not try to take too large a step since this may cause her to lose her balance or fall.
9. Note the patient's progress and report it to the therapist or your supervisor.
10. Replace the cane, as necessary, to its proper location.
11. Wash your hands.

♦♦♦

Procedure #52: Ambulating a Patient Using a Walker

1. Check the doctor's orders to obtain proper authorization for the walker.
2. Bring the walker to the patient.
3. Wash your hands.
4. Check the walker to ensure that it is in proper working condition. Make sure that the rubber suction tips are secured on all of the legs.
5. If possible, have the patient stand, using the wall or a chair to lean against. Make sure the patient is wearing sturdy shoes with heels no higher than one to one-and-one-half inches.
6. Check the height of the walker to make sure that the hand rests are level to the top of the patient's femur and that the patient's elbows are flexed at a 25 to 30 degree angle.
7. Start moving with the walker with the patient standing inside of it.
8. Instruct the patient to lift the walker and place it forward so that the back legs are even with his toes. Follow that command with instruction to transfer his weight forward slightly to the walker.
9. Tell the patient to use the walker for support and to walk into it.
10. Remain with the patient while he continues to practice using the walker. Since use of this ambulatory device may seem difficult at first, you should remain alert at all times and be ready to catch the patient if he starts to fall.
11. Determine the patient's progress and tolerance to the activity and report it to the therapist or your supervisor.
12. Replace the walker to its proper location.
13. Wash your hands.

♦♦♦

♦ ♦ ♦
SUMMARY OUTLINE

Assisting with Ambulation
- Defining ambulation
- Physical therapy aide's role
- Tips on preambulation teaching

Choosing the Appropriate Ambulatory Device
- Parallel bars
- Walker
- Crutches and crutch walking
- Canes
- Hemiwalker

CHAPTER REVIEW QUESTIONS

1. The term _____ means to walk.
2. The physical therapy aide may use _____ _____ to make walking easier for the patient.
3. The goal of the physical therapy team member is to _____ and _____ proper walking and gait movement to the patient.
4. The type of assistive device used by a patient depends greatly upon her _____.
5. _____ _____ are generally used as the first step toward teaching a patient to walk.
6. A _____ is almost always used after the patient becomes stable with his walking.
7. Two types of crutches that may be used as assistive devices include _____ crutches and _____ crutches.
8. In the standing position, the tips of the crutches should always be approximately _____ centimeters in front and _____ centimeters to the side of the toes.
9. If one leg is not affected and the patient can tolerate full weight bearing, she will use a _____ gait for crutch-walking.
10. In the _____ gait, only one leg or crutch is off the floor at one time.
11. The gait used with crutches that is closest to that of the natural rhythm of walking is called the _____ gait.
12. A patient suffering from paralysis of both lower extremities may use either the _____ gait or the _____ gait for crutch walking.

23

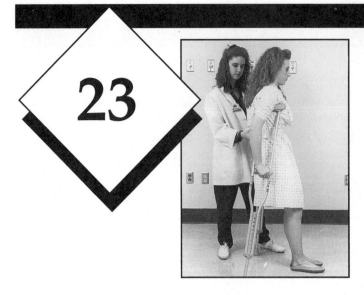

Gait Training and Gait Deviations

Objectives

After studying this chapter, you will be able to:

1. Define what is meant by the term *gait*.

2. Briefly explain what a normal gait is.

3. Discuss the differences between a normal gait and the following abnormal gaits: coxalgic gait, painful-knee gait, sacroiliac gait, and a flexed-hip gait.

4. Describe the gait of a patient with hemiplegia.

5. Describe the gait of a patient with Parkinson's Disease.

Having an understanding of the normal human gait provides the physical therapy aide with a basis for the treatment and management of gait deviations that may occur in patients with impairment of the function of the lower extremities.

The human gait is the result of a series of rhythmic alternating movements of the arms and legs and the trunk. These various movements create a forward motion of the body. They mainly occur between the legs, pelvis, and spine, as well as between the arms, shoulders, and spine. A person walking at a speed to which she is accustomed swings the arm and shoulder forward as the leg of the opposite side is brought forward. The same phase relationship between the arms and legs is present in running although the extent of the movement is greater.

Each human being has a slightly different walking pattern than that of other human beings. Differences in the walking pattern are relatively small, yet the principal pattern is the same for all of us. Generally speaking, individual particularities of the walking pattern do not mature until about the age of seven. Prior to that time, the youngster's body undergoes experimentation in order to find the best pattern for his own body build.

◆ THE NORMAL GAIT

The normal gait cycle consists of two major phases: the *stance phase* and the *swing phase.* The *gait cycle* is the time interval between successive heel strikes of the same foot. The stance phase begins when the heel of the shoe of one extremity strikes the floor and ends when the toes of the same foot leave the ground. The swing phase begins with lifting the toes off the floor and ends when the heel again strikes the ground after the leg has been brought forward.

The stance phase (see Figure 23-1), consists of the following components: the *heel strike,* when the heel contacts the floor; the *midstance,* when the sole of the foot is flat on the ground and the body weight is directly over the stance-phase leg; and the *toe push-off,* when the heel of the stance-phase leg rises from the floor and the body is pushed forward by the ball of the foot that is still in contact with the ground. At this exact moment, the body is propelled forward by the forceful action of the calf muscles and hyperextension of the hip.

The stance phase terminates and the swing phase begins when the entire foot rises from the ground. During the swing phase, the leg must be accelerated

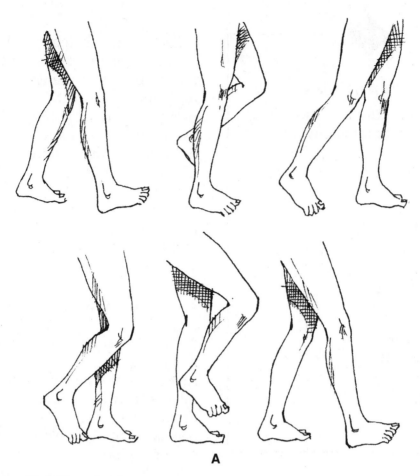

Figure 23-1 Normal gait.

in order to get in front of the body, ready for the next heel strike. To clear the ground in the swing phase, the leg has to be shortened by the hip and knee flexion. The leg is then brought in front of the body and in front of the leg of the other side. The swing phase ends at the exact moment of the heel strike.

There is also a rotation of the pelvis around the spine in the horizontal plane (see Figure 23-2). This rotation is generally six to eight degrees. The rotation comes to a complete stop at the exact time of the heel strike. As full weight is placed on the leg in the midstance phase, the rotation of the pelvis in the horizontal plane is reversed. As the leg of the other side goes into the swing

phase, the pelvis on the side starts to rotate forward.

The shoulder girdle moves in the horizontal plane with the same degree of excursion as the pelvis, the only difference being that the shoulder moves in reverse order. On the side where the pelvis rotates forward, the shoulder rotates backward.

There is one point in the gait cycle in which there is a period of double support when the two extremities are in contact with the ground at the same time. This occurs between the toe push-off on one side and the heel strike and midstance phase on the other. The length of time of double support is directly related to the speed of walking;

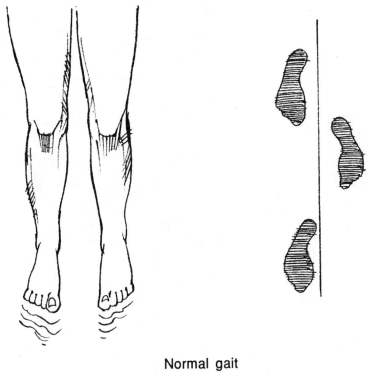

Normal gait

B

Figure 23-1 (*Continued*).

as the walking speed decreases, the length of time spent in double support increases. As speed increases, double support decreases; and as the person changes from walking to running, double support disappears.

As an individual ages, a decreased elasticity of the ligaments and muscles and loss of the smoothness of the joint surfaces bring about some change in the person's gait. Changes in the neurological system also contribute to gait alterations. As aging occurs, the gait loses the appearance of being effortless. The step becomes shorter and wider. The frequent need among the elderly to use a cane oftentimes resembles holding on to a firm object during a child's first attempts at walking. Also, certain diseases of the nervous and musculoskeletal systems may cause gait deviations. One such ailment, frequently found among the elderly, is **osteoarthritis** of the hip joint, which generally results in a painful hip or *coxalgic* gait.

♦ THE COXALGIC GAIT

In osteoarthritis of the hip, the smooth head of the femur becomes uneven. The motion of the hip joint, that is, the motion of the femoral head in the acetabulum, is hampered by

View of pelvis from above

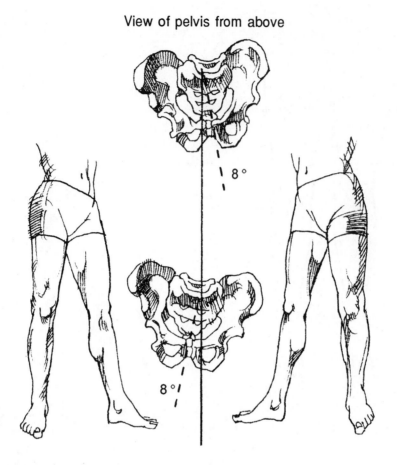

Figure 23-2 Pelvis rotation seen in a normal gait.

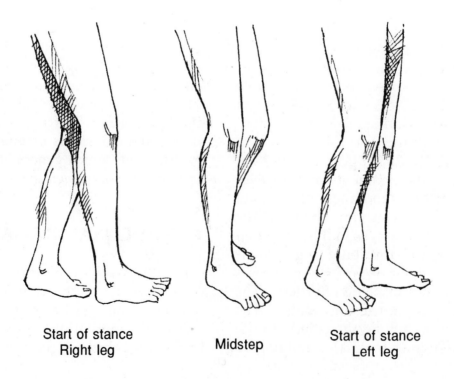

Start of stance
Right leg

Midstep

Start of stance
Left leg

Figure 23-3 The coxalgic gait.

increased friction and becomes restricted and painful. In the swing phase, when the hip and knee have to be flexed in order to bring the leg forward and in front of the other foot, flexion of the hip joint may be painful and restricted. The hyperextension of the hip at the end of the stance phase may be diminished; hence, the step becomes shorter.

In order to enable the swing phase leg to clear the ground in a very severe restriction of the hip flexion, the stance phase leg goes up on the toes (see Figure 23-3). The width of the step is reduced, depending on the degree of abduction limitation.

When there is pain in the hip joint on only one side, the weight-bearing period on the painful side tends to become shorter than on the normal side (see Figure 23-4). The person tries to shorten the burden of weight on the painful hip as much as possible. Therefore, the stance phase becomes shorter and the swing phase longer on the painful side.

The components of the normal gait that may be increased in the painful-hip or coxalgic gait are flexion and extension of the lumbar spine, and, with it, the backward and forward tilting of the pelvis. The lateral shift of the trunk is also oftentimes increased, mainly with one-sided hip pain and restriction. The cadence, or measurement of rhythmic motion, may become diminished.

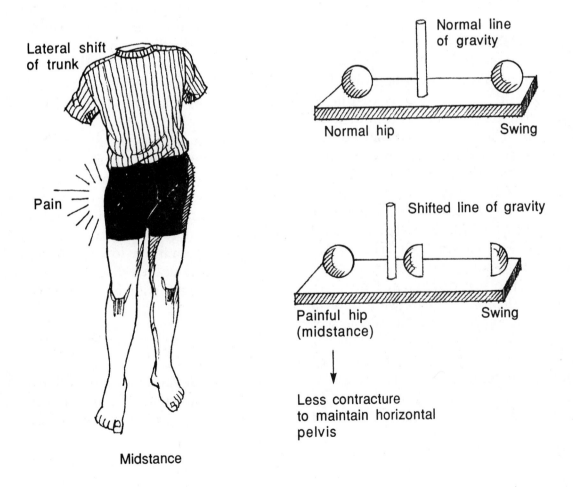

Figure 23-4 Weight shift seen in the painful–hip gait.

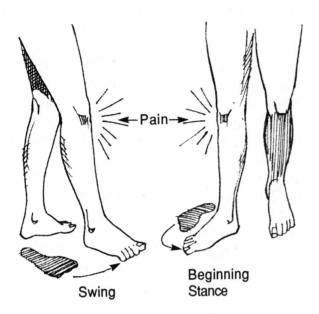

Figure 23-5 The painful–knee gait.

◆ THE PAINFUL-KNEE GAIT

A stiff or painful knee is not infrequent in old age. This may be due to osteoarthritis or other forms of joint affliction. Flexion and extension of the knee become painful. In order to protect the knee, the patient contracts the quadriceps to suppress any motion in the knee. The patient therefore assumes an outward rotation of the affected extremity (see Figure 23-5). The medial aspect of the knee and foot are pointed in the direction of forward motion. Thus, all flexion and extension play in the knee is avoided, and the whole sole can be placed on the ground. There is no heel-to-toe motion, and the outward rotation of the affected limb cannot be assumed by external rotation in the hip alone. There is also some increased rotation of the pelvis.

◆ THE SACROILIAC GAIT

During normal gait, there is a motion between the sacrum and the iliac bone. Both of these bones are connected firmly with ligaments. These connections, however, allow some motion during walking. With increased age, this motion becomes more difficult due to the increased friction and loss of elasticity of the ligaments. Persons who have an affliction or disorder within the sacroiliac joint, tend to walk slightly bent forward with a decreased motion of the pelvis. The gait has the appearance of being very cautious and does not have the features of complete relaxation that a normal gait shows. Pain in the sacroiliac region generally leads to a slight shortening of the step because there is no movement between the sacrum and the iliac bone.

◆ THE FLEXED-HIP GAIT

This type of gait (see Figure 23-6) is generally assumed by persons who suffer from flexion contractures of the hip joint capsule. Hip flexion contracture is frequently found in patients who are confined for long periods of sitting because of pain in the lower extremities. The pain does not necessarily have to be caused by an affliction of the hip joint.

◆ THE HEMIPLEGIC GAIT

This gait deviation is most often seen in elderly patients. It is usually caused by the neurological involvement seen in a stroke.

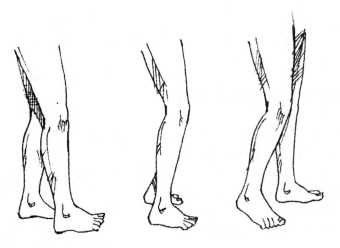

Figure 23-6 The flexed–hip gait.

The patient has loss of motion in the arm and leg on one side. Four to six weeks after the onset of the stroke, spasticity often sets in. The loss or partial loss of motion and the onset of the spasticity generally result in a rather severe gait deviation. When the hemiplegia is on the right side, the arm swing on the right is lost. The patient has the arm dangling if it is flaccid, or in a flexed-elbow point if spasticity has set in. In order to clear the ground during the swing phase, the hip has to be abducted and the trunk flexed to the healthy side to gain some elevation of the pelvis on the affected side (see Figure 23-7). At the beginning of the stance phase, there is no stride; the patient walks on the outside of her affected foot. The heel may never touch the ground, and when the affected leg is in the swing phase, the patient pushes up on the healthy side by

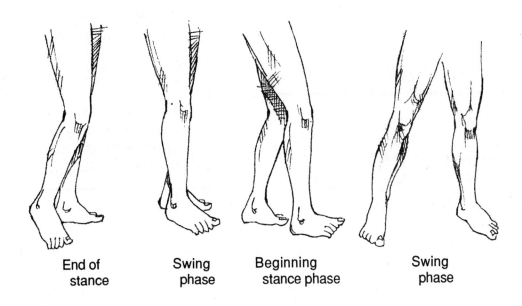

| End of stance | Swing phase | Beginning stance phase | Swing phase |

Figure 23-7 The hemiplegic gait.

elevating the heel. In essence, the patient actually throws the leg forward.

♦ THE PARKINSONIAN GAIT

One disease of the central nervous system that has a great affect on the patient's gait is Parkinson's Disease. It is an ailment that may be controlled through drug therapy and that occurs most often in the geriatric, or older, patient.

The patient suffering from Parkinson's Disease stands with a slightly forward-flexed trunk and flexed knees and hips. Sometimes there is also a continuous tremor. The base of the step is somewhat widened. When walking, there is generally no arm swing and the trunk oscillates from the right to the left in a block. The legs are advanced rigidly and with hesitation. The swing-phase heel does not pass the toes of the other leg, which is in a stance phase. Generally speaking, the severity of the gait deviation depends upon the severity of the disease.

♦ ♦ ♦
SUMMARY OUTLINE

Understanding Gait Training

The Normal Gait
- Major phases of the normal gait
- The gait cycle
- Pelvic rotation in the normal gait

The Coxalgic Gait
- Defining the coxalgic gait
- Differences between the normal gait and the coxalgic gait

The Painful-Hip Gait
- Defining the painful-hip gait
- Differences between the normal gait and the painful-hip gait
- Weight shift in the painful-hip gait

The Painful-Knee Gait
- Defining the painful-knee gait
- Differences between the normal gait and the painful-knee gait

The Sacroiliac Gait
- Defining the sacroiliac gait
- Differences between the normal gait and the sacroiliac gait

The Flexed-Hip Gait
- Defining the flexed-hip gait
- Differences between the normal gait and the flexed-hip gait

The Hemiplegic Gait
- Defining the hemiplegic gait
- Differences between the normal gait and the hemiplegic gait

The Parkinsonian Gait
- Defining the Parkinsonian gait
- Differences between the normal gait and the Parkinsonian gait

CHAPTER REVIEW QUESTIONS

1. The human gait is a result of _____ alternating movements of the _____, _____, and _____.
2. Generally speaking, walking patterns do not mature until about the age of _____.
3. The normal gait cycle consists of the _____ phase and the _____ phase.
4. The _____ phase consists of the _____, _____, _____, and the _____ _____.
5. In a normal gait, the pelvis _____.
6. Osteoarthritis generally results in a painful hip and _____ gait.
7. In the _____-_____ gait, the patient contracts the quadriceps in order to suppress any motion in the knees.
8. Patients suffering from disorders of the sacroiliac joint generally walk with a _____ gait.
9. The _____-_____ gait is generally assumed by patients suffering from flexion contractures of the hip joint capsule.
10. The gait deviation most frequently seen in elderly patients, usually caused by neurological involvement as seen in a stroke, is the _____ gait.
11. _____ _____ is almost always accompanied by an abnormal gait and a continuous tremor.

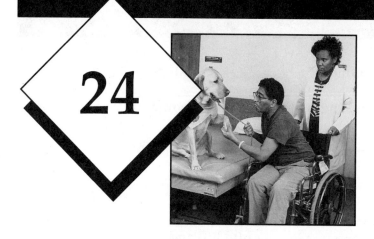

Specialized Therapies

Objectives

After studying this chapter, you will be able to:

1. Identify the different types of specialized therapies used for patients with specific physiological needs.

2. Define the term *reduction* and differentiate between open reduction and closed reduction.

3. Describe when a closed reduction may be used.

4. Describe when an open reduction may be used.

5. Discuss the concept of traction and identify various types of traction that can be used to maintain alignment and immobilization of a body part.

6. Discuss the purpose of a cast.

7. Describe instances when the administration of medications might be used as a therapeutic treatment.

8. Discuss how x rays and tomography are used as therapeutic treatments.

9. Identify specific specialized reflex tests and studies used in diagnosing physical disabilities and in administering therapeutic treatment.

10. Explain the purpose of a lumbar puncture.

11. Explain the purpose of an electroencephalogram.

12. Explain the purpose of magnetic resonance testing.

13. Briefly explain the use of pet therapy as a therapeutic treatment for patients suffering from a physical disability.

Depending upon the body part involved and the type of injury or disease sustained, the physical therapy aide may come in contact with any one of several different types of therapies or modalities. These therapies range from the use of immobilization by surgery to immobilization by traction. During this chapter, we will discuss some of the more frequently used of these specialized therapies.

◆ IMMOBILIZATION BY REDUCTION

Whenever a patient fractures a bone, depending upon the type of fracture involved, the physician must determine what type of therapy to use that will be promote the healing of the broken bone. It's important to note here that an untreated fracture begins to heal almost immediately. Therefore, the physician has two jobs in treating the break. The first is to place the broken bones so that the restored bone is in the right position to heal in the correct shape. The second is to keep the bone in place as it heals. Placing the bone in position is called **reduction.** It can be done in one of two ways, either by **closed reduction,** in which the physician manipulates the bone into place without opening up the skin, or in **open reduction,** in which an incision or cut into the site of the fracture is necessary to put the broken bone in place.

Holding the bone in place is called **immobilization.** It can usually be done with a cast or a strong bandage. However, in some cases the bone will not heal properly unless it is put in traction, an arrangement of weights and pulleys is set up to put enough tension on the bone and surrounding muscles to hold the bone in place as it begins to heal.

◆ TRACTION

Traction is defined as the pull provided by a series of weights, ropes, and pulleys that are connected to either a frame, wire, or pin or to straps applied over the skin of the patient. *Countertraction* is the force against the traction and is usually supplied by the weight of the patient's body. The application of traction is done by the physician. Maintenance of traction is absolutely necessary. Weights must hang free, ropes and pulleys must be free from interference, and splints and slings must be suspended without interference.

Several principles are involved in effective traction. First, the traction must be continuous. Second, counter-traction must be applied. Third, the traction apparatus must be correctly maintained.

Various types of traction can be used to maintain alignment and immobilization of a fracture or diseased body part. The two most common types are skin traction and skeletal traction. *Skin traction* uses tapes or traction strips attached to the skin, usually by elastic bandages. The tapes or strips are connected to a traction apparatus that consists of ropes, pulleys, and weights. Examples of skin traction are Hare traction (Figure 24-1), Russell traction, and Buck's extension. *Skeletal traction* uses a wire (Kirschner) or pin (Steinmann) inserted in the bone with pull (traction) applied to the pin or wire. The Thomas splint with the Pearson attachment is often used with the Kirschner wire or Steinmann pin to provide balanced skeletal traction. General anesthesia is required to insert these devices.

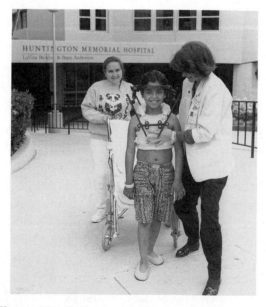

Figure 24-1 Patient with Hare traction.

◆ APPLICATION OF A CAST

Some disorders, such as those of the musculoskeletal system, may require the application of a cast as part of the therapeutic treatment and healing process. Casts hold the bone in place while it heals and permit early ambulation when a leg is broken. In some cases, a patient may be given a narcotic or general anesthetic before the cast is applied. Sometimes, a nerve block is performed, for example, infiltrating the brachial plexus with a local anesthetic agent for closed reduction of a fracture of the arm.

When applying the cast, the physician positions the patient in a way that ensures the proper alignment of the part to be immobilized. An aide holds the arm or leg exactly in place. A cast applied to an area that includes a joint usually is applied with the joint flexed to lessen stiffness.

◆ ADMINISTRATION OF MEDICATIONS

Many disorders of the musculoskeletal and nervous systems may require the administration of medications or drugs as part of therapeutic treatment. Some joint diseases, for example, may require the use of aspirin or other anti-inflammatory and pain-relieving drugs. Gout, another disease of the joints, can be virtually eliminated with medication. And osteoporosis, a common disorder of the bone, is always treated by providing the patient with supplements of vitamin D and calcium, pain-relieving drugs, and hormones to promote ossification and protection of the back.

A great many of the diseases affecting the muscles can also be treated through the administration of certain muscle relaxant medications, while other disorders of the nervous system generally use a number of drugs to relieve pain, treat bacterial infections, and reduce inflammation and swelling.

♦ SPECIALIZED THERAPIES USED IN DIAGNOSING

X Rays

Many specialized therapies and tests may be used in the diagnosing and treatment of disorders of the musculoskeletal and nervous systems. One of the most frequently used is x ray (see Figure 24-2).

X rays are often used to diagnose bone diseases and injuries. In general, they are only done when necessary to diagnose or treat a particular problem. The x ray machine bombards a photographic film with radiation through the part of the body that is injured. The rays can penetrate through the skin and connective tissue but not through bone, so wherever the bone intervenes between the rays and the film, which becomes dark when the rays penetrate it, stays white.

Computerized Axial Tomography (CAT) Scan

Computerized axial tomography, or the CAT scan, has largely replaced previous forms of x rays that were used to visualize specific structures and provides better information than ordinary x rays in many cases. The CAT scan gives a clear picture of the structure or organ being viewed. It does so by using a series of pictures of the cross-sections of the structure that were put together with a computer. The procedure is low-risk and gives information otherwise unobtainable except by surgery (Figure 24-3).

♦ SPECIALIZED REFLEX TESTS AND STUDIES

As a physical therapy aide, you may encounter certain specialized reflex tests

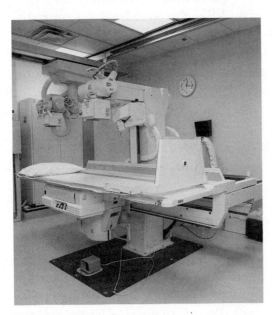

Figure 24-2 The x–ray machine.

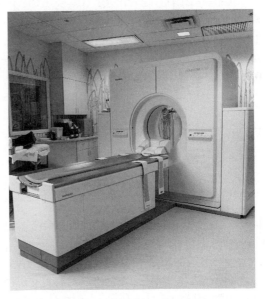

Figure 24-3 The CAT scan machine.

and diagnostic studies that may be used in the treatment of disorders of the musculoskeletal and nervous systems. Several reflexes can be tested quickly and easily to get general information about motor neuron function. In some facilities, the physical therapist or the physician may be responsible for conducting these tests. The role of the physical therapy aide is to assist the therapist or the physician in carrying out the tests.

The **patellar reflex,** or knee-jerk reflex, is tested by striking the patient's knee just below the kneecap, or patella. Normally the lower leg will automatically extend. This indicates a complete two-neuron reflex arc at the second, third, and fourth lumbar nerves and proper function of the related muscles.

The Babinski reflex is generally conducted by the physician and is performed by using a blunt object to stroke the outside of the sole of the patient's foot. Normally this causes the toes to flex immediately. An abnormal response is for the big toe to extend and the other toes to fan out. This is known as the positive *Babinski sign* and it usually indicates impairment of the spinocortical nerve pathways.

The **Achilles reflex,** or ankle jerk, is similar to the patellar reflex. On tapping the Achilles tendon in the ankle, the foot should flex. The centers for this reflex are in the first and second sacral nerves.

♦ OTHER TESTS

If it has been established that the patient is likely to have a neurological problem, other tests may be used to pinpoint the problem more exactly. The most common of these include the pre-

viously discussed CAT scan, lumbar puncture and examination of cerebrospinal fluid, electroencephalography (EEG), and nuclear magnetic resonance imaging (MRI).

Lumbar Puncture

A lumbar puncture is performed to measure pressure in the central nervous system and to obtain fluid for examination and laboratory testing. The fluid can be tested for blood, other foreign cells, infection, and chemical imbalances. The same technique is used to inject medications, anesthetics, or contrast media for x ray studies into the spinal canal.

Electroencephalograph (EEG)

The EEG is a painless procedure used for measuring the electrical activity of the brain. Electrodes are attached to both the patient's skull and a recording device that makes a tracing of electrical impulses from many areas of the brain. The patient should be awake, alert, and calm and should have eaten recently.

The EEG can also be used on patients in a coma to determine brain activity. A patient who has a "flat" EEG, that is, one that shows no activity, and who has no reflexes, breathing, or muscle activity for six hours or more is considered dead even if circulation can be mechanically maintained. This is because the brain tissue is almost all dead and cannot be regenerated.

Magnetic Resonance Imaging (MRI)

Magnetic Resonance Imaging is a relatively new technique and its usefulness in neurology and orthopedics has not been fully established. Using this proce-

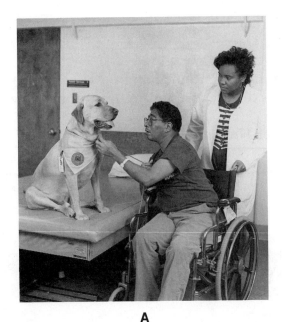 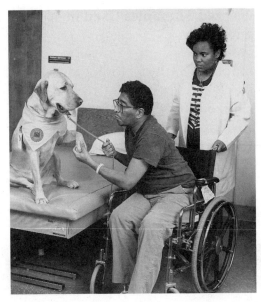

A B

Figure 24-4 Patient with a dog during a pet therapy session.

dure, it is possible to look at soft tissue rather than at bones or blood vessels; therefore, growths in the white or gray matter are easier to detect than they are with other tests.

♦ **PET THERAPY**

Another type of therapy being used more frequently than ever before because of its great physiological as well as psychological benefits, is pet therapy (see Figure 24-4). Physicians and physical therapists are discovering that pairing patients with disabilities with highly trained and emotionally socialized pets, results in a soothing, therapeutic effect on the patient's well-being. By doing so, such therapy has the ability to increase the patient's rehabilitative capacity, thereby making his recovery and ultimate healing process much more efficient.

♦ ♦ ♦
SUMMARY OUTLINE

Specialized Therapies
- Purpose and use of specialized therapies

Immobilization by Reduction
- Purpose of reduction
- Closed reduction
- Open reduction

Use of Traction
- Purpose of traction
- Principles of traction
- Types of traction

Application of a Cast
- Purpose of a cast

Administration of Medication

Specialized Therapies Used in Diagnosing
- X rays
- Computerized axial tomography scan

Specialized Reflex Tests and Studies
- Patellar reflex
- Babinski reflex
- Achilles reflex

Other Tests Used as Specialized Therapies
- Lumbar puncture
- Electroencephalogram
- Nuclear magnetic resonance imaging

pet Therapy

CHAPTER REVIEW QUESTIONS

1. Placing a bone in position is called _____.
2. _____ _____ involves manipulating a bone without opening the skin, and _____ _____ involves making an incision into the site and putting the broken bone in place.
3. Holding a bone in place is called _____.
4. Briefly define the term traction.
5. Briefly define the term countertraction.
6. List two types of traction frequently used in the hospital setting:
   a._____
   b._____
7. Briefly explain the purpose of applying a cast.
8. What disorder of the musculoskeletal system frequently calls for the administration of vitamin D as part of the treatment?
9. What diagnostic tool is often used to diagnose bone diseases and injuries?
10. Briefly define the difference between a CAT scan and an MRI.
11. What is the patellar reflex test used for?
12. The _____ is a painless procedure used for measuring the electrical activity of the brain.

SECTION IX

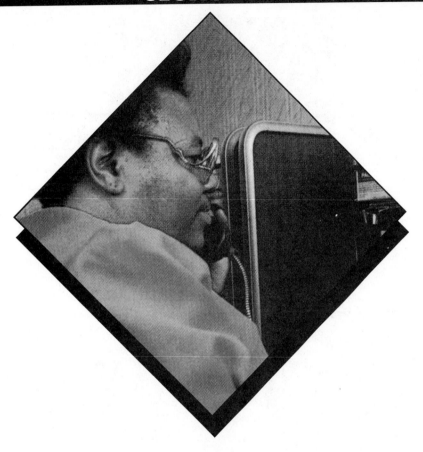

JOB SEEKING SKILLS

◆ ◆ ◆

25

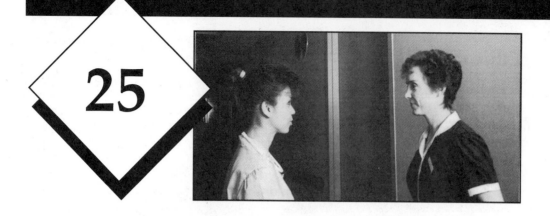

Job Seeking Skills

Objectives
After studying this chapter, you will be able to:

1. Identify where most jobs will occur by the year 2000.

2. Describe the steps and process involved in beginning a job search.

3. Explain how to fill out a job application form.

4. Discuss the purpose of a cover letter.

5. Define the function of a resume.

6. Identify the basic components of a resume.

7. Identify three types of resumes, when each should be used, and what components are in each.

8. List the proper guidelines for preparing a resume.

9. Discuss how to prepare for an interview.

10. Explain how to conduct oneself during the interview process.

11. Explain the follow-up process occurring after the interview.

◆ ◆ ◆

VOCABULARY

Learn the meaning and the correct spelling of the following words and abbreviations:

Labor
Employment
Employment agency
Job search
NA
DNA
Dun and Bradstreet, Inc.
Cover letter
Objective
Resume
Chronological resume
Functional resume
Combination resume
Interview

The United States Bureau of Labor Statistics estimates that by the year 2000 over half of the employment opportunities available will occur in professional, clerical, and service-oriented fields, with health care offering the brightest prospects. Physicians, nurses, physical therapists and physical therapy aides, medical assistants, technicians, and hospital administrators will be in high demand both in rural and urban communities, especially if a national health insurance program goes into effect. Key factors contributing to increased employment opportunities for physical therapy aides and other allied health care professionals include the need to staff medical offices for the increasing numbers of medical doctors being graduated from medical schools, public awareness of the need to provide quali-

ty health care, and an increase in the volume of paperwork emanating from insurance companies and from state and government regulatory agencies.

Research studies show that although the job-seeking person has all the skills to *do* a job, he often does not have the basic skills required to *get* a job. Therefore, before you begin actively seeking employment in a health care facility, there are specific steps you should take in order to *obtain* the best possible position.

First, you should consider the primary reasons employers give for rejecting job applicants. These include the applicant's showing little interest in or giving poor reasons for desiring a job. Showing a past history of "job hopping" and an inability to verify previous employment and/or educational background, tends to make a prospective employer hesitant to hire an individual. Demonstrating a lack of maturity or an inability to communicate effectively during the interview process are two additional reasons employers may not be interested in an applicant. Dressing unacceptably or showing a lack of professionalism or manners, are also reasons. Finally, providing the employer with a poorly completed job application form or resume or demonstrating a lack of job-related skills, are reasons employers shy away from hiring an individual for a position.

◆ BEGINNING THE JOB HUNT

When you are ready to begin your search for a position, you should try to follow through on all possible job leads. An individual who recently completed her education, might contact the school placement office and place her name on file. You might also attend physical therapy meetings and workshops that are open to the public. Those announcements are usually placed in a special section of your local newspaper. Because many jobs are never formally advertised, you should try to spread the word that you are looking for work to classmates, teachers, family, and acquaintances who work for physical therapists, physicians, or medical facilities. Hiring is often done through a network or grapevine of contacts, that is called the *hidden job market*. An employer passes the word of a specific job opening to friends and colleagues, who in turn spread the word and refer qualified persons they know. Because approximately 75 percent of the time a job opportunity derives from a personal contact, the most important job source is acquaintances (see Figure 25-1).

As you conduct your search for employment, you should visit public

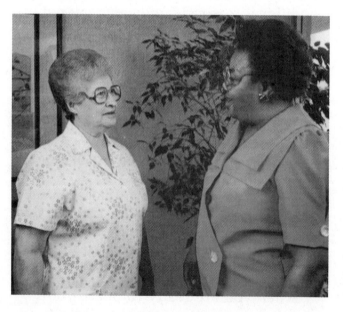

Figure 25-1 Friends, classmates, and colleagues are valuable sources of potential jobs. (From Hegner and Caldwell, *Nursing Assistant: A Nursing Process Approach,* 6th edition, copyright 1992 by Delmar Publishers Inc.)

and private employment agencies, fill out application forms, and take the required skills tests they administer. These agencies work as referral services and make their money by placing applicants in jobs. Often when a job applicant calls an employment agency about an advertised job opportunity, it will already have been filled, but the agency will suggest a visit to the office to talk about other openings. Before agreeing to an appointment, you should find out as much as possible about the other jobs because you may already have learned about them from another source since some positions are listed with more than one agency. Some agencies require that the job applicant sign a written binding contract before assisting in the job search. Before you agree to do this, make sure you read it carefully to determine whether you or the employer is required to pay the agency fee. Another source of leads is the help-wanted ads in the classified section of the newspapers. The advertisement explains how to make the initial contact, usually by telephone or written communication. Help-wanted advertisements appearing in newspapers cannot mention the age, sex, and race requirements of applicants, but situations-wanted ads can.

Another way in which to begin your job search is to visit personnel offices of hospitals, clinics, and medical facilities to find out if they keep files of potential job applicants and then fill out any questionnaires or forms they may provide for that purpose. It is important to study each question carefully before indicating an answer for the object of the question may be to see if the applicant can follow instructions. You should try to furnish as much information as possible, but if an item does not apply or cannot be answered, you should indicate that the question has not been overlooked by inserting *"no,"* *"none,"* *"NA (not applicable),"* or *"DNA (does not apply)."*

When filling out an application form, you should read the entire application because some instructions may be on the last line of the page. Make sure you read the fine print and take note of any special instructions such as *"please print"* or *"put last name first"* since doing so shows the employer your ability to follow instructions. Also, unless told to do otherwise, make sure you fill the application out in ink, and if your handwriting is illegible, you should block print. Never abbreviate words when there is ample space to write them out. Try to keep a completed application form on hand with you that has been checked for accuracy. You may use it as a "guide" to copy information onto each master application form. If the form asks for your experience using equipment, make sure you list each specific type of equipment. When listing your previous employment, make sure you

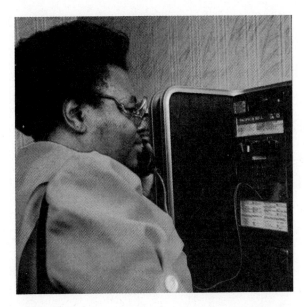

Figure 25-2 Get permission before using names for references. (From Hegner and Caldwell, *Nursing Assistant: A Nursing Process Approach,* 6th edition, copyright 1992 by Delmar Publishers Inc.)

are exact when listing the dates, because most employers will verify your employment history. If the form asks the reason why you left a position, this may be left blank for discussion during the interview. You will probably be asked to supply references. Get permission to use their names *before* you add them to any application form (Figure 25-2). And finally, make sure you sign the application upon its completion.

Occasionally a blind letter to an office where a possible job opportunity is discovered through a friend or where you would especially like to work may result in a positive response.

If you are planning to seek employment in a geographical area unfamiliar to you, advance planning will be necessary. Nothing is more discouraging to an unemployed person than a prolonged job search in unfamiliar surroundings. Dun and Bradstreet, Inc's *Million Dollar Directory* and *the Middle Market Directory* provide information on potential employers in many cities throughout the United States. Also, the *Yellow Pages* in your local telephone book provide listings of professional offices and hospitals. Chamber of Commerce publications also include membership directories, names of major professional employers in specific areas, and brochures describing regional facts. It is also a good idea to subscribe to the principal newspaper of a city where employment is desired since this is one way of *tuning in* to the local job market of that area and responding to their advertisements.

♦ THE COVER LETTER

A *cover letter* is like a personal introduction to a prospective employer (see Figure 25-3). It should be typed and addressed to the name of a person. If an advertisement provides a post office and/or telephone number for making an application, you should call and ask for the name of the personnel supervisor or person most likely to be doing the interviewing. This is done so that the cover letter can include that person's name. If the name is unknown, it is acceptable to use the salutation "Dear Sir or Madam," or "To Whom It May Concern," or a less formal, "Hello" or

18 Hireme Lane
Job City, Ohio 44444
June 3, 1993

Mr. Prospective Employer
Personnel Director
Health Care Facility
2 Nursing Lane
Dental City, Ohio 44833

Dear Mr. Employer:

In response to your advertisement in the _____ on _____, 19___, I would like to apply for the position of _____.

I recently graduated from_____. I majored in _____ and feel I am well qualified for this position. I enjoy working with people and have a sincere interest in additional training in_____.

My resume is enclosed. I have also enclosed a specific list of skills which I mastered during my school experience. I feel that previous positions noted on the resume have provided me with a good basis for meeting your job requirements.

Thank you for considering my application. If you desire additional information, or would like to interview me, please contact me at the above address or by telephone at 589-1111 after 2:00 P.M.

Sincerely,

Iamjob Hunting

Figure 25-3 The cover letter. (From Simmers, *Diversified Health Occupations*, 2nd edition, copyright 1988 by Delmar Publishers Inc.)

"Good Morning."

To attract the reader's interest, the first 20 words of the cover letter should state the reason you are applying for the position. It should also state your qualifications and how you learned about the position. Career objectives may then be mentioned. The concluding sentence paves the way for an interview appointment by calling attention to a telephone number. The cover letter should be a preview of the applicant's writing skill and should be free of any errors in spelling, punctuation, and grammar. A personal touch can also be added to make the letter stand out.

♦ THE RESUME

The primary purpose of the resume is to sell your job qualifications to a prospective employer in a brief and attractive format in order to obtain an interview. It should also summarize your educational and vocational history with an analysis of the problems effectively confronted and solved, emphasizing organizational, administrative, and clinical skills.

The ideal resume is a one-page document, written in language similar to a telegram. It should contain as many action words as possible and should avoid personal pronouns. If it is impossible to confine the resume to one page, it can be typed on a 10- by 14-inch page for reduction to standard letter size. Brevity is also important as long as it is possible to include all relevant information.

All data on the resume should be originally typed or printed on high quality, wrinkle-free bond paper, single spaced internally with double spacing between unrelated items, and with balanced spacing on all four margins. Headings should stand out and may be typed using a different style of type from the rest of the resume.

Types of Resumes

The three formats commonly used when typing a resume are *chronological*, *functional*, and *combination*.

The chronological resume (see Figure 25-4), is the most widely accepted and familiar to employers. It provides them with an interview script and is the easiest for the applicant to prepare. Specific dates and employers are listed in chronological order with either experience or education first, depending on the area of background to be emphasized. The chronological format stresses a steady employment record, but lack of experience is starkly revealed and skills are not highlighted. To counteract these weaknesses, the applicant sometimes encloses photocopies of certificates, emphasizing specific skills.

The functional resume (see Figure 25-5), usually the choice of the applicant just out of high school or college who has a spotty employment record, highlights qualifications and marketable skills. It does not list specific job titles or descriptions with dates, but rather, emphasizes growth and development in skills.

The combination resume emphasizes the applicant's work skills and lists employers with dates of work. This format shows an applicant's entire work and education background at a glance, particularly stressing the most relevant skills and work experience while minimizing less significant experience. A major weakness of this format, however, is that it tends to run on and on.

FLORENCE NURSE
22 South Main Street
Nursing, Ohio 33303
(419) 589-1111

PERSONAL DATA

Date of Birth:	June 3, 1962
Height:	5'4"
Weight:	118 pounds
Health:	Excellent
Social Security Number:	222-14-2343

EDUCATION

Career High School	Major: Health Occupations
5 Diamond Street	Grade Average: B
Nursing, Ohio 33302	

EMPLOYMENT OBJECTIVE: To work as a nurse assistant in a hospital facility

WORK EXPERIENCE

Summer 1979	Country King Fried Chicken
to Present	5 Southern Lane
	Mansfield, Ohio 44952
	Counterperson: operate register, record orders, promote sales

EXTRACURRICULAR ACTIVITIES
School Band: two years
Vocational Industrial Clubs of America: Class treasurer
Red Cross Club member
Red Cross Blood Mobile Volunteer Worker
March of Dimes Walkathon: three years
Church Youth Group member

REFERENCES

Mrs. Jane Smarto, R.N.	55 Education Lane
Teacher	School, Ohio 44595
Mrs. Jean Smith, L.P.N.	432 Geriatric Path
Happy Folks Home	Oldsville, Ohio 44592

Figure 25-4 The chronological resume. (From Simmers, *Diversified Health Occupations*, 2nd edition, copyright 1988 by Delmar Publishers Inc.)

TAMMY TOOTH

340 Dental Lane
Floss, Ohio 44598
(524) 333-2345

Born: January 2, 1964
Height: 5'6"   Weight: 124 pounds
Social Security: 234-45-3422

CAREER GOAL: Position as dental assistant in general practice.

EDUCATION: Ohio Joint Vocational School
678 Career Lane
Opportunity, Ohio 55432
Graduated in June, 1980
Major in two year Dental Assistant Program
Special skills in chairside assisting, radiology, dental
laboratory, and related knowledge

EXPERIENCE: Dental Laboratory Products
56 Model Street
Opportunity, Ohio 55433
Employed September, 1979 to present as dental lab
assistant; proficient in models, custom trays, prosthetic
devices
Druggist Stores, Inc.
8900 Pharmacy Lane
Opportunity, Ohio 56778
Employed as salesperson from June, 1978 to September,
1979; experience in customer relations, inventory,
register, and sales promotion

OTHER ACTIVITIES: Treasurer for Health Occupations Students of America
(H.O.S.A.)
First Place Regional Award in H.O.S.A.
Dental Assistant Contest
Volunteer worker during Dental Health Week, 1978
Member of School Pep Club
Hobbies include crafts, swimming, basketball

REFERENCES: Mr. John Palate, Dental Lab Technician
5567 Maxilla Road
Opportunity, Ohio 55433
Mrs. Smart Instructor, C.D.A., Teacher
43 Education Path
Opportunity, Ohio 55434
Rev. John Preacher, Pastor
St. Mark's Church
5789 Religion Street
Opportunity, Ohio 55433

Figure 25-5 The functional resume. (From Simmers, *Diversified Health Occupations*, 2nd edition, copyright 1988 by Delmar Publishers Inc.)

No matter which format is chosen, personal data such as your name, address, and telephone number is outlined briefly in a few lines at the beginning of the resume. According to a decision made in the Civil Rights Act of 1964 and enforced by the Equal Employment Opportunity Commission, comments on height, weight, birth date, marital status, social security number, and physical condition may be excluded from your resume.

Guidelines for Preparing the Resume

When preparing your resume, you will be much more successful in securing a position if you follow the guidelines set forth below.

1. Be brief, as to the purpose of your resume. Remember, you will get much better results if you do not detail all of your qualifications.
2. Explain job titles and duties, and mention awards, special interests, and activities.
3. Always emphasize positive points and avoid mentioning any weaknesses.
4. Enclose photocopies of certificates or diplomas only if they will be of value to the interviewer for recall purposes and indication of skills.
5. Indicate that references are available on request.
6. Always type, never handwrite, the data.
7. Unless requested to do so, always avoid mentioning a salary requirement.
8. List volunteer activities, especially if they are related to the medical field.

If the bulk of your resume is devoted to educational qualifications and skills, you should provide details of courses that relate to clinical and organizational skills. Awards may be mentioned as well as your grade average if it was good. The names of high schools and colleges attended are included with the degrees attained; the most recent school should be listed first. Work experience should include the name and address of the employer, the job title, the length of time employed, and a brief description of duties. Most recent employment is always listed first. Prospective employers usually verify the employment history of job applicants, so it is important that you are able to state the exact dates of previous employment.

Unless required, past salaries are never included in the resume or cover letter. Miscellaneous information, selectively chosen, belongs at the end of the resume. This information might include volunteer work, honors, awards, certificates, special language skills, and leadership positions in medical or professional organizations.

Because prospective employers usually ask for the names of people who can provide references, you should contact friends and former employers *before* an interview to ask if they will serve as references. This courtesy allows the person time to prepare a response before receiving an unexpected telephone call or communication from the prospective employer.

◆ PREPARING FOR THE INTERVIEW PROCESS

The interview process is so important that it often determines whether an applicant will be offered employment. Research studies have shown that when two applicants have similar skills and education, the choice of which candidate to hire is based almost entirely on physical appearance at the interview. The importance of good grooming in projecting a favorable first impression cannot be overemphasized. You should always wear immaculately clean, conservative clothing that fits the image of the job with coordinated accessories that show good taste. Looks speak louder than words and may reveal inner feelings. When the applicant knows she looks her best, she can be more confident and relaxed at the time of the interview.

Carrying a portfolio of information related to the current job opening to the interview, suggests that you are well organized and serious about obtaining the position. Such information might include letters of recommendation, school diplomas or degrees, transcripts, certificates, names and addresses of references, a copy of your resume, Social Security card, and items related to prior education.

It is important to find out as much as possible about the position before the interview. Because the interview appointment is the only time a physician or physical therapist will have to make a firsthand evaluation of your maturity, manners, personality, and verbal skills and to acquire information that does not appear on the resume, it is important that you take steps to prepare appropriate responses in order to project the best possible image. Being knowledgeable about the physician's or therapist's expectations makes it much easier to relax and to respond more intelligently to questions.

♦ THE JOB INTERVIEW

If contacted by an employer to be interviewed, you should always arrive promptly for your appointment and greet the interviewer by name. Always let the interviewer initiate a handshake and wait to be seated until he sits down or directs you to be seated. Listen attentively to each question and ask for clarification if there can be more than one interpretation. Remember, think before giving an answer; there is no need to hurry.

Do not answer questions about your personal life unless the answer will demonstrate an ability to perform the job. Always be discreet in reference to former employers. Make sure your responses are short but avoid one-word answers such as "yes" or "no."

A confident prospective employee always demonstrates interest in the position for which he is applying by asking questions about job specifications, continuing education policies, medical benefits, and to whom he will be responsible. Also, be prepared to reply to a question about the salary you expect. If you are unable to respond to a question, be honest and state that you are not able to reply. And, most important, always speak confidently to the interviewer without letting your eyes wander. You must appear relaxed, yet interested in the position.

There may be some questions that may be asked by the interviewer that legally do not have to be answered unless the information is job related. Jobs are to be offered on the basis of qualifications so questions related to marital status, religious preference, club memberships, height, weight, dependents, and age do not have to be answered. Inquiries dealing with credit ratings, home and automobile ownership, family planning, and pregnancy are all illegal.

Terminating the interview process is almost as important as getting it off to a good start. To indicate the end of the interview, the employer will probably stand, which is generally the applicant's cue to stand and prepare to leave. Let the interviewer take the lead in shaking hands at the conclusion of the interview process. Before departing, you should ask when you might expect to hear if the job is to be offered so that you will not miss the call, then leave with a "thank you" to both the interviewer and the receptionist.

♦ AFTER THE INTERVIEW

In today's employment market, a job offer is seldom initiated at an interview.

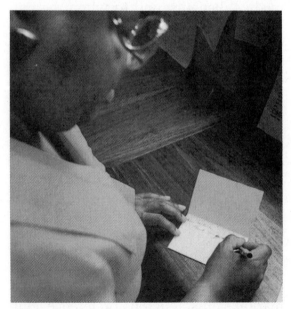

Figure 25-6 Write a thank you note after the interview; it helps the interviewer remember you. (From Simmers, *Diversified Health Occupations*, 2nd edition, copyright 1988 by Delmar Publishers Inc.)

Therefore, if there has been no word from the facility within a day or two, it is time for you to write a follow-up note of thanks (see Figure 25-6) or to place a call to express your continued interest in the position and to keep from being forgotten. The object of the reminder is to briefly restate your assets, emphasize any strong feelings you may have about obtaining the position, and reinforce the times you are available to be reached by telephone. Even if the position is not offered, you will learn from each interview until you are able to secure the right job.

Once a job has been secured it will be well for you to remember that, no matter what level you are hired at, you are still a beginner in that position with much to learn. It is a good idea to borrow the office or department's procedure manual to preview the facility's routines. Arriving for work the first day with a notebook to take notes saves the subsequent embarrassment of having to ask how to carry out tasks after they have been explained, and taking notes also reinforces procedures and demonstrates your genuine desire to do the best job possible.

♦ ♦ ♦
SUMMARY OUTLINE

Labor Market and Employment
• Careers and opportunities
• Employment by the year 2000

Beginning the Job Hunt
• Job leads and contacts
• Employment agencies
• Advertisements
• Visitations
• Location and geographic preference

The Cover Letter
- Purpose of the cover letter
- Parts of the cover letter

The Resume
- Purpose of the resume
- Creating the document
- Types of resumes
- Preparing the resume

Preparing for the Interview Process
- Purpose of the interview process
- Components of the interview

The Job Interview
- What to say and do
- Questions and answers
- Terminating the interview
- After the interview

CHAPTER REVIEW QUESTIONS

1. Identify at least three reasons an employer might reject a job applicant.
   a._____
   b._____
   c._____
2. Define resume.
3. Explain at least one way to demonstrate interest in a job interview.
4. Why should the physical therapy aide read the fine print of an employment agency contract before signing it?
5. Identify at least one weakness of the chronological resume.
6. If three days have passed since the physical therapy aide had an interview, and he has not heard from the prospective employer, what two follow-up steps should be initiated?
   a._____
   b._____
7. List three personal items that legally do not have to be included on a resume or answered during an interview.
   a._____
   b._____
   c._____
8. Which resume style stresses work experience dates?
9. What resume style highlights job skills?
10. List at least three steps the physical therapy aide would take to find a job opening.
   a._____
   b._____
   c._____

APPENDICES

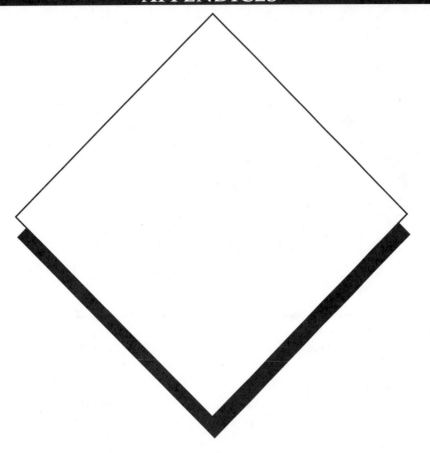

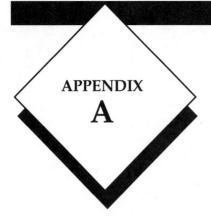

The Human Skeleton

I. **Divisions of the Skeleton**

A. **Axial skeleton:** section of the skeleton that includes the bony framework of the head and the trunk

B. **Appendicular skeleton:** section of the skeleton that forms the framework for the arms and legs, commonly referred to as the extremities

II. **The Framework of the Head: The Skull**

A. **Cranium:** a rounded box enclosing the brain and composed of eight cranial bones, including:
1. **Frontal bone:** forms the forehead
2. **Parietal bones:** form most of the top and side walls of the cranium
3. **Temporal bones:** form part of the sides and some of the base of the skull

4. **Ethmoid bone:** located between the eyes in the orbital cavities
5. **Sphenoid bone:** located at the base of the skull in front of the temporal bones
6. **Occipital bone:** forms the back and a part of the base of the skull

B. **Facial Portion**
1. **Mandible:** lower jaw; the only movable bone in the skull
2. **Maxillae:** forms the upper jaw
3. **Zygomatic bones:** forms the prominence of the cheek
4. **Nasal bones:** forms the bridge of the nose
5. **Lacrimal bones:** lies near the inside corner of the eye
6. **Vomer:** forms the lower part of the nasal septum
7. **Palatine bones:** paired, forming the back part of the hard palate
8. **Inferior nasal conchae:**

paired, lying alongside the lateral wall of the nasal cavities

III. Framework of the Trunk

A. **Vertebral column:** made up of a series of irregularly shaped bones, numbering 26 in the adult; named according to their location
   1. **Cervical:** seven in number, located in the neck
   2. **Thoracic:** 12 in number, located in the thorax
   3. **Lumbar:** five in number, located in the small of the back
   4. **Sacral:** five separate bones in the child, but eventually they fuse together in the adult, and is referred to as the Sacrum
   5. **Coccyx:** the tail bone, consisting of four or five tiny bones in the child, which fuse together in the adult to become one

B. **The Thorax**
   1. **True ribs:** the first seven pairs, attached directly to the sternum by costal cartilage
   2. **False ribs:** include the remaining five pairs; eighth, ninth, and tenth pairs attach to the cartilage of rib above; last two pairs have no attachment and are known as "floating ribs"

IV. The Bones of the Extremities

A. **Upper Extremities**
   1. **Shoulder girdle:** consists of two bones, the *clavicle*, or collar bone, and the *scapula*, or shoulder blade
   2. **Humerus:** the arm bone
   3. **Ulna and radius:** make up the forearm
   4. **Carpals:** eight small bones making up the wrist
   5. **Metacarpal bones:** make up the bones of the hand
   6. **Phalanges:** 14 bones, making up the bones of the fingers

B. **Lower Extremities**
   1. **Pelvic girdle:** strong bony ring forming the walls of the pelvis
   2. **Femur:** the thigh bone; longest and strongest bone in the body
   3. **Patella:** the kneecap
   4. **Tibia and fibula:** two bones making up the lower portion of the leg
   5. **Tarsal bones:** seven bones making up the ankle
   6. **Metatarsal bones:** form the framework of the instep
   7. **Phalanges:** bones of the toes

V. Joints

A. **Articulation (joint):** area or junction or union between two or more bones

B. **Kinds of joints**
   1. **Synarthroses:** referring to an immovable joint
   2. **Amphiarthroses:** referring to a slightly movable joint
   3. **Diarthroses:** referring to a freely movable joint

C. **Joint function**
   1. **Flexion:** bending motion that decreases the angle between bones
   2. **Extension:** straightening motion that increases the angle between bones
   3. **Abduction:** movement away from the midline of the body

4. **Adduction:** movement toward the midline of the body
5. **Rotation:** a twisting or turning of a bone on its own axis
6. **Supination:** turning the palm up or forward
7. **Pronation:** turning the palm down or backward
8. **Inversion:** turning the sole inward
9. **Eversion:** turning the sole outward

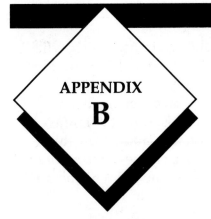

Major Muscles of the Body

I. Muscles of the Head and Neck

A. **Orbicularis oculi:** encircles the eyelids; function is to close the eye

B. **Levator palpebrae superioris:** located behind the orbit to the upper eyelid; function is to open the mouth

C. **Orbicularis oris:** encircles the mouth; functionis to close the lips

D. **Buccinator:** the fleshy part of the cheek; function is to flatten the cheek and help in eating

E. **Temporal:** located above and near the rear of the cheek; function is to close the jaw

F. **Masseter:** located at the ankle of the jaw; function is to close the jaw

G. **Sternocleidomastoid:** located along the side of the neck next to the mastoid process; function is to flex and rotate the head toward the opposite side

II. Muscles of the Upper Extremities

A. **Trapezius:** located at the back of the neck and upper back to the scapula; function is to raise shoulders and pull them back; also extends the head

B. **Latissimus dorsi:** middle and lower back to the humerus; function is to extend and adduct the arm behind the back

C. **Pectoralis major:** upper, anterior chest to the humerus; function is to flex and adduct arm across the chest and to pull the shoulders forward and downward

D. **Deltoid:** covers the shoulder joint to the lateral humerus; function is to abduct the arm

E. **Biceps brachii:** anterior arm to the radius; function is to flex the forearm and supinate hand

F. **Triceps brachii:** posterior arm to the ulna; function is to extend the forearm

G. **Flexor and extensor carpi groups:** located at anterior and posterior forearm to the hand; function is to flex and extend the hand

H. **Flexor and extensor digitorum groups:** located at anterior and posterior forearm to the finger; function is to flex and extend the fingers

III. Muscles of the Trunk

A. **Diaphragm:** dome-shaped partition located between the thoracic and abdominal cavities; dome descends to enlarge thoracic cavity from top to bottom

B. **External intercostals:** located between the ribs; function is to elevate the ribs and enlarge the thoracic cavity

C. **Rectus abdominis, obliquus, transversus:** located anteriolateral to the abdominal wall; function is to compress the abdominal cavity and expell substances from the body; also flexes the spinal column

D. **Levator ani:** the pelvic floor; function is to aid in defecation

E. **Sacrospinalis:** located deep in the back; function is to extend vertebral column and to assist in erect posture

IV. Muscles of the Lower Extremities

A. **Gluteus maximus:** the superficial buttock closest to the femur; function is to extend the thigh

B. **Gluteus medius:** the deep buttock closest to the femur; function is to abduct the thigh

C. **Iliopsoas:** crosses in front of the hip joint to the femur; function is to flex the thigh

D. **Adductor group:** the medial thigh to the femur; function is to adduct the thigh

E. **Sartorius:** winds down the thigh, ilium, and tibia; function is to flex the thigh and leg

F. **Quadriceps femoris:** the anteri or thigh to the tibia and fibula; function is to flex the leg

G. **Hamstrings group:** the posterior thigh to the tibia and fibula; function is to flex the leg

H. **Gastrocnemius:** the calf of the leg closest to the calcaneus; function is to extend the foot

I. **Tibialis anterior:** the anterior and lateral shin closest to the foot; function is to allow for dorsiflexion and inversion of the foot

J. **Peroneus longus:** the lateral leg, closest to the foot; function is to evert the foot

K. **Flexor and extensor digitorum groups:** the posterior leg, closest to the foot; function is to flex and extend the toes

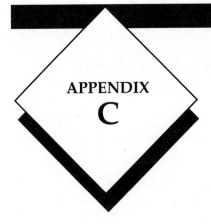

APPENDIX
C

Procedure Evaluations

**PROCEDURE
EVALUATION**   Student_____

PROCEDURE*	Satisfactory	Marginal	Unsatisfactory
Answering the Telephone			
Screening Telephone Calls			
Taking Callback Messages			
Scheduling an Appointment			
Completing a Medical Record			
Completing a 2-Minute Handwash			
Measuring Blood Pressure			
Measuring a Radial Pulse			
Obtaining a Respiratory Rate			
Descending and Ascending a Wheelchair from a Curb			
Turning Patient from Supine to Prone			
Turning Patient from Prone to Supine			
Turning Patient on a Floor Mat			
Turning Patient from a Supine to a Side-lying Position			

•Procedures required for HOSA evaluation are indicated by a >.

PROCEDURE EVALUATION

Student_____

PROCEDURE*	Satisfactory	Marginal	Unsatisfactory
Returning Patient from a Sitting to a Supine Position			
Assisting Patient from Bed to a Wheelchair			
Assisting Patient from Wheelchair to Parallel Bars			
Assisting Patient from Bed to a Wheelchair			
>Applying a Hot (hydrocollator) Pack			
>Applying a Cold Pack			
Performing Range of Motion on a Patient's Lower Extremities			
Performing Range of Motion on a Patient's Upper Extremities			
Assist a Patient to Ambulate Using a Walker			
>Assist a Patient with a 3-point Gait Using Crutches			
>Assist a Patient with a 2-point Gait Using Crutches			

•Procedure required for HOSA evaluation are indicated by a >.

**PROCEDURE
EVALUATION** Student_____

PROCEDURE*	Satisfactory	Marginal	Unsatisfactory
>Assist a Patient with a 4-point Gait Using Crutches			
>Assist a Patient with a Swing-to Gait Using Crutches			
>Assist a Patient with a Swing-through Gait Using Crutches			
Assist Patient to Walk Upstairs and Downstairs with Crutches			
>Assist a Patient to Walk Using a Standard Cane			
Prepare a Job Resume			

• Procedures required for HOSA evaluation are indicated by a >.

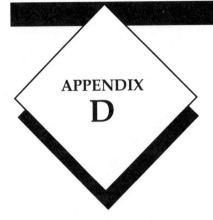

Practice Evaluation Test

Directions: For the questions given below, provide the answers you believe are most correct.

1. Define physical therapy.

2. Identify at least two goals of a physical therapy department.
   a.
   b.

3. Identify at least two goals of a rehabilitation department.
   a.
   b.

4. Of the agents listed below, circle at least four that would be used in a physical therapy department.

heat	radiology	antibiotics	asepsis
running	exercise	noise	anger
suntan oil	balance	energy	gas
electricity	light	water	enemas

5. Generally speaking, most physical therapy aides are employed in _____ and _____.

6. Identify at least six diseases or disabilities that are treated by the physical therapy department.

   a._____   d._____

   b._____   e._____

   c._____   f._____

7. Duties that could be performed by the physical therapy aide include all of the following, *except:* (circle the letters that do not below)

   a. acts as a receptionist

   b. tests patients for evaluation

   c. maintains equipment

   d. determines amounts of weights to be used for traction

   e. helps prepare patients for treatment

   f. transports patients to and from the physical therapy department in a hospital

8. Circle those professionals listed below who are members of the rehabilitation team:

   a. hygienist   f. cardiologist

   b. social worker   g. pediatrician

   c. psychologist   h. speech therapist

   d. orthotist   i. audiologist

   e. occupational therapist   j. gynecologist

9. Read the following statements. If the statement is more true than false, write true beside the statement; if the statement is more false than true, write false beside the statement

   _____a.   To be a physical therapy aide, the applicant must be a graduate of an accredited training program

   _____b.   The physical therapy aide should be in good health since the job requires a high level of energy

   _____c.   The physical therapy aide must be licensed to work in a physical therapy department

   _____d.   The physical therapy aide must work under the direction of a licensed physical therapist

10. Circle the desired qualities for a physical therapy aide:

   a. be in good health   f. be tactful

   b. be good in math   g. be attractive

   c. type at least 50 wpm   h. be strong

   d. have common sense   i. be tall

   e. be sincere with others

11. List at least two ways the physical therapy aide can prevent falls in the physical therapy department.
    a.
    b.

12. Guarding techniques and safety belts are used to

    _____.

13. List two safety observations the physical therapy aide can make while working with physical therapy equipment.
    a.
    b.

14. In case a fire breaks out, the physical therapy aide should know where the _____ is located, the _____ plan of the facility, and the _____ routes.

15. Briefly define the following terms:
    a. supination:_____
    b. erect: _____
    c. eversion: _____
    d. inversion: _____
    e. flexion: _____
    f. extension: _____
    g. proximal: _____
    h. inferior: _____
    i. distal: _____
    j. pronation: _____

16. What is another term for the back-lying position?

17. What is another term for the face-lying position?

18. What is another term for the side-lying position?

19. Turning the palm of the hand downward is called _____.
    a. supination   c. pronation
    b. rotation   d. adduction

20. Identify at least five modalities that the physical therapy aide might use in the treatment of patients. For each modality listed, briefly explain what the treatment is trying to accomplish:

Modality	**Result of Modality**
a. _____	_____
b. _____	_____
c. _____	_____
d. _____	_____
e. _____	_____

21. Explain the difference between passive and active range of motion exercises.

22. List three methods of applying heat for physical therapy treatments.
    a.
    b.
    c.

23. Briefly explain hydrotherapy.

24. Briefly explain the procedure for applying a paraffin bath.

25. Matching: Place the correct letter in the space beside the correct answer:
    ____ 1. heat therapy
    ____ 2. cryotherapy
    ____ 3. massage
    ____ 4. traction
    ____ 5. active-assistive exercise

    A. patient performs the exercise with an aide's assistance
    B. examples are ice packs and cold water immersion
    C. reduces pain and increases circulation
    D. involves squeezing and pressing the muscles
    E. reduces pain and restores ROM using weights and pulleys

26. List two goals of the guarding techniques.
    a.
    b.

27. Briefly describe the purpose of a gait belt

28. In your own words, briefly discuss why it is important to use good body mechanics when guarding a patient.

29. Identify three safety factors to be considered while guarding a patient.
    a.
    b.
    c.

30. **Matching:** Place the letter of the correct standing position in front of the correct number.
    ___ 1. guarding on level ground
    ___ 2. guarding a patient with a weak side and balance problems
    ___ 3. guarding a patient going up a staircase
    ___ 4. guarding a patient going down a staircase
    ___ 5. guarding while transferring a patient

    A. Standing in front of the patient
    B. Standing behind the patient

31. If a patient begins to fall, the physical therapy aide should try to control certain parts of the body. The _____, hips, and _____ are the best body points to control.

32. In your own words, briefly describe the "gait" or "walking" belt.

33. If a patient does fall, it is important to protect her _____ from hard or sharp objects.

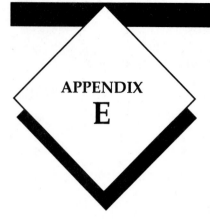

APPENDIX
E

Glossary

Abduction: pertaining to movement away from the midline of the body, as in moving the arms straight out to the sides.

Adduction: pertaining to movement toward the midline of the body, as in bringing the arms back to their original position.

Alignment: the positioning and supporting of the body in such a way that all body parts are in correct anatomical position.

Amphiarthroses: pertaining to a slightly movable joint.

Anterior: referring to the front.

Aponeurosis: a tendon-like expansion that connects a muscle with the parts that it moves.

Appendicular skeleton: the section of the skeleton that forms the framework for those parts usually referred to as the arms and legs, but are commonly called the extremities.

Arthritis: inflammation of a joint.

Articulation: pertaining to the place of a union, as in the union of a joint.

Atrophy: pertaining to a wasting or decrease in the size of a muscle when it cannot be used.

Axial skeleton: the section of the skeleton that includes the bony framework of the head and the trunk.

Axilla: pertaining to the armpit or the area under the arms.

Body mechanics: a term used to refer to the way in which the body moves and maintains its balance by the most efficient use of all of its parts.

Caudal: pertaining to something being inferior or away from the head.

Contractility: the capacity of a muscle fiber to become shorter in its response to a stimuli.

Contracture: a tightening or shortening of a muscle.

Cranial: meaning nearest the head.

Diarthroses: pertaining to a freely movable joint.

Dislocation: a derangement of the parts of a joint.

Distal: pertaining to being farthest from a point of reference.

Dorsal: pertaining to near the back of the body.

Endosteum: a thin membrane that lines the marrow cavities of bone and is a source of cells that aid in the growth and repair of bone tissue.

Epimysium: pertaining to a fibrous sheath surrounding a muscle.

Eversion: pertaining to turning the sole outward, away from the body.

Excitability: the capacity of a muscle to respond to a stimuli.

Extension: a straightening motion that increases the angle between bones, as in straightening the fingers in order to open the hand.

Flexion: a bending motion that decreases the angle between the bones, as in bending the fingers in order to close the hand.

Foramen: a natural opening or passageway; used as a general term for describing a passage into or through a bone.

Fracture: a break, usually referring to a break in a bone.

Insertion: the place of attachment of a muscle to the bone that it moves.

Inversion: pertaining to the act of turning the sole inward so that it faces the opposite foot.

Irritability: the capacity of a muscle to respond to a stimulus.

Isometric contraction: contractions in which there is no change in muscle length, but there is a great increase in muscle tension.

Isotonic contraction: contractions in which the tone or tension within the muscle remains the same, but the muscle as a whole, shortens, producing movement.

Joint: an articulation or area of junction or union between two or more bones.

Ligament: a band of fibrous tissue connecting bones.

Medial: pertaining to near the midline of the body.

Muscle tone: refers to a partially contracted state of the muscles that is normal even though the muscles may not be in use at the time.

Origin: pertaining to the less movable attachment of a muscle.

Orthopedics: the study or branch of medicine or surgery that deals with the treatment of diseases and deformities of the bones, muscles, and joints.

Osteoblast: a cell involved in the production of bone.

Osteoclast: a large cell involved in the absorption and removal of bone.

Physical Therapy: treatment by physical means such as heat, cold, water, massage, and electricity.

Posterior: referring to the back.

Process: referring to a prominence or part extending from an organ.

Pronation: the act of turning the palm down or backward.

Prone: the position in which a person is lying with the face down or on the abdomen.

Prosthesis: replacement of a natural part with an artificial part such as a limb.

Proximal: nearest to a point of reference.

Radiology: branch of medicine dealing with X rays and radioactive substances.

Sprain: pertaining to an injury of a joint with stretching or tearing of the ligaments.

Strain: pertaining to an injury caused by excessive stretching, overuse, or misuse of a muscle.

Superior: meaning above, or being in a higher position.

Supination: the act of turning the palm up or forward.

Supine: lying flat on the back with the face upward.

Synarthroses: pertaining to an immovable joint.

Tendon: a fibrous cord that attaches a muscle to a bone.

Therapy: pertaining to treatment of a disease or disorder, as in physical therapy.

Ultrasonic unit: a piece of equipment that uses sound waves as treatment.

Ventral: meaning the same as anterior; pertaining to something being located near the belly surface or front of the body.

Xiphoid process: the small bony projection at the lower end of the sternum or breastbone.

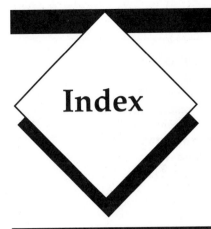

Index

Note: page numbers in bold type refer to non–text material.

A